Skip: Have fun reading the book
+ happy holidays

Hab Kaul

Dec 2011

Body MR Imaging at 3 Tesla

Body MR Imaging at 3 Tesla

Edited by

Ihab R. Kamel
Johns Hopkins School of Medicine, Baltimore, Maryland, USA

Elmar M. Merkle
Duke University School of Medicine, Durham, North Carolina, USA

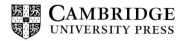

CAMBRIDGE UNIVERSITY PRESS
Cambridge, New York, Melbourne, Madrid, Cape Town,
Singapore, São Paulo, Delhi, Tokyo, Mexico City

Cambridge University Press
The Edinburgh Building, Cambridge CB2 8RU, UK

Published in the United States of America by
Cambridge University Press, New York

www.cambridge.org
Information on this title: www.cambridge.org/9780521194860

First published 2011

Printed in the United Kingdom at the University Press, Cambridge

A catalog record for this publication is available from the British Library

Library of Congress Cataloging-in-Publication Data
Body MR imaging at 3 Tesla / edited by Ihab R. Kamel, Elmar M.
Merkle
    p.   ;   cm.
  Includes bibliographical references and index.
  ISBN 978-0-521-19486-0 (Hardback)
  1. Magnetic resonance imaging.   I. Kamel, Ihab R., editor.
II. Merkle, Elmar M., editor.
  [DNLM: 1. Magnetic Resonance Imaging–methods. WN 185]
  RC78.7.N83B63 2011
  616.07′548–dc22
                                                        2010050337

ISBN 978-0-521-19486-0 Hardback

Contents

The color plate section found between pp. 180 and 181.

Contributors

Susan M. Ascher, MD
Georgetown University Hospital,
Washington, DC, USA

Regina G. H. Beets-Tan, MD, PhD
Department of Radiology, Maastricht
University Medical Centre, Maastricht,
The Netherlands

Rafael O. P. de Campos, MD
Department of Radiology, University of North
Carolina at Chapel Hill, NC, USA

Kevin J. Chang, MD
Brown University Alpert Medical School,
Providence, RI, USA

Byun Ihn Choi, MD
Department of Radiology, Seoul National University,
College of Medicine, Seoul, South Korea

Christopher J. François, MD
Department of Radiology, University of Wisconsin –
Madison, Madison, WI, USA

Jurgen J. Fütterer, MD, PhD
Department of Radiology, Radboud University
Nijmegen Medical Centre, Nijmegen,
The Netherlands

Elizabeth M. Hecht, MD
Department of Radiology, Hospital of the University
of Pennsylvania, Philadelphia, PA, USA

Ihab R. Kamel, MD, PhD
The Johns Hopkins University School of Medicine,
The Russell H. Morgan Department of Radiology
and Radiological Science,
Baltimore, MD, USA

Daniel R. Karolyi, MD PhD
Clinically Applied Research Body MR imaging
Program, Department of Radiology, Emory
University School of Medicine, Atlanta,
GA, USA

Hiroumi D. Kitajima, PhD
Department of Radiology, Emory Healthcare, Inc.,
Atlanta, GA, USA

Doenja M. J. Lambregts, MD
Department of Radiology, Maastricht
University Medical Centre, Maastricht,
The Netherlands

Chang Hee Lee, MD
Department of Radiology, University of North
Carolina at Chapel Hill, NC, USA, and Korea
University Guro Hospital, Korea University
College of Medicine, South Korea

Jeong Min Lee, MD
Department of Radiology, Seoul National University,
College of Medicine, Seoul, South Korea

Constance D. Lehman, MD, PhD
Section of Breast Imaging, University of
Washington Medical Center, Seattle Cancer Care
Alliance, Seattle, WA, USA

John R. Leyendecker, MD
Department of Radiology and Magnetic Resonance
Imaging, Wake Forest University School of Medicine,
Winston-Salem, NC, USA

Monique Maas, MD
Department of Radiology, Maastricht University
Medical Centre, Maastricht, The Netherlands

Katarzyna J. Macura, MD, PhD
The Russell H. Morgan Department of Radiology
and Radiological Science,
Johns Hopkins University,
Baltimore, MD, USA

Daniele Marin, MD
Department of Radiology, Duke University
Medical Center, Durham, NC, USA

Diego R. Martin, MD, PhD
Clinically Applied Research Body MR Imaging
Program, Department of Radiology, Emory
University School of Medicine, Atlanta, GA, USA

Elmar M. Merkle, MD
Department of Radiology, Duke University School
of Medicine, Durham, NC, USA

Henrik J. Michaely, MD
Institute of Clinical Radiology and Nuclear Medicine,
University Medical Center Mannheim, Medical
Faculty Mannheim – University of Heidelberg,
Mannheim, Germany

Aart J. Nederveen, PhD
Department of Radiology, Academic Medical Center,
University of Amsterdam, Amsterdam,
The Netherlands

Savannah C. Partridge
Section of Breast Imaging, University of Washington
Medical Center, Seattle Cancer Care Alliance, Seattle,
WA, USA

Habib Rahbar
Section of Breast Imaging, University of Washington
Medical Center, Seattle Cancer Care Alliance, Seattle,
WA, USA

Scott B. Reeder, MD, PhD
Departments of Radiology, Medical Physics,
Biomedical Engineering, and Medicine, University of
Wisconsin – Madison, Madison, WI, USA

Richard C. Semelka, MD
Department of Radiology, University of North
Carolina at Chapel Hill, NC, USA

Puneet Sharma, PhD
Department of Radiology, Emory Healthcare, Inc.,
Atlanta, GA, USA

Sang Soo Shin, MD
Department of Radiology, University of
North Carolina at Chapel Hill, NC, USA, and
Chonnam National University Medical School,
Gwangju, South Korea

Jaap Stoker, MD, PhD
Department of Radiology, Academic Medical
Center, University of Amsterdam, Amsterdam,
The Netherlands

Bachir Taouli, MD
Department of Radiology, The Mount Sinai
Medical Center, New York, NY, USA

Marije P. van der Paardt, MD
Department of Radiology, Academic Medical Center,
University of Amsterdam, Amsterdam,
The Netherlands

Oliver Wieben, PhD
Departments of Medical Physics and Radiology,
Wisconsin Institutes for Medical Research,
University of Wisconsin – Madison, Madison,
WI, USA

Darcy J. Wolfman, MD
Georgetown University Hospital,
Washington, DC, USA

Manon L. W. Ziech, MD
Department of Radiology, Academic Medical Center,
University of Amsterdam, Amsterdam,
The Netherlands

Foreword

As the use of 3T systems evolves into the standard of care for body MR imaging, an in-depth understanding of the differences between body imaging at 3T versus 1.5T becomes critical for all diagnostic imagers. Up until now, a thorough knowledge of protocols, physics, and potential pitfalls in 3T MR imaging of the body has been limited to those radiologists with extensive experience at this higher field strength. Fortunately, with the publication of *Body MR Imaging at 3 Tesla* by Drs. Ihab Kamel and Elmar Merkle, this knowledge and insight is now available to a wide audience of diagnostic radiologists and other clinical imaging physicians. Drs. Merkle and Kamel are truly authorities in high-field body MR imaging; in this book, they have gathered additional experts from around the world to lend their own proficiency in MR imaging at 3T. The editors have done an outstanding job of choosing clinicians and scientists involved in the development and early adoption of 3T MR imaging of the body, and have created a compendium that will truly impact the field for years to come. It is a particular pleasure for me to write this introduction, as I have had the honor of working closely with Dr. Merkle for over 12 years and with Dr. Kamel for the past 7 years. Watching them produce this textbook is a pleasure only equaled by the satisfaction of reading its content. To you, the reader, I wish many hours of enjoyment and learning in your reading of this book, and I am certain your future patients will benefit from much that you learn in the process!

Jonathan S. Lewin, MD, FACR

Preface

The intent of *Body MR Imaging at 3 Tesla* is to provide a closer look at various MR applications within the chest, abdomen, and pelvis with specific emphasis on the effects of a higher 3T magnetic field strength.

Since the inception of MR imaging in the 1970s, radiologists have intensively searched for the optimal magnetic field strength, and this quest continues. In the early 1980s, a magnetic field strength of 0.3T was considered optimal. During the 1990s, we saw a shift toward 1T and 1.5T; and over the last ten years, we have seen a substantial trend toward 3T MR imaging. The search for higher field strength has been driven by the desire for an increase in signal-to-noise ratio, which can be kept to improve image quality, or traded for increased spatial resolution, improved temporal resolution, or both. Besides a gain in signal-to-noise ratio, other factors such as safety issues, image artifacts, and efficiency of contrast agents, to name a few, also have to be considered.

For this book, we are fortunate to have the contributions of many colleagues, all of whom were chosen as clinicians and scientists involved in the early adoption of 3T scanners in their practice. In the first chapter of this book, Dr. Kevin Chang and Dr. Ihab Kamel cover the basic concepts of MR physics and safety aspects relevant to the switch from 1.5T to 3T. Following this chapter, Dr. Diego Martin's group discusses novel acquisition techniques that are facilitated by 3T. Dr. Connie Lehman's group contributed the chapter on breast MR imaging, where early results at 3T have been both promising as well as challenging. Two cardiovascular research groups based in Madison/Wisconsin and Mannheim/Germany discuss cardiac as well as thoracoabdominal vascular MR. These chapters are followed by organ-specific contributions that examine in greater detail MR imaging of the liver, biliary system, pancreas, adrenals, kidneys, small bowel, large bowel and rectum. Finally, Dr. Katarzyna Macura and Dr. Susan Ascher's groups provide their insights of the advantages of 3T MR imaging of the male and female pelvis, respectively.

As you read this book, it is our hope that you realize how little is scientifically proven about the advantages of 3T over 1.5T MR imaging. None of the contributors had a wealth of scientific literature to rely on, and there are topics such as renal MR imaging, where not a single comparison study is currently available. This is surprising since the US Food and Drug Administration (FDA) approved 3T MR systems for clinical use in 2002. Thus, despite the mostly marketing-driven hype about 3T, it currently remains unclear whether body MR imaging at 3T is superior to standard 1.5T MR imaging. Notwithstanding radiologists' continued faith in the advantages of 3T, perhaps this book will provide the necessary guidance to make an informed choice between 3T and 1.5T body MR imaging rather than simply following the all-too-common "bigger must be better" approach.

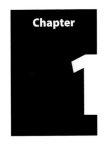

Chapter

1

Body MR imaging at 3T: basic considerations about artifacts and safety

Kevin J. Chang and Ihab R. Kamel

Introduction

Three Tesla magnetic resonance (MR) imaging scanners have been seeing steadily increasing use recently as hardware has matured and pulse sequences have become more optimized for a higher field strength. This increase in popularity has been more pronounced for neurologic and musculoskeletal imaging than for body imaging, however, due to the fact that 3T imaging with the larger field of view required for the torso tends to be more susceptible to artifacts and energy absorption limits than the imaging of smaller body parts.

Imaging artifacts at 3T tend to be more numerous and/or more pronounced than at lower field strengths [1]. While most of these artifacts are the same ones encountered at lower field strengths (e.g., flow artifacts, motion artifacts, Gibbs ringing), many are more peculiar to high-field imaging. This chapter will discuss these field strength-related artifacts at 3T as they apply to body imaging with specific comparisons made to 1.5T. The differences in relaxation times, chemical shift effects, and issues related to field inhomogeneity will also be discussed. Various approaches to mitigating artifacts peculiar to an increase in field strength at 3T will also be addressed.

Signal-to-noise ratio

MR signal relates directly to the ratio of protons aligned parallel rather than anti-parallel to the static magnetic field (B0). This ratio varies by the square of the magnetic field strength so a doubling of field strength from 1.5T to 3T should result in a quadrupling of MR signal. However, the doubling of field strength is also accompanied by a doubling of noise. The net effect of these changes results in an overall theoretical doubling of the signal-to-noise ratio (SNR). Thus, the theoretical SNR varies directly with the increase in magnetic field strength. It is this promised gain in SNR from an increase in field strength that allows for a boost in spatial resolution, temporal resolution, or some combination of the two. An increase in SNR also promises to improve MR spectroscopy and diffusion-weighted imaging. In practice, however, moving from 1.5T to 3T usually results in a less than twofold realized gain in SNR due to physiologic noise and limitations in energy deposition as well as other factors such as inadequate optimization of scanner hardware and software, radiofrequency (RF) field (B1) inhomogeneity, and increased magnetic susceptibility effects.

T1 relaxation times

For most physiologic tissues an increase in magnetic field strength leads to a prolongation of T1 relaxation times [2]. When attempting to generate soft tissue contrast at 3T, a longer repetition time (TR) may be required to obtain a similar imaging appearance that one may be accustomed to at 1.5T and lower field strengths (Figures 1.1 and 1.2) [3]. The downside of a longer TR is a concomitant increase in imaging time. T1 relaxation times tend to be approximately 20–40% longer at 3T when compared with 1.5T [2].

Approaches to addressing this problem with unenhanced T1-weighted images include the addition of an inversion recovery preparatory pulse to accentuate T1 contrast (e.g., T1 fluid-attenuated inversion recovery [FLAIR]). Other possibilities include the use of magnetization preparation pulses, short echo time (TE) gradient echo pulses, as well as parallel imaging techniques to decrease overall imaging time [4, 5].

Body MR Imaging at 3 Tesla, ed. Ihab R. Kamel and Elmar M. Merkle. Published by Cambridge University Press.

Gadolinium contrast effects

While the T1 relaxation time of unenhanced soft tissues is longer at 3T compared with lower field strengths, the T1 relaxation time of gadolinium chelate-based contrast agents is relatively unaffected. As a result, post-contrast imaging at 3T yields a more conspicuous degree of contrast enhancement. This

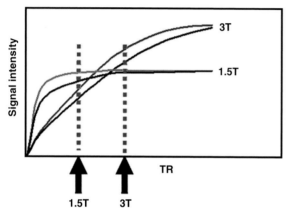

Figure 1.1 Signal intensity–time curves show longer T1 relaxation times at MR imaging in liver (black curves) and tumor tissue (gray curves) at 3T than at 1.5T. To generate a level of T1 contrast between the two tissue types at 3T commensurate with that at 1.5T, longer repetition times (TR, represented by dotted vertical lines) are required. Reproduced with permission from Chang KJ, Kamel IR, Macura KJ, Bluemke DA. 3T MR imaging of the abdomen: comparison with 1.5T. *RadioGraphics* 2008; **28**: 1983–98. © Radiological Society of North America.

wider dynamic range of effect leads to an increase in the contrast-to-noise ratio (CNR), an effect illustrated in Figures 1.3 and 1.4.

An increase in CNR at 3T leads to increased target conspicuity on post-contrast imaging, improved vessel delineation and visualization on MR angiography (MRA), as well as the possibility of decreasing contrast dose compared with 1.5T [6–8] This latter option is becoming increasingly relevant due to the heightened awareness of the risks of nephrogenic systemic fibrosis (NSF). In fact, for imaging of brain tumors, a half dose of gadolinium-based contrast at 3T approximates the CNR of a full dose of contrast at 1.5T [8].

T2 and T2* relaxation times (magnetic susceptibility)

The effects of an increase in field strength on the T2 relaxation times of tissues are less predictable than the changes in T1 relaxation times. While for lattice-fixed protons, T2 relaxation times may be similarly prolonged with an increase in field strength, most tissues experience an increase in efficiency of chemical exchange mechanisms at 3T which tends to result in a net shortening of T2 relaxation times (the efficiency of proton exchange between molecules varies with the square of the magnetic field strength). While for most soft tissues, T2 relaxation times are slightly shorter, T2 relaxation times for adipose tissues remain slightly

(a)

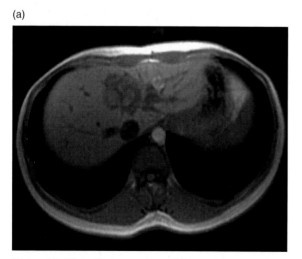

(b)

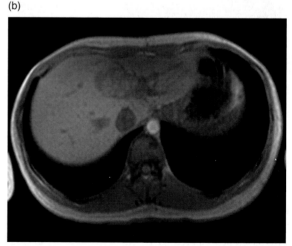

Figure 1.2 Effect of higher magnetic field strength on the visibility of a colon adenocarcinoma metastasis in the liver of a 32-year-old woman. Unenhanced T1-weighted gradient echo images obtained at 1.5T with 180/4.4 (TR ms/echo time [TE] ms), 90° flip angle, and 8-mm section thickness (a) and at 3T with 263/2.3, 75° flip angle, and 8-mm section thickness (b) show higher SNR but decreased lesion conspicuity in (b).

(a) (b)

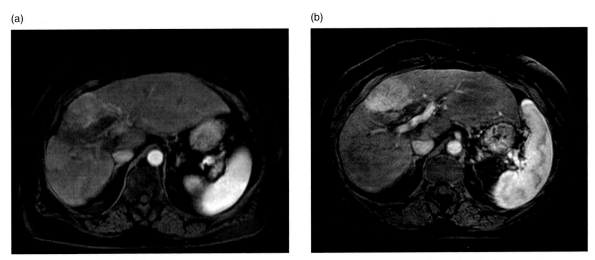

Figure 1.3 Increased conspicuity of lesions at 3T MR. Gadolinium-induced contrast enhancement of a moderately differentiated cholangiocarcinoma in an 82-year-old woman is less pronounced on the 1.5T three-dimensional (3D) volumetric interpolated breath-hold examination (VIBE; 4.9/2.5, 10° flip angle) image (a) than on the 3T 3D T1-weighted high-resolution isotropic volume examination (THRIVE; 3.3/1.6, 10° flip angle) image (b) because of lower CNR at 1.5T compared with 3T, even allowing for equipment differences.

(a) (b)

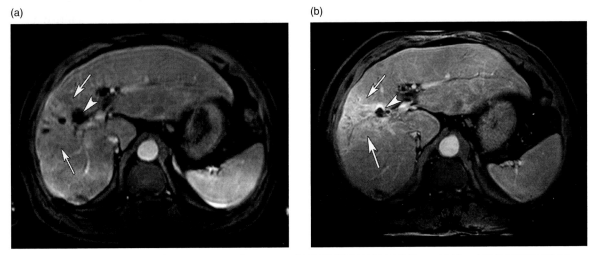

Figure 1.4 Increased conspicuity of lesions at 3T MR. Comparison of 1.5T 3D VIBE (4.9/2.5, 10° flip angle) (a) and 3T 3D THRIVE (3.3/1.6, 10° flip angle) (b) MR images in a 68-year-old man with hepatitis C-related cirrhosis shows greater contrast of a wedge-shaped region of hyperperfusion (transient hepatic signal intensity difference) (arrows) at 3T than at 1.5T. Magnetic susceptibility artifacts related to a surgical clip (arrowheads) also are partially mitigated in (b) because of the use of a shorter TE.

longer and T2 relaxation times for fluids are largely unchanged [2].

Nevertheless, there is a significant perceived improvement in image quality on T2-weighted images with a move to a higher field strength (Figure 1.5). This is chiefly related to an increase in SNR and is more pronounced on T2-weighted imaging than T1-weighted imaging as the longer TR of T2-weighted pulse sequences allows for more recovery of longitudinal magnetization than on T1-weighted sequences. Sequences such as single-shot fast spin echo (SSFSE), half-Fourier acquisition single-shot turbo spin echo (HASTE), as well as three-dimensional (3D) turbo spin echo (such as in 3D MR cholangio-pancreatography) stand to benefit the most from a higher field strength.

T2* relaxation times are affected much more predictably with a move to 3T and vary inversely

(a) (b)

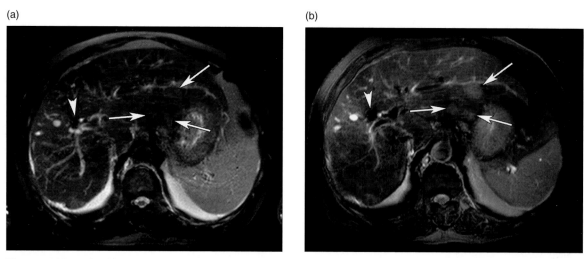

Figure 1.5 T2-weighted fast spin echo images in a 68-year-old male with hepatocellular carcinoma in the setting of hepatitis C-associated cirrhosis (same patient as Figure 1.4 but at a slightly different level) at 1.5T (a) and 3T (b). Multiple T2-intense metastases (white arrows) are more apparent at 3T than 1.5T (3T examination 1 month prior to 1.5T examination). Also note the increased susceptibility related to a metallic clip (white arrowhead) in the central right lobe at 3T which is barely perceptible at 1.5T. Parameters: (a) 1.5T 4000/103/90°. (b) 3T 2053/100/90°.

(a) (b)

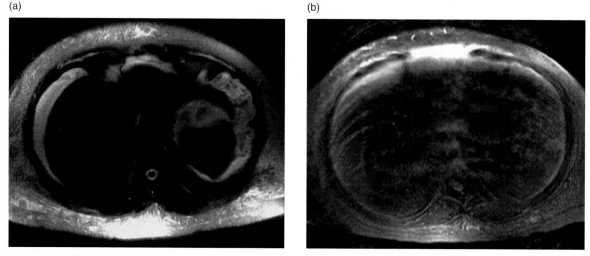

Figure 1.6 Field inhomogeneity and standing wave effects. T2-weighted images through the liver at 1.5T (2416/180) (a) and at 3T (2052/100) (b) show diffuse hepatic iron deposition and ascites in a 49-year-old woman with hepatitis C–related cirrhosis. In (b), there is increased susceptibility artifact and decreased signal intensity in the liver because of iron deposition, standing wave effects with signal drop-off related to ascites (seen in the central abdomen), and significant respiratory motion artifact. Reproduced with permission from Chang KJ, Kamel IR, Macura KJ, Bluemke DA. 3T MR imaging of the abdomen: comparison with 1.5T. *RadioGraphics* 2008; **28**: 1983–98. © Radiological Society of North America.

with the strength of the magnetic field [9, 10]. Thus, a doubling of field strength from 1.5T to 3T results in a doubling of magnetic susceptibility artifact and a larger area of "blooming" related to paramagnetic effects. This has a particularly profound effect on gradient echo images and echo planar pulse sequences such as those commonly used in diffusion-weighted imaging and functional MR imaging. When used in conventional imaging, the more pronounced magnetic susceptibility at air–soft tissue interfaces and areas adjacent to paramagnetic materials such as metals can lead to significant localized variations in magnetic field homogeneity (inhomogeneous B0 field, Figure 1.6). This results in larger artifactual signal voids than at 1.5T. This effect does, however, allow for higher sensitivity to

(a)

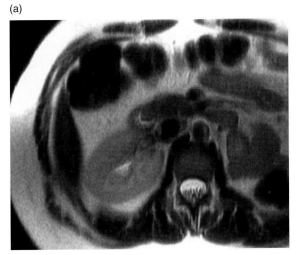

(b)

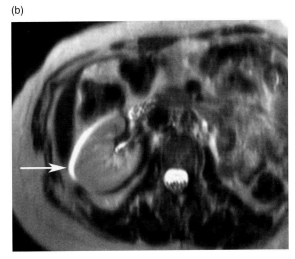

Figure 1.7 Chemical shift artifact at 1.5T (a) and 3T (b) in normal kidneys. Note increased water–fat misregistration at the renal cortex at 3T (white arrow). Parameters: (a) 1.5T SSFSE 1759/88, slice thickness 8 mm. (b) 3T SSFSE 4500/90, slice thickness 8 mm. Reproduced with permission from Chang KJ, Kamel IR, Macura KJ, Bluemke DA. 3T MR imaging of the abdomen: comparison with 1.5T. *RadioGraphics* 2008; **28**: 1983–98. © Radiological Society of North America.

the detection of gas, items such as surgical clips, and areas of iron deposition in solid organs. This effect, in fact, makes 3T imaging more sensitive to superparamagnetic iron oxide contrast agents (SPIO) as well as the blood oxygen level-dependent (BOLD) phenomenon used extensively in functional MR imaging [11–13].

Approaches to minimizing magnetic susceptibility artifacts include shortening TE, using parallel imaging to shorten imaging time and decrease echo train length, and increasing receiver bandwidth to decrease the echo spacing of the readout train. These approaches have already shown significant success in reducing artifacts on diffusion-weighted imaging in the brain [14, 15].

Chemical shift effects

Just as with magnetic susceptibility effects, chemical shift effects also directly vary with an increase in the magnetic field strength. For chemical shift effects of the first kind, the difference in precession frequency of water protons and fat protons holds steady at 3.5 ppm. With a doubling of field strength from 1.5T to 3T the Larmor frequency doubles from 64 MHz to 128 MHz, respectively. Accompanying this doubling of Larmor frequency is a chemical shift separation between water and fat which also doubles from approximately 220 Hz to 440 Hz, respectively

(Larmor frequency × 3.5 ppm). This means at a constant bandwidth, the misregistration artifacts between fat voxels and water voxels in the frequency-encoding direction doubles in conspicuity with a doubling in field strength (Figure 1.7). While this misregistration artifact is more pronounced at 3T, this wider spectral separation between fat and water also allows for improved spectral resolution in MR spectroscopy as well as improved fat suppression limited only by the degree of magnetic field inhomogeneity [16, 17].

There are various approaches to decreasing the conspicuity of the misregistration artifact associated with chemical shift effects of the first kind. An increase in bandwidth will counteract an increase in chemical shift at the cost of SNR. For example, a doubling of bandwidth to fully offset a doubling of field strength will result in a 29% decrease in relative SNR. This ability to increase bandwidth is limited by gradient coil strength. Another approach to mitigating fat–water misregistration is utilizing fat suppression.

Chemical shift artifacts of the second kind are also significantly affected by an increase in magnetic field strength. These phase cancellation or "India ink" artifacts are seen in voxels sharing both fat and water protons at specific TEs corresponding to times when fat and water protons precess out of phase with each other resulting in signal cancellation. This is most commonly seen at the edges of solid organs where

(a)

(b)

(c)

(d)

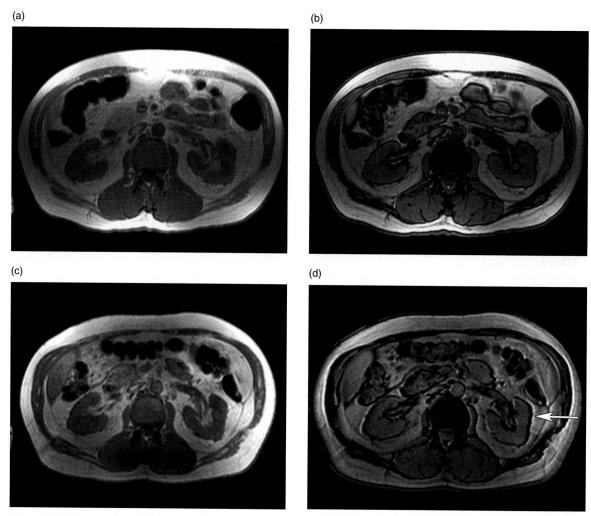

Figure 1.8 In-phase and out-of-phase imaging at 1.5T and 3T. (a) 1.5T in-phase TE 4.6 ms. (b) 1.5T out-of-phase TE 2.3 ms. (c) 3T in-phase TE 2.3 ms. (d) 3T out-of-phase TE 1.15 ms. Note increased chemical shift at 3T (white arrow).

they interface with surrounding fat. A doubling of field strength will double the precession frequency of these protons and, correspondingly, halve their out-of-phase and in-phase TEs from approximately 2.3 and 4.6 ms respectively at 1.5T to approximately 1.15 and 2.3 ms at 3T (Figure 1.8) [18]. When gradient coils are incapable of imaging with a TE as short as 1.15 ms, significant changes may need to be incorporated when obtaining T1-weighted in- and out-of-phase images routine in abdominal imaging. If the next shortest out-of-phase TE of 3.45 ms is obtained, if compared with an in-phase image at TE 2.3 ms, magnetic susceptibility effects related to a longer TE cannot be differentiated from signal dropout related to chemical shift effects of the second kind. An

alternative approach is obtaining two separate image acquisitions rather than using a dual-echo pulse sequence; however, this introduces problems related to imperfect image co-registration of the two acquisitions and necessitates longer imaging time. Another approach is the use of a dual-echo 3D fast spoiled gradient echo pulse sequence [19].

Field inhomogeneity (B0, B1, and dielectric shading)

One of the most apparent challenges faced with MR imaging at 3T relates to significant variations in signal intensity that are often encountered across the field of

(a)

(b)

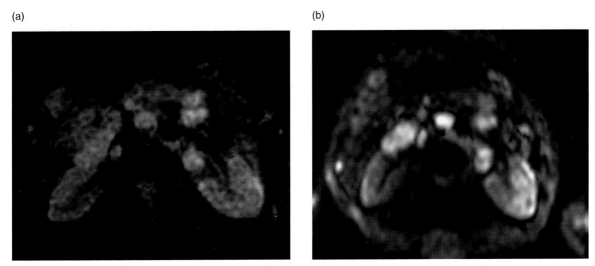

Figure 1.9 Diffusion-weighted imaging of normal kidneys in the axial plane at 1.5T (a) and 3T (b), B = 750 s/mm². Higher SNR at 3T increases sensitivity for areas of restricted diffusion. Image quality may be limited by increased sensitivity to magnetic susceptibility artifact. Reproduced with permission from Chang KJ, Kamel IR, Macura KJ, Bluemke DA. 3T MR imaging of the abdomen: comparison with 1.5T. *RadioGraphics* 2008; **28**: 1983–98. © Radiological Society of North America.

view, especially with the larger field of view required in imaging the human torso. Multiple factors can account for these signal intensity variations across an image. As has been discussed above, increased sensitivity to T2* effects can lead to pronounced magnetic susceptibility effects, especially in areas adjacent to air or the skin surface. This effect is commonly seen in the upper abdomen adjacent to the lung bases as well as around gas-filled loops of bowel. Gradient echo and echo planar acquisitions such as those typically used in diffusion-weighted imaging can be quite susceptible to these effects (Figure 1.9), although, when combined with the use of parallel imaging, diffusion-weighted imaging at 3T can be performed more quickly and with higher SNR [15]. In addition, underlying B0 field inhomogeneities have been a challenge addressed with some success on newer-generation 3T scanners, with improvements in B0 field homogeneity through better shimming and magnet design. Other approaches to limiting B0 field inhomogeneity are similar to limiting susceptibility artifact and include shortening TE (which may require an increase in bandwidth and resultant decrease in SNR), using parallel imaging to shorten imaging time, and decreasing voxel size to limit intra-voxel dephasing.

Another major factor accounting for signal intensity variations on 3T images is inhomogeneity in the B1 or RF field. Particularly with larger fields of view

such as in the abdomen and pelvis, standing wave or dielectric effects become a significant source of RF field inhomogeneity at 3T. The reason why these effects are so much more pronounced at 3T than at lower field strengths is related to the RF wavelength corresponding to the resonant frequency (Larmor frequency) of water protons. While at 1.5T a Larmor frequency of 64 MHz corresponds to an RF wavelength of 52 cm, at 3T a higher Larmor frequency of 128 MHz corresponds to a shorter wavelength of 26 cm, which is much closer in dimension to the human abdomen or pelvis. These wavelengths lead to areas of constructive and destructive interference within the torso, termed standing wave or "dielectric shading" effects, which can lead to large variations in local signal intensity across an image [20]. This finding is more apparent in those with a wider body habitus or more ellipsoid body cross section [21]. Similar-appearing artifacts can be even more troublesome in patients with a large volume of conductive intra-abdominal fluid such as ascites or amniotic fluid. Rapid alterations in the magnetic field caused by changing RF currents tend to induce circulating currents within large volumes of conductive fluid that counteract or "shield" the RF field and attenuate signal intensity within the central torso (Figure 1.10) [22]. This "black-hole" artifact tends to be more noticeable with fast spin echo pulse sequences than gradient echo sequences.

(a)

(b)

(c)

(d)

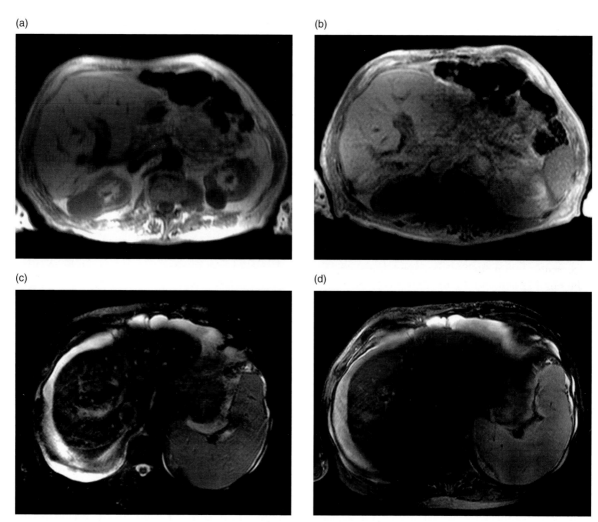

Figure 1.10 Standing wave artifacts. T1-weighted images at 1.5T (a) and 3T (b). Standing wave effects in the upper abdomen cause significant artifact at 3T. Note inhomogeneity around the spine in (b). T2-weighted images in a patient with ascites at 1.5T (c) and 3T (d). Note large region of signal dropout in the central abdomen at 3T accentuated by ascites in (d). Parameters: (a) 1.5T T1 gradient echo in-phase 200/4.4/90°, (b) 3T T1 GRE in-phase 263/2.3/75°, (c) 1.5T T2 FSE 4000/103, (d) 3T T2 FSE 2053/100.

There are many ways to attempt to alleviate the issues related to standing wave artifacts and B1 field inhomogeneity. One of the simplest ways to decrease dielectric shading is through the use of dielectric pads or "RF cushions," pads or bags of conductive fluid or gel which are placed on the region of interest in an attempt to change the shape of the torso or partially mitigate standing waves within the torso [23]. Many recent hardware advances have also resulted in significant improvements in B1 field homogeneity through more efficient and homogeneously designed RF coils as well as the use of multi-transmitter coils "tuned" to fit the body part to be imaged [24].

Combined transmit–receive coils are also in development to improve RF transmission and signal detection efficiency at 3T. These alternative coil designs are of particular importance as well, given the specific absorption rate (SAR) intensity of pulse sequences at 3T.

Specific absorption rate

The US Food and Drug Administration and the International Electrotechnical Commission limit the SAR to 4 W/kg over 15 minutes or 8 W/kg over 5 minutes, a limit intended to prevent tissues from heating more than $1\,^{\circ}$C. This limit holds regardless of the field strength of a magnet. When compared with 1.5T, a doubling of field strength to 3T is accompanied by a quadrupling of the SAR. At 3T, SAR limits become a much more realistic limitation to the use of pulse sequences such as fast spin echo, 3D gradient echo, and steady-state free precession sequences. As SAR also directly relates to the imaged volume, SAR limitations become more of an issue with body MR imaging than with the imaging of smaller body parts.

$$SAR \propto B_0^2 \alpha^2 DV$$

The relationship of SAR to various imaging parameters can be illustrated with the above equation where **B0** represents the magnetic field strength, **α** represents the flip angle, **D** represents the duty cycle (the number and spacing of RF pulses), and **V** represents the volume imaged. While doubling B0 quadruples SAR, altering the other parameters can mitigate these effects to avoid exceeding SAR restrictions. Decreasing flip angles can lead to significant decreases in SAR at the potential expense of prolonged acquisition time and decreased T1 contrast. More sophisticated techniques for varying flip angles include the use of RF refocusing pulse sequences such as flip angle sweep and hyperechoes at a slight cost of SNR [25, 26]. Techniques related to reducing the duty cycle of a pulse sequence include increasing TR (at the expense of prolonging scan time), decreasing the number of phase-encode or slice-select steps (at the cost of decreased spatial resolution, slice thickness, or field of view), alternating high and low SAR pulse sequences during the course of an examination, and using parallel imaging (at a slight cost of SNR – an effect which is less noticeable at 3T than at 1.5T). Imaging volume is less easily varied but can be affected by the use of more RF efficient transmit–receive coils or with the use of a shorter magnet bore.

Safety

Safety considerations remain a significant consideration when moving to a higher magnetic field strength. Implanted medical devices that are deemed MR compatible at 1.5T or lower are not necessarily approved for MR imaging at 3T. Metallic devices require further testing in the 3T environment prior to 3T approval as there is a proportional increase in translational attraction and torque upon these implanted devices with an increase in magnetic field strength [27]. This is especially true in the latest generation of wider- and shorter-bore magnets due to their increased spatial gradients and higher associated deflection angles [28]. With an ever-expanding clinical experience with 3T MR imaging, more devices will eventually gain 3T approval.

In addition to device safety, MR imaging siting issues are also important to consider with a higher field strength. A higher field strength results in a larger magnetic fringe field. This requires either a wider 5 Gauss safety margin increasing the 3T MR suite's "footprint" or the use of active shielding to counteract the larger fringe field (not without additional installation and maintenance cost). Acoustic noise concerns are also an issue with higher field strength imaging although this has been mitigated on newer scanners with improved acoustic shielding.

Conclusion

MR imaging at 3T is becoming more popular, more widespread, and increasingly accepted as the current "cutting edge" in clinical MR imaging. This is especially the case for neurologic and musculoskeletal imaging. However, the adoption of 3T in body imaging has been comparatively slower and much of this is related to the imaging challenges that a higher field strength presents in the abdomen and pelvis.

There are many differences in the behavior of protons at 3T compared with lower field strengths and this accounts for many of the artifacts encountered at 3T MR imaging. T1 relaxation times are longer with a significant effect on soft tissue contrast, particularly on pre-contrast imaging. T2* effects are more pronounced with an increase in magnetic susceptibility artifacts as well as difficulties in maintaining a homogeneous B0 field. Chemical shift artifacts of both the first and second kind are also predictably different at 3T and require adjustments in imaging parameters and changes in pulse sequence timing. And last, but definitely not least, standing wave artifacts ("dielectric shading") are a source of significant local variation in signal intensity across the larger imaging field of view utilized in the abdomen and pelvis. Many options exist in addressing these artifacts at 3T including changes in TE, use of parallel imaging, changes in bandwidth, as well as more hardware-oriented solutions such as the use of dielectric pads and various strategies employed to generate a more homogeneous B0 and B1 field. Only when pulse sequences and image quality can be sufficiently optimized for 3T imaging can the promise of an increased SNR truly yield perceptible improvements in spatial and temporal resolution.

Acknowledgements

Special thanks to David A. Bluemke, MD, PhD and Katarzyna J. Macura, MD, PhD for their additional help and guidance during the preparation of this topic.

References

1. Vargas MI, Delavelle J, Kohler R, Becker CD, Lovblad K. Brain and spine MRI artifacts at 3 Tesla. *J Neuroradiol* 2009; **36**(2): 74–81.

2. de Bazelaire CM, Duhamel GD, Rofsky NM, Alsop DC. MR imaging relaxation times of abdominal and pelvic tissues measured in vivo at 3T: preliminary results. *Radiology* 2004; **230**(3): 652–9.

3. Bushberg J. *The Essential Physics of Medical Imaging*, 2nd edn. Philadelphia, PA, Lippincott Williams & Wilkins, 2002. pp. xvi, 933.

4. Lee JH, Garwood M, Menon R, *et al.* High contrast and fast three-dimensional magnetic resonance imaging at high fields. *Magn Reson Med* 1995; **34**(3): 308–12.

5. Wolff SD, Eng J, Balaban RS. Magnetization transfer contrast: method for improving contrast in gradient-recalled-echo images. *Radiology* 1991; **179**(1): 133–7.

6. Elster AD. How much contrast is enough? Dependence of enhancement on field strength and MR pulse sequence. *Eur Radiol* 1997; 7 Suppl 5: 276–80.

7. Fukatsu H. 3T MR for clinical use: update. *Magn Reson Med Sci* 2003; **2**(1): 37–45.

8. Krautmacher C, Willinek WA, Tschampa HJ, *et al.* Brain tumors: full- and half-dose contrast-enhanced MR imaging at 3T compared with 1.5T – initial experience. *Radiology* 2005; **237**(3): 1014–19.

9. Lewin JS, Duerk JL, Jain VR, *et al.* Needle localization in MR-guided biopsy and aspiration: effects of field strength, sequence design, and magnetic field orientation. *AJR Am J Roentgenol* 1996; **166**(6): 1337–45.

10. Olsrud J, Latt J, Brockstedt S, Romner B, Bjorkman-Burtscher IM. Magnetic resonance imaging artifacts caused by aneurysm clips and shunt valves: dependence on field strength (1.5 and 3T) and imaging parameters. *J Magn Reson Imaging* 2005; **22**(3): 433–7.

11. Chang JM, Lee JM, Lee MW, *et al.* Superparamagnetic iron oxide-enhanced liver magnetic resonance imaging: comparison of 1.5T and 3T imaging for detection of focal malignant liver lesions. *Invest Radiol* 2006; **41**(2): 168–74.

12. Simon GH, Bauer J, Saborovski O, *et al.* T1 and T2 relaxivity of intracellular and extracellular USPIO at 1.5T and 3T clinical MR scanning. *Eur Radiol* 2006; **16**(3): 738–45.

13. Li LP, Vu AT, Li BS, Dunkle E, Prasad PV. Evaluation of intrarenal oxygenation by BOLD MRI at 3T. *J Magn Reson Imaging* 2004; **20**(5): 901–4.

14. Kuhl CK, Textor J, Gieseke J, *et al.* Acute and subacute ischemic stroke at high-field-strength (3.0-T) diffusion-weighted MR imaging: intraindividual comparative study. *Radiology* 2005; **234**(2): 509–16.

15. Kuhl CK, Gieseke J, von Falkenhausen M, *et al.* Sensitivity encoding for diffusion-weighted MR imaging at 3T: intraindividual comparative study. *Radiology* 2005; **234**(2): 517–26.

16. Gruetter R, Weisdorf SA, Rajanayagan V, *et al.* Resolution improvements in in vivo 1H NMR spectra with increased magnetic field strength. *J Magn Reson* 1998; **135**(1): 260–4.

17. Katz-Brull R, Rofsky NM, Lenkinski RE. Breathhold abdominal and thoracic proton MR spectroscopy at 3T. *Magn Reson Med* 2003; **50**(3): 461–7.

18. Wehrli FW, Perkins TG, Shimakawa A, Roberts F. Chemical shift-induced amplitude modulations in images obtained with gradient refocusing. *Magn Reson Imaging* 1987; **5**(2): 157–8.

19. Cornfeld DM, Israel G, McCarthy SM, Weinreb JC. Pelvic imaging using a T1W fat-suppressed three-dimensional dual echo Dixon technique at 3T. *J Magn Reson Imaging* 2008; **28**(1): 121–7.

20. Collins CM, Liu W, Schreiber W, Yang QX, Smith MB. Central brightening due to constructive interference with, without, and despite dielectric resonance. *J Magn Reson Imaging* 2005; **21**(2): 192–6.

21. Hussain S. *Body MR Imaging: Current Practice and Future Horizons*. Scientific Assembly and Annual Meeting of Radiological Society of North America, Chicago, IL, 2006.

22. Merkle EM, Dale BM, Paulson EK. Abdominal MR imaging at 3T. *Magn Reson Imaging Clin N Am* 2006; **14**(1): 17–26.

23. Franklin KM, Dale BM, Merkle EM. Improvement in B1-inhomogeneity artifacts in the abdomen at 3T MR imaging using a radiofrequency cushion. *J Magn Reson Imaging* 2008; **27**(6): 1443–7.

24. Tomanek B, Ryner L, Hoult DI, Kozlowski P, Saunders JK. Dual surface coil with high-B1 homogeneity for

deep organ MR imaging. *Magn Reson Imaging* 1997; 15(10): 1199–204.

25. Hennig J, Scheffler K. Hyperechoes. *Magn Reson Med* 2001; **46**(1): 6–12.

26. Hennig J, Weigel M, Scheffler K. Multiecho sequences with variable refocusing flip angles: optimization of signal behavior using smooth transitions between pseudo steady states (TRAPS). *Magn Reson Med* 2003; **49**(3): 527–35.

27. Shellock FG. Biomedical implants and devices: assessment of magnetic field interactions with a 3.0-Tesla MR system. *J Magn Reson Imaging* 2002; **16**(6): 721–32.

28. Shellock FG, Tkach JA, Ruggieri PM, Masaryk TJ. Cardiac pacemakers, ICDs, and loop recorder: evaluation of translational attraction using conventional ("long-bore") and "short-bore" 1.5- and 3.0-Tesla MR systems. *J Cardiovasc Magn Reson* 2003; 5(2): 387–97.

Novel acquisition techniques that are facilitated by 3T

Hiroumi D. Kitajima, Puneet Sharma,
Daniel R. Karolyi, and Diego R. Martin

Introduction

Compared with lower field strength systems, magnetic resonance (MR) at 3T has many theoretical and real advantages. Included in the advantages are higher signal-to-noise ratios (SNRs) as well as larger spectral separation of fat, water, and various metabolites which can be used to improve fat saturation techniques as well as MR spectroscopy methods. In addition to these advantages that can be applied to already routine clinical imaging, 3T systems also provide advantages that can be exploited for novel techniques. This chapter will outline the advantages of 3T systems in terms of basic physics considerations, application, and advantages in routine sequences as well as potential application in novel imaging techniques such as MR spectroscopy, diffusion-weighted imaging (DWI), arterial spin labeling (ASL), susceptibility-weighted imaging (SWI), as well as magnetic resonance elastography (MRE).

Basic science considerations

Larmor frequency and chemical shift

The Larmor frequency is directly proportional to magnetic field strength (B0) as defined by the gyromagnetic ratio of nuclei. This relation has implications both in MR imaging and MR spectroscopy when exciting various tissues. In MR imaging, a larger difference in frequency theoretically allows better fat suppression, water excitation, and other chemically specific pulses. In addition, a higher frequency at higher field strength means that fat and water will be in-phase or in opposed-phase sooner, allowing for shorter echo times (TEs) and faster imaging. Spectroscopy benefits significantly from chemical shift with improved differentiation of various nuclei.

The resonance frequency of fat and water are directly related to the external magnetic field strength [1]. At 1.5T, these resonant frequencies are separated by approximately 210 Hz as compared to a 420 Hz separation at a 3T field strength [2]. This difference can cause a misregistration artifact in the phase-encoding direction. Keeping other parameters such as bandwidth and voxel size constant, the misregistration artifact will be approximately twice as large at the 3T field strength compared with the 1.5T field strength. Although this artifact rarely causes an issue with clinical interpretation, the alterations in signal adjacent to fat–fluid interfaces could obscure subtle findings. To minimize these effects, the receiver bandwidth can be increased or the field of view (FOV) can be decreased, but at the cost of SNR. One important application of this phenomenon is with in- and opposed-phase imaging. At the 3T field strength, the TEs at which these images are acquired must be adjusted. At 3T, the opposed-phase image should be acquired at a TE of 1.2 ms while the in-phase image should be acquired at a TE of 2.4 ms. The increase in separation of the fat and water frequencies can also be advantageous in the application of certain fat saturation and spectroscopy techniques. More accurate spectroscopic analysis can be performed due to less overlap between spectroscopic fat and water peaks and the increased SNR. The greater separation can also be used to create more uniform and faster fat saturation when spectroscopic techniques are utilized.

Magnetization, signal, and signal-to-noise ratio (SNR)

Magnetization is directly proportional to field strength as governed by the number of excited nuclei. Although magnetization is linearly related to field strength,

Body MR Imaging at 3 Tesla, ed. Ihab R. Kamel and Elmar M. Merkle. Published by Cambridge University Press.
© Cambridge University Press 2011.

(a)

(b)

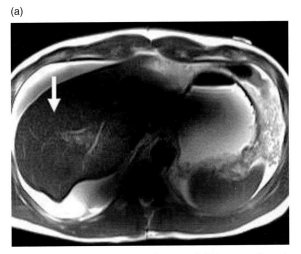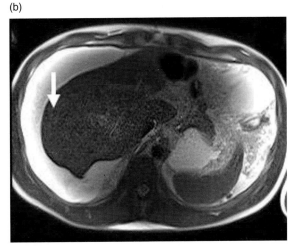

Figure 2.1 Higher SNR at 3T (a) than at 1.5T (b) in a two-dimensional (2D) single-shot fast spin echo (SSFSE) axial series. Note grainy central band overlying liver (b, arrow) due to SNR being lower at 1.5T.

signal is related to the electromotive force (EMF) induced in a receive coil and the square of field strength [3]. While signal increases quadratically in relation to field strength, noise at field strengths higher than 0.5T increases in a linear relation; at 3T one can expect a fourfold increase in signal with a twofold increase in noise, resulting in a twofold net SNR gain (Figure 2.1). In practice, however, the 100% increase in SNR is not attained when moving from 1.5T to 3T because of radiofrequency (RF) heating. As a consequence, flip angle must often be decreased because of International Electrotechnical Commission (IEC) specific absorption rate (SAR) limits of 8 W/kg in tissue over 5 minutes or 4 W/kg in a whole body over 15 minutes [1]. The US Food and Drug Administration (FDA) limits SAR to 2 W/kg in normal mode and 4 W/kg at a first-level controlled mode [4]. Alternatively, increasing repetition time (TR), decreasing echo train length, or increasing delays between sequences can be implemented as techniques that improve SNR, but at the expense of longer scan times. The advantages of increasing SNR using a higher field strength 3T system may be traded for shorter acquisition time or increased spatial resolution. Typical SNR gains at 3T are about 1.7–1.8 that of 1.5T systems [5, 6].

B0 inhomogeneities

B0 inhomogeneities can present limitations at higher field strengths. Dephasing due to B0 inhomogeneity

impacts T2* weighted sequences and further necessitates the use of refocusing pulses. However, dephasing in DWI cannot be restored by a refocusing pulse, but rather by a reversed gradient. A decrease in TE can minimize dephasing as well, often by also increasing bandwidth. Dephasing also can create flow voids in moving fluids, particularly when flow compensation is not used. Flow pulsatility can lead to ghosting artifacts, even with flow compensation, because of time-varying inflow effects. Dephasing can also create errors in phase contrast magnetic resonance angiography (MRA). B0 inhomogeneity can also cause distortion in the read direction in Cartesian imaging, or as a radial smear in radial imaging. Bandwidth can be increased to limit distortion without a significant penalty in SNR due to higher field strength. Image distortion is more severe in gradient echo (GRE) than in spin echo (SE) imaging, but is minimized with improved shimming. Distortion due to local field differences caused by susceptibility is usually not corrected completely, however. Phase images can be used to generate field maps to visualize B0 inhomogeneities. As such, phase imaging such as in flow quantification is particularly sensitive to artifacts from field homogeneity. Phase imaging is also sensitive to ghosting, more so than magnitude images, but ghosting is usually caused by errors in the receiver, transmitter, or gradient subsystems rather than from B0 inhomogeneities. Undesired phase dispersion can be minimized by flow velocity compensation and by a short TE. The B0 inhomogeneities encountered at

(a)

(b)

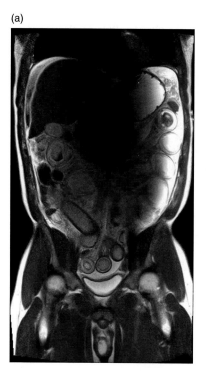
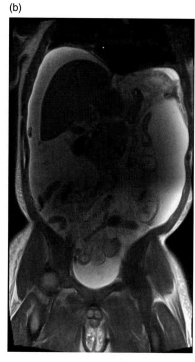

Figure 2.2 More prominent standing wave artifact shown at 3T (a) than at 1.5T (b) in a 2D SSFSE coronal series in a patient with ascites.

higher field strengths particularly affect steady-state free precession (SSFP) sequences. Because transverse magnetization is allowed to evolve without spoiling, T2* effects contribute to off-resonance banding artifacts. These artifacts are suppressed by shimming and by minimizing TR.

B1 inhomogeneities and radiofrequency (RF) wavelength

At higher field strengths, B1 inhomogeneity becomes a greater issue. Although usually a consideration with transmit and receive coil RF fields, tissues have higher permittivity and conductivity at high frequencies and therefore change the RF wavelength and create eddy currents. The reduced wavelength generates RF field pattern changes and decreased penetration, where signal is diminished and shading artifacts may develop (Figure 2.2).

The coils utilized at 3T field strength operate at 128 MHz rather than the 64 MHz utilized at the 1.5T field strength [4]. Although the wavelength of the RF field outside of the body is approximately 234 cm, this value is decreased to approximately 30 cm due to the high dielectric constant of water which reduces both the speed and wavelength of electromagnetic

radiation [4, 7]. The 30 cm wavelength is on the order of the FOV which can result in standing wave artifacts. These artifacts are manifested by areas of increased and decreased signal caused by constructive and destructive interference. While T1-weighted GRE imaging is usually not compromised by B1 inhomogeneity artifacts, this kind of artifact often occurs in T2-weighted imaging, especially with fat suppression [4, 6]. These artifacts also become more problematic the larger the FOV is relative to the wavelength. Shimming, dielectric pads filled with ultrasound gel, and B1-insensitive adiabatic pulses can minimize artifacts [5]. Improved RF transmitters may also help RF penetration.

Radiofrequency (RF) heating and specific absorption rate (SAR)

The SAR is a specific measure of energy deposition which is regulated by the FDA in the United States to avoid excessive tissue heating. The SAR is related to the square of the electric field, pulse duration, as well as TR. As the electric field is directly proportional to the magnetic fields, the SAR is quadrupled at the 3T field strength compared with the 1.5T field strength of the same pulse sequence. Increases in flip angle also cause quadratic increases in SAR. These limitations are particularly important when utilizing SE sequences that require at least two RF pulses per TR and in sequences that require large flip angles that also increase energy deposition. To compensate for increased SAR at 3T, pulse sequences must often decrease flip angle, decrease echo train length, or increase bandwidth to stay within allowable limits. Sequences with intense RF pulses such as fast spin echo (FSE) and fluid-attenuated inversion recovery (FLAIR) have high SAR, as well as GRE sequences with short TR such as SSFP and MRA sequences. Several novel approaches have been developed to overcome this limitation. Included in these approaches are variable-rate selective excitation (VERSE) sequences as well as variable flip angle refocusing techniques. These can lower RF deposition by an order of 2.5–6.0 [6]. Parallel imaging has also significantly contributed to the overall decrease in energy deposition at high-field imaging by reducing the number of repetitions. Transmit–receive coils can also reduce SAR. Short-bore MR imaging scanners have also decreased SAR because of the smaller transmitting body coils.

T1 relaxation

The resonant frequency of spins at 3T is double compared with 1.5T field strength. This higher resonant frequency diminishes the efficiency of energy transfer to the adjacent lattice which causes an increase in T1 relaxation times. In addition, the relaxation for protons in different organs is not linearly related. For example, the reported relaxation time in the liver increases approximately 40% compared with a 73% increase in renal tissue [5]. Therefore, both absolute and relative contrast between tissues is different at the 3T field strength. Generally, lower contrast is seen at 3T with pulse sequence parameters optimized for 1.5T. Traditional T1-weighted SE sequences are particularly affected. To generate a similar level of T1 contrast, a longer TR is required, which also causes an overall longer scan time. In addition, increases in T1 relaxation times also cause a decrease in SNR. When T1 contrast is still insufficient, T1 FLAIR sequences can also be considered. The longer T1 relaxation times can also be used to improve certain imaging techniques including contrast-enhanced and time-of-flight (TOF) MRA. Longer T1 relaxation times improve suppression of background tissues compared to the contrast-enhanced arterial and venous structures. Although the relaxivity of gadolinium-based contrast agents also decreases 5–10%, the contrast-to-noise ratio (CNR) between contrast-enhanced vasculature and unenhanced tissue is increased [6]. As a result, some centers elect to administer smaller doses of gadolinium at 3T [1, 6]. Increased T1 relaxation times also improve ASL techniques. Protons in blood are labeled magnetically and imaged as they flow through vascular structures and perfuse organs. This magnetic labeling of blood lasts for longer periods of time in 3T field strengths, resulting in greater SNR as well as more anatomical coverage utilizing this technique.

T2 relaxation and susceptibility

T2 relaxation times slightly decrease as field strength increases, accounting for a 10% decrease when comparing 3T with 1.5T [5]. Therefore, SNR decreases for long TE sequences such as magnetic resonance cholangiopancreatography (MRCP) in addition to standard T2-weighted sequences and must be adapted for 3T.

T2* decay times are shorter in 3T systems compared with 1.5T largely due to main field inhomogeneities that increase linearly with field strength [8]. Shortened T2* decay times can have both detrimental as well as advantageous effects. Areas of signal loss, geometric distortion, and inhomogeneous fat saturation are increased at higher field strength systems (Figure 2.3). Although susceptibility does not affect traditional SE sequences significantly, GRE and echo planar imaging (EPI) sequences are particularly sensitive to susceptibility. These artifacts can be minimized by using larger bandwidths and shorter TEs as well as smaller voxel sizes [1, 8]. The introduction of routine parallel imaging has also decreased these artifacts because of decreased echo spacing, but at a cost of SNR. More advanced methods have also been described, such as slice resolution corrections, postprocessing with B0 field maps, and spiral k-space acquisitions. Areas of localized susceptibility can also degrade images from sequences utilizing magnetization preparation pulses. These areas of increased susceptibility can cause incomplete inversion of spin magnetization since the local spins may lie outside of the pulse bandwidth. This can result in areas of inhomogeneous and incomplete fat saturation. However, the increased T2* shortening can also be used

(a)

(b)

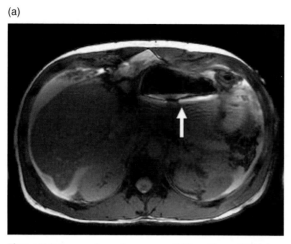
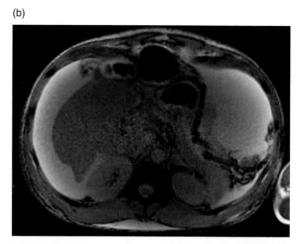

Figure 2.3 Increased gas–tissue susceptibility artifact at 3T (a) than at 1.5T (b) in a SSFP axial series. This is evident along the posterior margin of the gas-containing stomach (a, arrow). Note also that there is greater shading effect at 3T (seen as a drop in signal) but greater noise at 1.5T (seen as graininess), both features appearing through the central parts of the images.

advantageously in certain applications such as blood oxygen level-dependent (BOLD) functional magnetic resonance imaging (fMRI) and SWI. The BOLD technique uses the differences in magnetic properties of oxygenated and deoxygenated hemoglobin to create images related to tissue pO_2 levels. The different magnetic properties of these two states of hemoglobin affect the $T2^*$ relaxation times of regional water molecules, which creates contrast in the $T2^*$-weighted images. Studies have reported a signal increase by a factor of 1.7–3.2 when comparing BOLD fMRI at 1.5T and 4T, although inflow effects because of longer T1 relaxation and increased susceptibility are additional considerations [8]. These techniques have been applied to study disease states in native as well as allograft kidneys. Increased susceptibility also improves visualization of hemorrhage, paramagnetic contrast agents, and hemosiderosis. In the liver, iron overload is of interest to monitor hepatic fibrosis, and SWI is currently under investigation.

Parallel imaging

At higher field imaging, parallel magnetic resonance imaging (pMRI) is critically important. The application of pMRI can be used to improve temporal resolution which can be used for faster imaging in patients who cannot comply with breath-hold times, faster time-resolved MRA, and improved perfusion studies. The advantages of pMRI can also be used to improve spatial resolution by increasing matrix sizes or acquiring thinner slices. pMRI can also decrease effective inter-echo spacing resulting in less image blurring and image distortion in echo-train spin-echo and EPI. The SAR can also be significantly reduced utilizing pMRI techniques. Despite the 40% reduction in SNR with an acceleration factor of 2, the SNR increase at 3T makes the shorter acquisition worthwhile for many sequences. The first successful in-vivo implementation of pMRI was demonstrated by Sodickson and Manning based on the simultaneous acquisition of spatial harmonics (SMASH) and coil sensitivities [9]. Currently, sensitivity encoding (SENSE) is the most versatile method of pMRI. There are several differences between these two methods. Whereas SENSE is an image-domain method, SMASH is considered a k-space-based method. Sensitivity profiles needed for final image reconstruction are measured more precisely in SENSE than in SMASH.

Acoustic noise

Advances in gradient performance at 3T have also created an increase in acoustic noise. In addition, short-bore scanners have less acoustic shielding and dampen noise less. The IEC and FDA limit ambient noise to 99 dB [1]. To stay within this limit, additional noise shielding/cancellation methods such as ear plugs, headphones, and destructive interference techniques may be necessary.

(a)

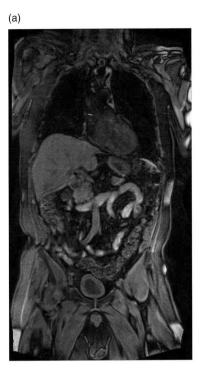

(b)

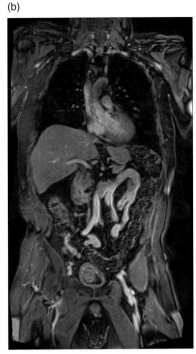

Figure 2.4 3D T1-weighted GRE coronal series at pre- (a) and post-contrast (b) at 3T.

Spatial resolution

Signal in MR imaging is proportional to voxel size. Therefore, when the SNR at 1.5T for an application is sufficient, at 3T voxel size can be reduced to increase spatial resolution. An increase in spatial resolution is beneficial for MR spectroscopy to prevent contamination from partial volume effects. This is important when analyzing small or irregularly shaped structures as occurs with applications for prostate, brain, or for pediatric applications.

Temporal resolution and acquisition time

When SNR and spatial resolution suffice at 1.5T, temporal resolution can be increased at 3T. Theoretically, SNR is proportional to the square root of scan time. Thus, a fourfold decrease is expected, but in practice, longer T1 relaxation rates, limits on gradient performance, slices per TR, and SAR diminish time savings. However, when combined with parallel imaging, perfusion scanning and dynamic MRA become more feasible. Similarly, for sequences with multiple numbers of acquisition and sufficient SNR at 1.5T, acquisition time can theoretically be reduced by a factor of 4 at 3T because doubling the number of acquisition scales leads to an SNR gain of $\sqrt{2}$ [2].

However, other factors such as the benefits of higher SNR, chemical shift and RF wavelength artifacts, SAR limitations, relaxation times, and susceptibility effects all limit how much acquisition time can truly be minimized. Reduced acquisition time is seen the most for MR spectroscopy, whole-body MR imaging, DWI, and three-dimensional (3D) imaging. One comparison reports the total imaging time for whole-body MR imaging at 52 minutes for 1.5T and at 43 minutes for 3T with unchanged image resolution [10].

Application to body imaging sequences
3D T1-weighted gradient echo (GRE)

Perhaps the sequence that has the most to gain from higher field imaging is the 3D T1-weighted GRE sequences (Figures 2.4 and 2.5). These images are often acquired both pre-contrast administration as well as during dynamic post-contrast imaging. This sequence benefits from the higher field strength by taking advantage of higher SNR. The higher SNR can be used to increase spatial resolution as well as to accelerate the imaging time (decrease the breath-hold time) for patients that have difficulty breath-holding. In addition, 3D acquisitions are generally performed with fat suppression, particularly when acquired with

(a)

(b)

(c)

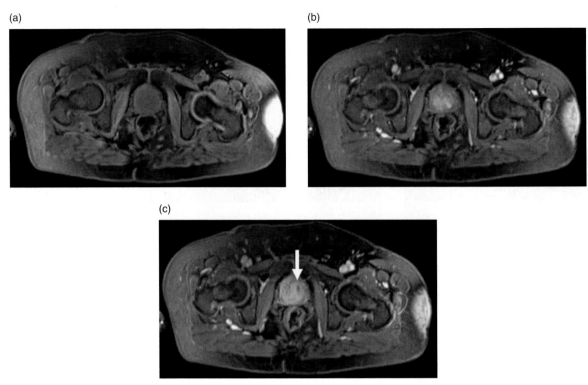

Figure 2.5 Prostate carcinoma (c, arrow) in 3D T1-weighted GRE axial series pre-contrast (a), 20 seconds post-contrast (b), and 3 minutes post-contrast (c) at 3T.

gadolinium-chelate contrast enhancement. Fat suppression should be superior at 3T due to improved spectral separation of the major water and fat peaks. A limitation may be seen in the setting of susceptibility factors around gas–water interfaces or metallic structures such as surgical clips. This adverse effect, however, may be counteracted by utilizing the higher SNR achievable at 3T to allow for a larger bandwidth and shorter TR. This achieves two effects: (1) a reduction in the overall scan time that can be converted to higher resolution, more slice coverage in the out-of-plane direction, or shorter breath-hold time; and (2) a reduction in susceptibility effects.

2D T1-weighted gradient echo (GRE)

As previously discussed, the Larmor frequency is 128 MHz at 3T, which is double that found at 1.5T. The difference between lipid and water is 3.25 ppm, which accounts for a 420 Hz difference at 3T. Because of this difference, the in- and opposed-phase TEs are different at 3T and at 1.5T. At 1.5T, in-phase TEs are at 4.8 ms, 9.6 ms, 14.4 ms, etc. and opposed-phase TEs are at 2.4 ms, 7.2 ms, 12 ms, etc., whereas at 3T in-phase TEs are sooner at 2.4 ms, 4.8 ms., 7.2 ms, etc. and opposed-phase TEs are at 1.2 ms, 3.6 ms, 6 ms, etc. Minor variations are due to slight differences in field strengths between scanners. Because TEs are sooner at 3T, bandwidth must often be increased at the expense of SNR. Some centers have found it best to acquire the first in-phase echo and the second opposed-phase echo at 3T to maintain SNR [11], but this is not advisable as differentiation between lipid and susceptibility effects, namely tissue iron, will not be possible. Alternatively the two echoes may be acquired as separate single echo acquistion using optimal image quality factors and optimal first in/opposed-phase TEs, but this will add to the overall scan time. During in-phase TEs, lipid and water are additive and positively contribute to signal. However, at opposed-phase TEs, lipid and water have a canceling effect and produce a black boundary (or India ink) artifact. Although signal drops at lipid–water interfaces when the relative fraction is 50%, this artifact can be exploited to compute a lipid fraction within voxels of a tissue of interest (Figure 2.6).

(a)

(b)

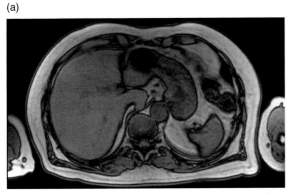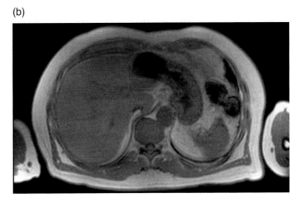

Figure 2.6 Opposed- (a) and in-phase (b) dual-echo 2D T1-weighted GRE axial series at 3T. Note that these images were acquired in one breath-hold with the shortest echo corresponding to the first opposed-phase TE (1.2 ms) and the longer echo corresponding to the first in-phase TE (2.4 ms).

However, $T2^*$ decay must also be taken into account. At 1.5T, in-phase TEs at 4.8 ms and 9.6 ms do not produce the same image primarily because of $T2^*$ decay. At 3T, since $T2^*$ is shorter, the effect is further pronounced. Particular clinical significance concerns patients with steatohepatitis and hemosiderosis. Methods involving spectroscopy have been developed to quantify lipid fraction independent of this $T2^*$ decay [12]. Approaches with low flip angles have also been described.

Single-shot partial Fourier T2

Single-shot T2 represent one of the major pillars for reproducible high-quality abdominal–pelvic MR imaging, regardless of field strength (Figure 2.7). These images should be acquired both without and with fat suppression: without fat suppression to facilitate structural anatomical visualization with lower signal tissues outlined by higher signal intensity mesenteric and retroperitoneal fat; and fat-suppressed images improving conspicuity of fluid-containing processes such as tissue edema and collections. At 3T specific considerations include SAR limitations resulting from the high number of RF echoes applied in the long echo trains and longer tissue T1 resulting in greater cross-talk effects and decreased SNR. The acquisition may be kept within SAR limits by reducing the echo-train flip angle from 180°, used at 1.5T to maximize SNR, to a lower value around 150° at 3T. While reducing the flip angle diminishes the SNR we rely on the intrinsic higher SNR achievable on 3T to compensate for the signal loss. Additional gains in SNR are achieved by use of parallel processing that leads to a significant shortening of the echo train length. Compensation for the longer T1 at 3T may be achieved by using respiratory triggering that will lengthen the effective TR to approximately 4000 ms (assuming 16 breaths per minute). Respiratory triggering may be achieved using either a mechanical device, applied at the time of coil placement during initial patient setup, which detects patient movement, or using an automated tool that detects diaphragmatic excursion by real-time imaging.

Fat suppression is critically important and represents another advantage at 3T. The main consideration is the improved spectral separation of the water and fat signal. Optimal fat suppression for single-shot partial Fourier T2 imaging is achieved using a spectral attenuated inversion recovery (SPAIR) technique due to the ability of this sequence to achieve motion and susceptibility-insensitive fat suppression while preserving water signal [13].

Steady-state free precession (SSFP)

SSFP sequences are valuable additions to body MR imaging given their relative motion insensitivity as well as providing excellent contrast in vascular structures. However, these sequences are also affected by off-resonance effects that result in banding artifacts. The higher field strength of 3T results in even greater B1 inhomogeneities as well as susceptibility effects that contribute to the banding artifacts (Figure 2.8). These artifacts can be shifted to the more peripheral aspects of the image by reducing the TR or minimized by optimized shimming. However, this approach is not as practical at higher field strengths due to the associated increased T1 values. Because of SAR limits, flip angle must often be decreased, which reduces the

(a)　　　　　　　　　　　　　　　(b)

(c)　　　　　　　　　　　　　　　(d)

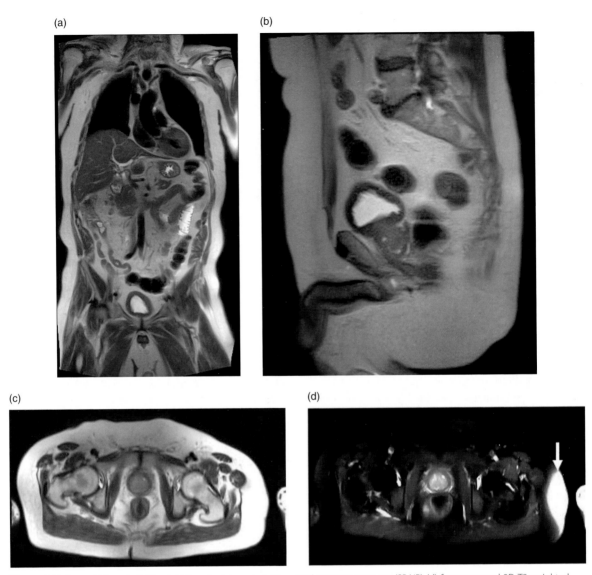

Figure 2.7 Coronal (a), sagittal (b), axial (c), and axial spectral attenuated inversion recovery (SPAIR) (d) fat-suppressed 2D T2-weighted SSFSE images show high-quality single-shot imaging feasible at 3T with excellent fat suppression showing uniform elimination of the fat signal while the water signal is preserved. Severe disturbance of the field due to susceptibility from a device lying beside the patient caused breakdown in fat suppression on the left flank (d, arrow).

contrast of blood, which may become more problematic when using SSFP for vessel delineation, especially in cardiac applications.

Magnetic resonance cholangiopancreatography (MRCP)

Breath-hold heavily T2-weighted single-shot FSE (SSFSE) remains the technique of choice for acquiring MRCP images at 3T. The breath-hold technique is preferred due to less respiratory motion artifact as well as overall decreased scan time. A respiratory-triggered multislice 3D turbo spin echo technique can also be employed when greater detail regarding the pancreatic or biliary systems is desired. Both of these techniques benefit from the greater SNR provided at the higher 3T field strength. However, both imaging techniques can be significantly affected by the increased susceptibility effects at 3T due to the significantly prolonged TEs. Artifacts from surgical

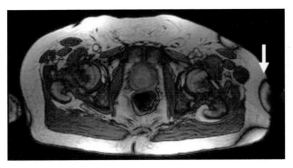

Figure 2.8 Several banding artifacts shown in an SSFP axial series at 3T (arrow).

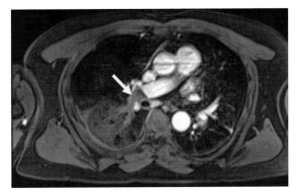

Figure 2.9 Arterial phase 3D GRE showing a right pulmonary artery saddle embolus (arrow) with good contrast and resolution. Note that the susceptibility effect from lung is well-controlled using short TR/TE of under 4 ms/2 ms.

clips, surgical debris, and blood products as well as intrinsic iron deposition from hemochromatosis can all significantly degrade MRCP images due to increased susceptibility effects.

Magnetic resonance angiography (MRA)

Because of longer T1 relaxation times, improved background suppression is possible at 3T. Because of the additional gain in SNR, TOF and contrast-enhanced MRA imaging improve significantly. In addition, MRA can be acquired faster at 3T, allowing for dynamic time-resolved MRA in applications such as renal perfusion [14].

Lung imaging for pulmonary emboli may be improved at 3T due to intrinsic advantages for 3D GRE imaging (Figure 2.9). Breath-holds can be achieved in a shorter time and with higher spatial resolution, characteristics favorable to imaging a tachypnic patient who has pulmonary emboli.

Pediatric imaging

Shorter acquisition, shorter breath-holds, and higher resolution with young patients who cannot hold breath as long and are small represent advantages of 3T over 1.5T. The shorter timing creates a potential to image neonates without sedation. Otherwise, the same limitations are considerations including dielectric effects and signal gradients causing nonuniformity of image signal.

Specific novel applications

Advantages of MR spectroscopy at 3T relate to the improved SNR and improved separation of spectral peaks. The increased SNR can be applied to the acquisition of smaller voxels to more accurately isolate a region of interest. The additional SNR also makes MR spectroscopy of phosphorus and carbon more feasible. Prostate MR imaging also benefits from higher SNR achievable at 3T. It has been proposed that the endorectal coil has a number of disadvantages for routine prostate scanning and that the need for an endorectal coil is diminished [15–17] (Figure 2.10). This has been based on the demonstration that similar MR spectroscopy accuracy for prostate carcinoma may be obtained on a 3T scanner with a surface coil as compared with scanning the same patient on a 1.5T system with an endorectal coil [15] (Figure 2.11). Advantages of 3T imaging without an endorectal coil also include avoiding anatomical distortion, which precludes use of the images for radiation planning. Other advantages include improved patient acceptance, faster scan setup time, diminished motion effects from coil movement, improved field uniformity, and larger FOV. Additional benefits of 3T imaging of the prostate and pelvis include the ability to achieve higher SNR T2-weighted high-resolution 3D imaging of the pelvis that facilitates both local staging with delineation of transcapsular extension of disease, and for facilitating radiation planning (Figure 2.12). Spectroscopy obtained in the prostate gland also benefits with 3T.

Diffusion-weighted imaging (DWI)

DWI remains a developmental tool with yet-to-be-proven benefits for routine clinical application at most centers. At institutions studying these methods there have been reported potential applications for

(a)

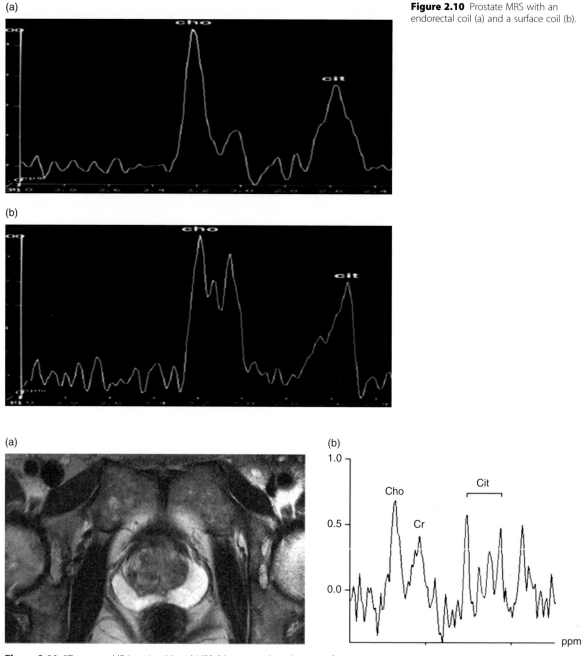

(b)

Figure 2.10 Prostate MRS with an endorectal coil (a) and a surface coil (b).

(a)   (b)

Figure 2.11 3T prostate MR imaging (a) and MRS (b) using a phased-array surface coil. A T2-weighted image was obtained with 0.4 mm in-plane resolution in 5 minutes and a corresponding single voxel size 12 mm³ acquired in 8 minutes. Note that spectral details of the citrate peaks (for example) are achievable at 3T even when using a surface coil.

tumor detection and for characterization of post-therapy tumor response. Tissues and tumors of interest have included lymphoma and solid tumors of the liver, pancreas, and prostate [15]. Considerations at 3T include higher b-values ($> 1000 \, s/mm^2$), thinner

slices, and imaging in multiple directions because of higher SNR [1, 5]. The higher SNR can also in turn be used for easier breath-holding [18]. Because EPI is more sensitive to susceptibility, improved volume shimming, parallel imaging, and bandwidth

(a)

(b)

(c)

(d)

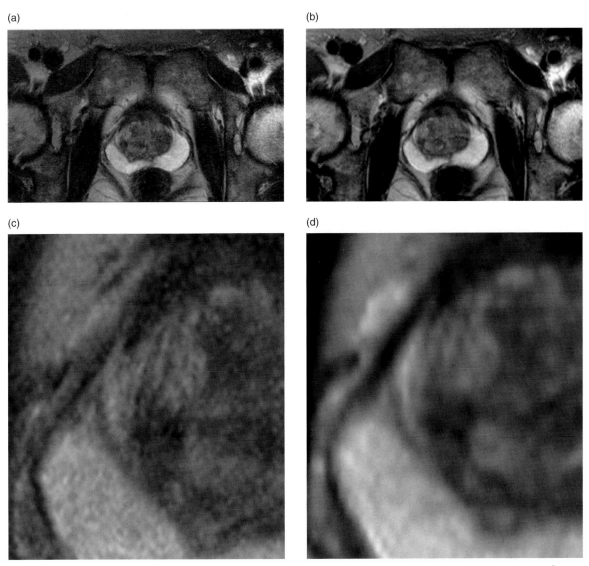

Figure 2.12 Wide (a, b) and tight (c, d) zoom of the prostate acquired at comparable acquisition times at 3T ($512 \times 512 \times 4\,mm^{-3}$) (a, c) versus 1.5T ($256 \times 256 \times 4\,mm^{-3}$) (b, d).

optimization should be used for DWI at 3T. Imaging in the liver can also be difficult because of susceptibility effects with air because of lung and bowel gas. Some studies have also shown improved sensitivity and specificity for prostate cancer using diffusion tensor imaging (DTI) [17].

Arterial spin labeling (ASL)

Although applications have not developed to the extent of neuroimaging, ASL imaging has recently been investigated in body MR imaging. Due to increased T1 relaxation times, blood labeling persists longer and can potentially improve image quality [19]. However, the SSFP sequence used for acquisition has B1 inhomogeneity considerations that must be taken into account when optimizing ASL for 3T.

Susceptibility-weighted imaging (SWI)

SWI has become a mainstay of neuroimaging and is used routinely for common conditions such as examination for blood products resulting from traumatic brain injury. However, SWI has yet to show similar diagnostic useful application for common indications for MR imaging of abdominal–pelvic diseases. SWI has been suggested as a possible tool for the evaluation of diffuse liver diseases. Chronic liver disease and fibrosis has been one suggested application, but this remains questionable. A more validated role is for the measurement of elevated liver iron in the setting of iron deposition disease including hemochromatosis.

Magnetic resonance elastography (MRE)

MRE is an evolving technique that is used to examine the physical properties of tissues. In this method, a known stress is applied to an organ or soft tissue element and the degree of resulting deformation is measured using MR methods. These data are then used to calculate the elastic modulus of the medium. Recent implementations of this technique have used harmonic low-frequency sound waves to mechanically stress the tissues. The mechanical stress results in shear waves that may be measured by employing sensitizing gradients to detect the small cyclic motion of the protons based on phase shifts. Potential applications for this method are currently being investigated and include quantification of liver fibrosis as well as tumor detection and characterization. Several improvements to this technique have been investigated taking advantage of the higher SNR at 3T. These improvements include using second harmonic imaging which permits image acquisitions with shorter TEs and greater signal retention, applying shorter RF pulses, using stronger gradient magnitudes to compensate for the second harmonic imaging, and increasing the echo train length to reduce overall scan time. This may also result in higher resolution.

Conclusion

The advantages and improvements of 3T imaging have made MR imaging increasingly attractive in comparison to diagnostic imaging with ionizing radiation and iodinated contrast agents for certain applications. Vascular imaging at 3T has improved the quality of MRA, diminished the needed contrast load, and has further diminished the need for digital subtraction angiography (DSA) or computed tomography (CT) angiography. While lesion detection in the abdomen and pelvis may shift toward MR imaging at 3T from CT, the improvements in MR imaging have been mostly a result of advances in RF coil design, gradient performance, and electronics to improve readout and k-space reconstruction. The additional advantages of 3T have been incremental in this regard. Further potential improvements in 3T applications will continue with increases in the number of coil elements and parallel imaging acceleration factors, improved electronics and computational systems, and further refinements in special applications as discussed in this review. These developments must be implemented while managing SAR limits and maintaining safety in the clinical environment with the numerous medical devices currently in use. The advantages of 3T will always have to be measured by assessing the relative diagnostic benefits over less expensive and more commonly available 1.5T systems.

References

1. Tanenbaum LN. Clinical 3T MR imaging: mastering the challenges. *Magn Reson Imaging Clin N Am* 2006; **14**(1): 1–15.

2. Machann J, Schlemmer HP, Schick F. Technical challenges and opportunities of whole-body magnetic resonance imaging at 3T. *Phys Med* 2008; **24**(2): 63–70.

3. Haacke EM. *Magnetic Resonance Imaging: Physical Principles and Sequence Design*. New York, Wiley, 1999.

4. Hussain SM, van den Bos IC, Oliveto JM, Martin DR. MR imaging of the female pelvis at 3T. *Magn Reson Imaging Clin N Am* 2006; **14**(4): 537–44, vii.

5. Dagia C, Ditchfield M. 3T MR imaging in paediatrics: challenges and clinical applications. *Eur J Radiol* 2008; **68**(2): 309–19.

6. Soher BJ, Dale BM, Merkle EM. A review of MR physics: 3T versus 1.5T. *Magn Reson Imaging Clin N Am* 2007; **15**(3): 277–90, v.

7. Merkle EM, Dale BM, Paulson EK. Abdominal MR imaging at 3T. *Magn Reson Imaging Clin N Am* 2006; **14**(1): 17–26.

8. Lin W, An H, Chen Y, *et al.* Practical consideration for 3T imaging. *Magn Reson Imaging Clin N Am* 2003; **11**(4): 615–39, vi.

9. Sodickson DK, Manning WJ. Simultaneous acquisition of spatial harmonics (SMASH): fast imaging with radiofrequency coil arrays. *Magn Reson Med* 1997; **38**(4): 591–603.

10. Schmidt GP, Reiser MF, Baur-Melnyk A. Whole-body MR imaging for the staging and follow-up of patients with metastasis. *Eur J Radiol* 2009; **70**(3): 393–400.

11. Guiu B, Loffroy R, Ben Salem D, *et al.* [Liver steatosis and in-out phase MR imaging: theory and clinical applications at 3T]. *J Radiol* 2007; **88**(12): 1845–53.

12. Pineda N, Sharma P, Xu Q, *et al.* Measurement of hepatic lipid: high-speed T2-corrected multiecho acquisition at 1H MR spectroscopy – a rapid and accurate technique. *Radiology* 2009; **252**(2): 568–76.

13. Lauenstein TC, Sharma P, Hughes T, *et al.* Evaluation of optimized inversion-recovery fat-suppression techniques for T2-weighted abdominal MR imaging. *J Magn Reson Imaging* 2008; **27**(6): 1448–54.

14. Lohan DG, Saleh R, Tomasian A, Krishnam M, Finn JP. Current status of 3-T cardiovascular magnetic resonance imaging. *Top Magn Reson Imaging* 2008; **19**(1): 3–13.

15. Villers A, Lemaitre L, Haffner J, Puech P. Current status of MR imaging for the diagnosis, staging and prognosis of prostate cancer: implications for focal therapy and active surveillance. *Curr Opin Urol* 2009; **19**(3): 274–82.

16. Puech P, Huglo D, Petyt G, Lemaitre L, Villers A. Imaging of organ-confined prostate cancer: functional ultrasound, MR imaging and PET/computed tomography. *Curr Opin Urol* 2009; **19**(2): 168–76.

17. Kurhanewicz J, Vigneron D, Carroll P, Coakley F. Multiparametric magnetic resonance imaging in prostate cancer: present and future. *Curr Opin Urol* 2008; **18**(1): 71–7.

18. Naganawa S, Kawai H, Fukatsu H, *et al.* Diffusion-weighted imaging of the liver: technical challenges and prospects for the future. *Magn Reson Med Sci* 2005; **4**(4): 175–86.

19. Deibler AR, Pollock JM, Kraft RA, *et al.* Arterial spin-labeling in routine clinical practice, part 1: technique and artifacts. *AJNR Am J Neuroradiol* 2008; **29**(7): 1228–34.

Breast MR imaging

Savannah C. Partridge, Habib Rahbar, and Constance D. Lehman

Introduction

The move to higher magnetic field strength holds promise for advancing magnetic resonance (MR) imaging of the breast. Potential benefits include higher signal-to-noise ratio (SNR), contrast, and spectral resolution, which could translate into higher spatial and temporal resolution than previously possible. However, technical, physical, and safety considerations present challenges for fully realizing these benefits for breast MR imaging.

Background on clinical utility of breast MR imaging

MR imaging has proven to be a valuable imaging tool in detecting, characterizing, and assessing the extent of breast cancer. However, due to the relatively higher costs of MR imaging when compared to mammography and ultrasound, judicious use for specific clinically proven applications is essential. Current evidence-based clinical applications of breast MR imaging include screening high-risk patients (including patients with a known genetic mutation such as BRCA or with a greater than 20% lifetime risk based on family history), evaluating patients with a new diagnosis of breast cancer, monitoring response to neoadjuvant chemotherapy, evaluation of patients with metastatic axillary adenocarcinoma of unknown primary, and evaluation of silicone implants suspected of rupture.

The power of breast MR imaging is in its ability to provide not only useful morphologic information but also functional information. Breast MR examinations typically involve a dynamic contrast-enhanced scan to identify malignant tumors based on abnormal vascularity. Enhancement kinetics provided by dynamic contrast-enhanced breast MR imaging provide

information regarding a lesion's perfusion. Diffusion-weighted imaging (DWI) and MR spectroscopy are two advanced functional breast MR imaging techniques that can provide complementary information to conventional contrast-enhanced MR imaging and are currently under investigation for use as part of the clinical breast MR imaging protocol. High-field imaging may improve the clinical utility of each of these functional breast imaging techniques.

Potential advantages of 3T over 1.5T for breast imaging

Imaging at 3T can provide a potential doubling of SNR over 1.5T, which can be used to obtain higher spatial resolution images at comparable imaging times to 1.5T or to shorten imaging times. Contrast-enhanced breast MR examinations can benefit from increased spatial resolution (Figure 3.1), faster imaging times, and improved fat suppression owing to the greater spectral separation of fat and water at 3T. The increased spatial resolution enables the acquisition of small isotropic voxels, which may be preferable as it allows reformations of equal resolution in any plane. Imaging at higher field strength and higher spatial resolution holds particular promise for improved visualization of small-volume processes, with implications for earlier detection of disease in MR imaging screening and improved detection of ductal carcinoma *in situ*.

Review of 3T breast MR imaging literature
Lesion detection, morphology, and kinetics

It is well established that breast MR imaging is a highly sensitive imaging modality for breast cancer

---

Body MR Imaging at 3 Tesla, ed. Ihab R. Kamel and Elmar M. Merkle. Published by Cambridge University Press.

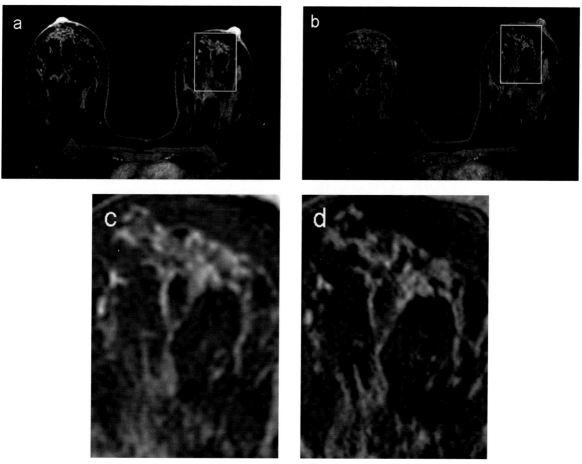

Figure 3.1 Comparison of breast MR images acquired at 1.5 (a) and 3T (b) in the same patient. Imaging parameters were optimized at each field strength for maximal spatial resolution with comparable image quality in a scan time of 3 minutes or less. Both acquisitions incorporated a three-dimensional (3D) T1-weighted gradient echo sequence with parallel imaging and active fat suppression. An 8-channel phased-array breast coil was used for 1.5T imaging and a 7-channel coil for 3T imaging. At 1.5T, the acquired imaging resolution was 0.9 mm in-plane with 1.6-mm slice thickness. Higher spatial resolution was achieved at 3T, with 0.5 mm in-plane and 1-mm slice thickness. The improved clarity of the 3T images for assessing fine detail is demonstrated in the magnified sections of the 1.5 (c) and 3T (d) images.

detection, but continues to experience moderate specificity, ranging from 37% to 88%. As a result, recent research exploring the advantages of 3T MR imaging over 1.5T have primarily focused on improved differentiation of benign lesions from malignant lesions. As the current clinical breast MR imaging approach is to assess lesion morphology and lesion kinetics for diagnostic classification, initial research has centered on potential improvements that higher field strength may provide for these two parameters.

Lesion identification is primarily dependent on the contrast-to-noise ratio (CNR), which is dependent upon relaxation times of breast tissue and gadolinium-based contrast agents used for breast MRI. At 3T, the T1 relaxation time is increased for both fat and glandular tissue in the breast by approximately 21% and 17% respectively [1] but T1 relaxation of gadolinium is increased to a lesser extent [2]. As a result, gadolinium-enhanced tissues demonstrate an increase in conspicuity at 3T, which can be traded for a reduction of the gadolinium dose [3]. However, an initial 3T study demonstrated a lower enhancement of breast lesions than at 1.5T, which was attributed to a reduction of the flip angle necessitated by power deposition limitations and increased B1 field inhomogeneity at 3T [4]. Another study further showed the B1 field inhomogeneity issue persisted across varying breast coils and was correlated to increasing body size [5]. These findings showed that further refinement of imaging parameters is necessary to realize the potential CNR benefit at 3T.

Improvements in assessment of lesion morphology have perhaps demonstrated the most initial promise in 3T breast MR imaging. The increased SNR achieved at 3T when compared with 1.5T can be used to acquire images of higher spatial resolution for a fixed time period, which could theoretically improve anatomical detail and morphologic description of lesions. At higher field strength, smaller voxel sizes are obtainable without the cost of extending scan time to perform extra signal averaging that is necessary at lower field strengths to boost SNR and achieve adequate image quality. In practice, higher spatial resolution is achieved by employing multichannel coils and higher parallel imaging factors to acquire the greater matrix size in a clinically feasible time frame.

A recent study by Kuhl et al. compared the appearance of 53 lesions prospectively at both 1.5 and 3T field strengths, utilizing the increased SNR at 3T to improve spatial resolution and assess improvement of subtle morphologic detail [6]. They demonstrated that a statistically significant higher diagnostic confidence was achieved at a higher field strength, with a total of 11 unique lesions being classified differently. The improved confidence was due to the ability to better resolve morphology, particularly evident in four biopsy-proven fibroadenomas that were prospectively classified as BI-RADS 3 lesions on the 1.5T scan but were definitively classified as BI-RADS 2 lesions on the 3T scan due to the ability to resolve dark internal septations characteristic of fibroadenomas not seen at the lower field strength.

There is also potential for improvement in dynamic kinetic information with 3T imaging of the breast. Imaging at 3T affords increased temporal resolution, which could be utilized to obtain more detailed enhancement information to better characterize breast lesions. While increasing temporal resolution could limit spatial resolution benefits, a recent report has described a protocol in which both factors are optimized, creating improvements in both spatial and temporal resolution, and producing sensitivity and specificity greater than most published 1.5T protocols [7].

Addressing specific challenges at 3T for breast imaging

While 3T holds strong potential advantages for breast imaging, particular challenges to imaging at higher field strengths must be addressed to facilitate routine clinical implementation of 3T breast MR imaging.

Need for new higher channel breast coils

Perhaps first and foremost, breast radiofrequency (RF) coils with higher numbers of coil elements and increased parallel imaging capability must be utilized in order to translate the higher SNR to higher spatial resolution or shorter scan times. Higher numbers of coil elements will increase the acceleration factor R and reduce MR imaging times and resulting RF power deposition. The scan length can then be shortened or kept to a reasonable limit while increasing the number of slices and pixels acquired for high spatial resolution. In addition to the number of coil elements, the layout of the coil elements affects the maximum R for each orthogonal direction, important for three-dimensional (3D) breast MR imaging acquisitions where parallel imaging can be employed in multiple directions simultaneously. Although R is typically limited to 4 or less at 1.5T due to SNR limitations, considerably higher R is possible at higher field strengths [8]. Newer MR imaging systems available typically support up to 32 simultaneous RF channels [9]. At present, 16-channel phased-array breast coils provide the highest potential acceleration factor for 3T imaging with commercially available hardware, but new higher channel coils are under development. Figure 3.2 shows a comparison of maximal spatial resolution achieved at 3T using a 7-channel versus 16-channel breast coil within the same scan time.

Specific absorption rate limitations

The specific absorption rate (SAR) is the rate at which RF energy is absorbed by tissue and quantifies power deposition in the person during an MR imaging scan. SAR-induced temperature changes of a human body are a significant safety issue of high-field MR imaging. SAR increases with field strength, and the energy deposited in a patient's tissues is fourfold higher at 3T than at 1.5T. As a result, SAR constraints necessitate some tradeoffs in image acquisition rates, resolution, and slice coverage to reduce power deposition. In particular, T2-weighted fast spin echo (FSE) based sequences typical of standard breast MR imaging protocols can produce high SAR. To limit SAR for breast imaging, effective approaches are to use smaller flip angles along with parallel imaging techniques to reduce RF exposure and scan time.

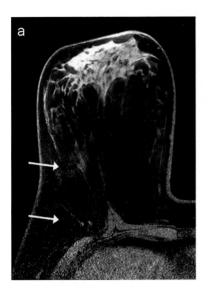
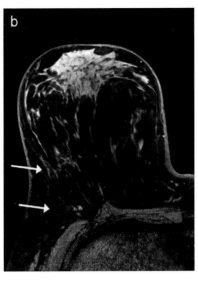

Figure 3.2 Comparison of breast MR images acquired at 3T using 7-channel (a) and 16-channel (b) RF breast coils. Both acquisitions incorporated a 3D T1-weighted gradient echo sequence with parallel imaging and active fat suppression, with the same scan time of 2:50 minutes. Higher spatial resolution was achieved within the same scan time using the 16-channel coil; acquired voxel sizes were $0.5 \times 0.5 \times 0.1.3\,\text{mm}^3$ with the 16-channel coil and $0.7 \times 0.7 \times 1.5\,\text{mm}^3$ with the 7-channel coil. Furthermore, the 16-channel coil afforded increased SNR particularly near the chest wall (arrows) compared to the 7-channel coil.

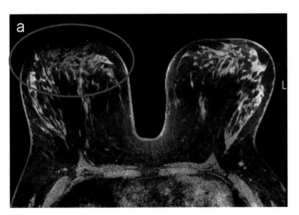
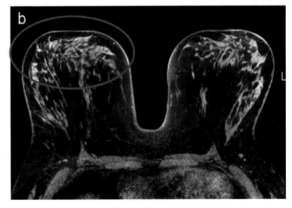

Figure 3.3 Comparison of breast MR images acquired at 3T using a standard rectangular volume shim technique (a) and a "patient-adaptive" image-based shim technique (SmartExam Breast, Philips Healthcare, Best, The Netherlands) (b). Images were acquired using a 3D T1-weighted gradient echo sequence with parallel imaging and active fat suppression, 16-channel coil, and scan time of 2:50 minutes. In this example, improved image quality was obtained at air–tissue interfaces (circled region) using the image-based shim due to improved B0 homogeneity (b). See plate section for color version.

B0 inhomogeneity/susceptibility artifacts

Accurate undistorted imaging with good-quality fat suppression requires the magnetic field (B0) to be homogeneous throughout the entire region of interest. For breast MR imaging, magnetic susceptibility effects often occur at the interfaces between soft tissue (breast) and air as a result of B0 variations. Susceptibility artifacts scale linearly with increasing field strength and are therefore twice as prominent at 3T compared with 1.5T [10]. Achieving adequate B0 homogeneity for breast imaging at 3T requires improved shimming techniques over 1.5T. New image-based higher order shimming methods can dramatically improve B0 homogeneity for bilateral breast imaging (Figure 3.3). Parallel imaging also reduces image artifacts and distortions caused by susceptibility effects, such as those associated with echo planar imaging, by shortening echo train lengths.

B1 inhomogeneity

Another technical issue associated with high-field imaging is spatial inhomogeneity of the applied RF magnetic field (B1). This results from an interaction

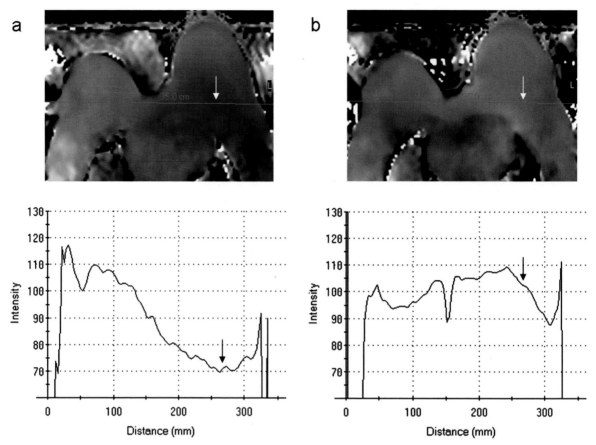

Figure 3.4 Improvement in B1 homogeneity using an adaptive parallel RF transmission technique. B1 maps acquired with conventional single source RF transmission (a) and with parallel transmission (Multi-Transmit, Philips Healthcare, Best, The Netherlands) (b) are compared. Shown below the B1 maps are corresponding flip angle profiles measured across the field of view as indicated by the red line. Signal intensity relates to the delivered excitation, expressed as percent of intended flip angle or B1. B1 maps were calculated using an interleaved dual-TR T1-weighted gradient echo sequence. Improved bilateral B1 homogeneity can be appreciated on both the parallel RF transmission B1 map and corresponding plot (b), particularly in the left breast (arrows). Flip angle variation across the image ranged from 70% to 115% of the intended flip angle with conventional imaging, compared with only 90% to 110% using parallel transmission. See plate section for color version.

between the coil inducing and receiving the signal and the electromagnetic properties of the tissue being imaged, known as the dielectric effect. B1 inhomogeneities cause the flip angle and signal measured in the breast to be nonuniform across the field of view (Figure 3.4a), which can result in a loss of tissue contrast and diagnostic power depending on location. New parallel transmission techniques have largely overcome this issue for breast imaging (Figure 3.4b). Parallel RF transmission is a new adaptive excitation technique that uses multiple transmit coils and is able to independently control the RF waveforms and compensate for patient-induced B1 inhomogeneities. Parallel RF transmission can provide improved consistency in image quality (contrast, signal

homogeneity, and fat suppression), improved RF uniformity, and reduced RF energy deposition.

T1 relaxation differences

Extended T1 relaxation times at higher field strength may affect tissue contrast and visibility of breast lesions on breast MR imaging. However, the increase in T1 of contrast agents in tissue is much lower than the increase in tissue T1. Therefore, in theory, enhancing breast tumors should be more easily distinguished from normal nonenhancing breast tissue at 3T than at lower field strengths based on T1-weighted signal intensity. However, other factors as described earlier can also affect the visibility of lesions at 3T.

Advanced functional breast MR imaging techniques at 3T

Diffusion-weighted imaging

Diffusion-weighted imaging (DWI) is a non-contrast-enhanced technique that has shown promise in oncologic imaging. As tumors tend to be of higher cell density than surrounding tissue, they often demonstrate restricted diffusion with a corresponding lower apparent diffusion coefficient (ADC) value. Thus, DWI provides functional information regarding the cellularity of a lesion, which several studies have shown to be useful for differentiating carcinomas from normal breast tissue and benign lesions [11, 12]. Further, a recent study has demonstrated that the positive predictive value of lesion characterization improves significantly when DWI is used as an adjunct to the standard dynamic contrast-enhanced breast MR imaging protocol [13].

Because DWI is inherently associated with limited SNR, it may be advantageous to perform DWI at higher field strength to obtain a valuable increase in both SNR and CNR, which could aid in the detection of smaller lesions. Theoretically, ADC values should remain constant with increasing field strength. Preliminary study results are promising and have supported these proposed advantages. An initial study directly comparing the visibility of lesions on DWI and their ADC values at 1.5 and 3T demonstrated that ADC values are not affected by increasing field strength, but smaller lesions (≤ 1 cm) were significantly more visible at 3T [14]. A study by Lo *et al.* in which a total of 31 lesions were assessed with dynamic contrast-enhanced MR imaging (DCE-MR imaging), qualitative DWI, and quantitative DWI with ADC thresholds independently both at 1.5 and 3T, found similar sensitivities for the three methods (95%, 95%, and 90%, respectively) and that quantitative DWI with ADC thresholds was equivalent in specificity (91%) to DCE-MR imaging [15].

MR spectroscopy

MR spectroscopy is another non-contrast-enhanced technique that detects proton-containing metabolites. MR spectroscopy has been shown to improve the specificity of lesion characterization both alone and when used in conjunction with dynamic contrast breast MR imaging [16]. Breast cancers have been shown to have increased choline levels owing to increased cellularity and cell turnover; however, ductal carcinoma *in situ* (DCIS) and infiltrating breast cancers with a large DCIS component have shown to often be negative for elevated choline levels, somewhat limiting the sensitivity of this technique [17]. Recent research has also demonstrated promise for MR spectroscopy in the realm of monitoring treatment of patients on neoadjuvant chemotherapy.

Although MR spectroscopy measurement of breast tumor choline levels can be successfully performed on 1.5T MR scanners, increases in both SNR and spectral resolution at higher field strength can improve choline detectability, decrease measurement errors, and enable the assessment of smaller lesions [18]. In general, for breast MR spectroscopy at 1.5T, qualitative detection of the presence of a choline peak at 3.2 ppm is indicative of malignancy, whereas at higher field strengths, more quantitative methods must be used because choline also becomes detectable in normal breast tissue. It has also recently been reported that changes measured in breast tumor choline levels detectable at higher field strengths may be an early predictive marker of treatment response. In a preliminary study of patients undergoing neoadjuvant therapy, reduction of choline levels as early as 24 hours after the first dose of chemotherapy correlated with response as measured by final change in tumor size [19].

Clinical perspective

In practice, the improved SNR afforded by 3T should translate to improvement in spatial resolution that facilitates evaluation of morphology of small lesions and improved assessment of margins of all lesions. In our experience, scanning at 3T can provide high-quality dynamic contrast-enhanced breast MR images with higher spatial resolution than that achievable at 1.5T (Figure 3.5). The imaging protocols employed at our institution for DCE-MR imaging at 1.5T and 3T are compared in Table 3.1, with smaller voxel sizes achieved at 3T within the same time frame using a higher parallel imaging factor, larger acquisition matrix, and smaller field of view.

However, imaging at higher field strength also creates some practical clinical challenges. The increased spatial resolution leads to an increased number of image slices per series, which ultimately increases the number of images the radiologist must review. In addition, the larger data sets require

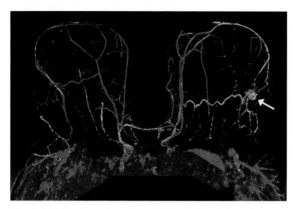

Figure 3.5 Maximum intensity projection (MIP) of dynamic contrast-enhanced breast MR images acquired at 3T. The MIP was created from subtraction images (post-contrast minus pre-contrast) to demonstrate enhancing structures. Delayed phase contrast kinetics are represented in color, with red, green, and blue representing washout, plateau, and persistent enhancement, respectively. In this example case, a lesion with suspicious enhancement characteristics is visible in the left breast (arrow). See plate section for color version.

Table 3.1 Comparison of T1-weighted imaging parameters for 1.5T and 3T breast protocols

Field strength	1.5T	3T
Breast coil type	8-Channel	16-Channel
Plane	Axial	Axial
Mode	3D	3D
Sequence type	Fast gradient echo	Fast gradient echo
Parallel imaging factor	**1.5**	**2.7 R/L, 2.0 S/I**
TR	5.6 ms	5.9 ms
TE	3 ms	3 ms
Flip angle	10°	10°
FOV	$36 \times 36\,cm^2$	$22 \times 33\,cm^2$
Slice thickness	**1.6 mm**	**1.3 mm**
Matrix	420×420	440×660
In-plane voxel size	**0.85 mm**	**0.5 mm**
Scan time (min)	2:53	2:51

R/L = right/left, S/I = superior/inferior, TR = repetition time, TE = echo time, FOV = field of view. Bold indicates differences in spatial resolution.

increased storage capacity, and can place increased demands on scanner and offline computer-aided detection (CAD) post-processing programs commonly used with breast MR imaging. Furthermore, as technology continues to improve, it will be important to re-evaluate predictors of malignancy as assessment of lesion morphology and in particular lesion margins will improve with increased spatial resolution.

There is a paucity of data assessing potential differences in kinetic curves when moving from 1.5 to 3T. While there have been some anecdotal reports that there is an increase in benign background enhancement and significant effects on the kinetic curves at 3T, these issues have not been a significant factor to date in our experience. Further study of the effects on kinetics and benign background enhancement is needed.

MR imaging-guided breast biopsy techniques have been refined greatly over the past decade; however, some mild adjustments may be needed in biopsy technique at higher field strength. Breast biopsies are generally performed with larger-gauge biopsy needles, typically at least 14 gauge, in order to ensure adequate tissue sampling of a lesion. However, as susceptibility artifact increases both with higher field strength and larger biopsy needle sizes, there can be an increase in the signal void of biopsy devices at 3T. A study by Peters *et al.* reported a signal void that was over twice the size of that at 1.5T for a 14-gauge

needle; however, they noted that despite this difference, diagnostic accuracy of the biopsies was not affected [20]. If necessary, alterations to the imaging protocol such as increasing bandwidth or reducing echo time may help to compensate for this difference in susceptibility and reduce the signal void of a biopsy device at 3T.

Conclusion

Breast MR imaging with 3T scanners provides both potential benefits of increased SNR, as well as added challenges of increased SAR and magnetic field inhomogeneities. Perhaps most importantly, scanning at 3T can provide breast MR images with higher spatial resolution than that achievable at 1.5T. However, these improvements can be realized only through optimization of a variety of technical factors including use of a multichannel breast coil, parallel RF transmission, and high order shimming. More research is necessary to determine the added clinical value of 3T for breast imaging.

References

1. Rakow-Penner R, Daniel B, Yu H, Sawyer-Glover A, Glover GH. Relaxation times of breast tissue at 1.5T and 3T measured using IDEAL. *J Magn Reson Imaging* 2006; **23**: 87–91.

2. Rohrer M, Bauer H, Mintorovitch J, Requardt M, Weinmann HJ. Comparison of magnetic properties of MRI contrast media solutions at different magnetic field strengths. *Invest Radiol* 2005; **40**: 715–24.

3. Barth MM, Smith MP, Pedrosa I, Lenkinski RE, Rofsky NM. Body MR imaging at 3.0 T: understanding the opportunities and challenges. *Radiographics* 2007; **27**: 1445–62; discussion 1462–4.

4. Kuhl CK, Kooijman H, Gieseke J, Schild HH. Effect of B1 inhomogeneity on breast MR imaging at 3.0 T. *Radiology* 2007; **244**: 929–30.

5. Azlan CA, Di Giovanni P, Ahearn TS, *et al.* B1 transmission-field inhomogeneity and enhancement ratio errors in dynamic contrast-enhanced MRI (DCE-MRI) of the breast at 3T. *J Magn Reson Imaging* 2010; **31**: 234–9.

6. Kuhl CK, Jost P, Morakkabati N, *et al.* Contrast-enhanced MR imaging of the breast at 3.0 and 1.5 T in the same patients: initial experience. *Radiology* 2006; **239**: 666–76.

7. Pinker K, Grabner G, Bogner W, *et al.* A combined high temporal and high spatial resolution 3Tesla MR imaging protocol for the assessment of breast lesions: initial results. *Invest Radiol* 2009; **44**: 553–8.

8. Wiesinger F, Van de Moortele PF, Adriany G, *et al.* Potential and feasibility of parallel MRI at high field. *NMR Biomed* 2006; **19**: 368–78.

9. Ladd ME. High-field-strength magnetic resonance: potential and limits. *Top Magn Reson Imaging* 2007; **18**: 139–52.

10. Rakow-Penner R, Hargreaves B, Glover GH, Daniel B. Breast MRI at 3T. *Appl Radiol* 2009; **38**(3): 6–13.

11. Guo Y, Cai YQ, Cai ZL, *et al.* Differentiation of clinically benign and malignant breast lesions using diffusion-weighted imaging. *J Magn Reson Imaging* 2002; **16**: 172–8.

12. Woodhams R, Matsunaga K, Kan S, *et al.* ADC mapping of benign and malignant breast tumors. *Magn Reson Med Sci* 2005; **4**: 35–42.

13. Partridge SC, DeMartini WB, Kurland BF, *et al.* Quantitative diffusion-weighted imaging as an adjunct to conventional breast MRI for improved positive predictive value. *AJR Am J Roentgenol* 2009; **193**: 1716–22.

14. Matsuoka A, Minato M, Harada M, *et al.* Comparison of 3.0- and 1.5-tesla diffusion-weighted imaging in the visibility of breast cancer. *Radiat Med* 2008; **26**: 15–20.

15. Lo GG, Ai V, Chan JK *et al.* Diffusion-weighted magnetic resonance imaging of breast lesions: first experiences at 3T. *Comput Assist Tomogr* 2009; **33**(1): 63–9.

16. Bolan PJ, Nelson MT, Yee D, Garwood M. Imaging in breast cancer: magnetic resonance spectroscopy. *Breast Cancer Res* 2005; **7**: 149–52.

17. Sinha S, Sinha U. Recent advances in breast MRI and MRS. *NMR Biomed* 2009; **22**: 3–16.

18. Haddadin IS, McIntosh A, Meisamy S, *et al.* Metabolite quantification and high-field MRS in breast cancer. *NMR Biomed* 2009; **22**: 65–76.

19. Meisamy S, Bolan PJ, Baker EH, *et al.* Neoadjuvant chemotherapy of locally advanced breast cancer: predicting response with in vivo (1)H MR spectroscopy – a pilot study at 4 T. *Radiology* 2004; **233**: 424–31.

20. Peters NH, Meeuwis C, Bakker CJ, *et al.* Feasibility of MRI-guided large-core-needle biopsy of suspiscious breast lesions at 3 T. *Eur Radiol* 2009; **19**: 1639–44.

Cardiac MR imaging

Christopher J. François, Oliver Wieben, and Scott B. Reeder

Introduction

Cardiac magnetic resonance (CMR) imaging is routinely used for the diagnosis and management of patients with ischemic and nonischemic heart disease because it can provide a comprehensive, noninvasive evaluation of cardiac morphology, function, perfusion, and viability [1]. In fact, CMR is widely considered the clinical gold standard for assessing right and left ventricular function using balanced steady-state free precession (bSSFP) [2] and determining myocardial viability in patients with ischemic heart disease using inversion recovery (IR) prepared spoiled gradient echo [3]. Technical advances that have improved the spatial and/or temporal resolution of magnetic resonance (MR) imaging have led to improvements in the ability of this modality to visualize pathologic changes in the heart. This has led to an increase in the use of 3T MR imaging scanners for CMR studies.

Specifically, increases in signal-to-noise ratio (SNR) performance and changes in nuclear magnetic resonance (NMR) relaxation parameters (T1, T2) present the opportunity to improve our ability to characterize the changes that occur with a variety of cardiac diseases. However, CMR at 3T also presents particular challenges compared with 1.5T, including increased radiofrequency (RF)-induced energy deposition, higher demands on shimming requirements to compensate for amplified susceptibility artifacts, and increased B1 field inhomogeneities. This chapter will review technical considerations for performing CMR at 3T, including the impact of 3T on SNR, relaxation times, chemical shift and susceptibility, specific absorption rate (SAR), dielectric effects (magnetic field inhomogeneity), bSSFP imaging, and parallel imaging. This is followed by a discussion of specific CMR sequences and their performance at 3T.

Technical considerations for CMR at 3T
Signal-to-noise ratio (SNR)

The increase in SNR is one of the most appealing reasons for imaging at a higher field strength. The noise in most MR imaging applications is dominated by the intrinsic noise caused by the random motion of electrons within tissue. With current MR imaging scanners, electrical noise from the receiving circuit and other external noise contributions are minimal. When the magnetic field strength is greater than 1T, the noise has a linear dependence on the static magnetic field (B0) while the MR imaging signal exhibits quadratic growth with respect to B0. Consequently, one would expect a doubling of SNR when scanning at 3T compared with 1.5T, with all other factors being equal. However, the MR imaging signal, contrast, and image quality are heavily influenced by other parameters also affected by changes in magnetic field strength – including the longitudinal and transversal relaxation times (T1 and T2), RF coil design, artifacts from off-resonances and B1 field inhomogeneities, and pulse sequence adjustments that may be required due to safety constraints regarding the allowable energy deposition from the RF pulses.

Relaxation times

The transverse relaxation time (T2) in most tissues experiences only a small decrease when increasing the field strength from 1.5T to 3T. The longitudinal relaxation time (T1), however, increases approximately by the third root of the magnetic field strength [4]. For oxygenated blood, the T1 increases from 1200–1600 ms at 1.5T to 1500–1900 ms at 3T and the T2 decreases from 200–325 ms at 1.5T to 140–275 ms at 3T. For normal myocardium, the T1 increases from

Body MR Imaging at 3 Tesla, ed. Ihab R. Kamel and Elmar M. Merkle. Published by Cambridge University Press.

870–1070 ms at 1.5T to 1115–1470 ms at 3T and the T2 decreases from 40–60 ms at 1.5T to 40–50 ms at 3T. While the T1 and T2 values of oxygenated blood and normal myocardium vary from study to study, the trends are similar across the studies: slight decreases in T2 and larger increases in T1. The variability in the reported changes in relaxation times is likely related to differences in measurement techniques, tissue sources, and other factors.

The relaxation rates R1 and R2 of gadolinium-based contrast agents are reported to decrease when scanning at higher magnetic field strengths [5]. While lower relaxivity rates reduce the T1 shortening caused by the contrast agent, our experience has been that this effect is rather small and has not been an issue.

Chemical shift and susceptibility

The precession frequency, or Larmor frequency, varies linearly with the magnetic field strength. For protons, the precession frequency increases from 64 MHz at 1.5T to 128 MHz at 3.0T. This also leads to a greater separation in the precession frequencies of different metabolites. For example, protons in fat precess 210 Hz slower than free protons at 1.5T. This difference increases to 420 Hz at 3T. While increased chemical shift is beneficial for all MR spectroscopy applications, including cardiac MR spectroscopy [6], the increased chemical shift leads to greater chemical shift artifacts and amplifies off-resonance artifacts from susceptibility at tissue interfaces. The decreased B0 inhomogeneity leads to increased banding artifacts with bSSFP sequences. These effects can be minimized by identifying the optimal synthesizer frequency or by improving the shimming with a smaller field-of-view shim or with higher order shimming corrections [7].

Specific absorption rate (SAR)

The RF pulse used to excite the magnetic spins leads to energy deposition within the object imaged. Regulatory agencies mandate specific patient safety guidelines for SAR thresholds for human imaging. This is to minimize any potential rise in global and local body temperature. At 1.5T, these SAR guidelines typically do not limit CMR applications. This is not the case when performing CMR at 3T.

The flip angle (α) for a given RF pulse is proportional to the integral of the amplitude of the alternating B1 field for the time during which it is applied (Eq. 4.1):

$$\alpha \propto \int B1 \, dt \approx B1 \Delta T. \tag{4.1}$$

In CMR, where rapid sequences are used to image cardiac motion, high B1 fields are employed to minimize pulse duration (ΔT), repetition time (TR), and the echo time (TE). However, the SAR is proportional to the integral of the square of the amplitude of the alternating B1 field over the time during which it is applied (Eq. 4.2):

$$SAR \propto \int B1^2 \, dt \approx B1^2 \Delta T. \tag{4.2}$$

Therefore, the B1 amplitude required to achieve a given flip angle doubles at 3T, which leads to a fourfold increase in SAR for the same RF pulse design when scanning at 3T compared with 1.5T. To maintain SAR within patient safety guidelines requires that sequences with rapidly repeating high flip angles be appropriately adjusted to maintain a safe SAR. For CMR, this affects black-blood fast spin echo sequences, three-dimensional (3D) gradient echo sequences with short TRs that are used for magnetic resonance angiography, and, most importantly, bright-blood bSSFP sequences that require very short TRs with relatively high flip angles (i.e., 50–70° at 1.5T). Although reducing the flip angle is a simple and effective way to reduce the SAR, this can lead to undesired tissue contrast alterations. Because tissue contrast is less strongly dependent on flip angle for bSSFP sequences, the overall effect for bSSFP sequences is relatively minor.

SAR can also be reduced by using parallel imaging to reduce the number of RF pulses necessary to complete image acquisition, lengthening the duration of the RF pulse, and using RF pulses with more constant B1 amplitudes (VERSE, variable-rate selective excitation).

Dielectric effects: B1 inhomogeneity

To change the state of the magnetic spins in MR imaging, the frequency of the RF pulses must match the resonance frequency. The wavelength of the RF pulse is inversely proportional to that frequency. The actual wavelength also depends on the electrical permittivity of the medium through which the RF wave is propagating. At 1.5T, the wavelength is larger than the human body being imaged. At 3T, however, the wavelength is less than 1 m and is typically less than the size of the human body through which it is propagating, causing "dielectric effects" [8]. This leads

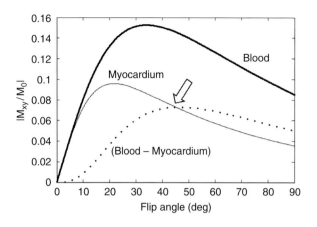

Figure 4.1 Magnitude of the transverse magnetization for blood (solid line), myocardium (thin line), and their difference (dotted line) as a function of the flip angle for imaging with a bSSFP sequence at 3T. This simulation assumes steady-state conditions with the following parameters: TR = 3.8 ms; TE = 1.9 ms; T1 = 1512 ms and T2 = 141 ms for blood; and T1 = 1115 ms and T2 = 41 ms for the myocardium, similar to the parameters used by others [9, 10]. Optimal blood–myocardial contrast is achieved with 40–45° flip angle (arrow).

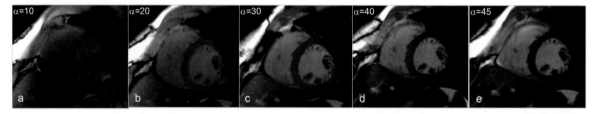

Figure 4.2 Short-axis views obtained at 3T with a bSSFP sequence and varying flip angles. Within the range from 0° to 45° flip angles, the blood-to-myocardium contrast increases with increasing flip angles. The SAR increases with the square of the flip angles, limiting the maximum allowable flip angle. As demonstrated in Figure 4.1, this contrast ratio also reaches a plateau.

to standing wave patterns that cause an inhomogeneous B1 field and subsequently result in nonuniform flip angles across the imaging volume. For bSSFP sequences, these B1 inhomogeneities are less of a concern because of the relative insensitivity of bSSFP signal and contrast to flip angle variations. Inversion recovery spoiled gradient echo sequences, used for delayed myocardial enhancement imaging, however, do require highly uniform inversion pulses to ensure robust inversion of magnetization across the heart. This can result in areas of inadequately nulled myocardium because of nonuniform flip angle of the inversion pulse. Adiabatic pulses can partially alleviate this problem by providing a more homogeneous flip angle for delayed myocardial enhancement and coronary imaging.

bSSFP imaging at 3T

Cardiac morphology and function are primarily assessed with MR imaging using bSSFP. Understanding of the challenges of performing bSSFP at 3T is critical to performing high-quality cardiac MR imaging at 3T. This includes increased banding

artifacts from off-resonances and suboptimal options for flip angle due to SAR restrictions. In Figure 4.1, we show results from a simulation showing the blood and myocardium signal as a function of the flip angle. As the flip angle increases, there is an increase in the blood-to-myocardium contrast (Figure 4.2). The in-vivo signal behavior of the blood is likely somewhat different because of additional inflow effects that are not accounted for here, but this simulation demonstrates the large blood–myocardial signal contrast achievable with bSSFP imaging. Despite the challenges faced when using bSSFP, the very large CNR and improvement in SNR is highly motivating to address these challenges rather than reverting to using spoiled gradient recalled acquisition in the steady state (SPGR) sequences at 3T. For example, it can be shown that the bSSFP signal for normal myocardium is more than twice the signal from the spoiled gradient echo sequence for optimized flip angle choices. Importantly, Figure 4.1 also demonstrates how the bSSFP contrast is relatively constant for flip angles exceeding 35°, with an optimal flip angle at 40–45° in order to maximize the contrast between blood and myocardium. Therefore, the bSSFP sequence is

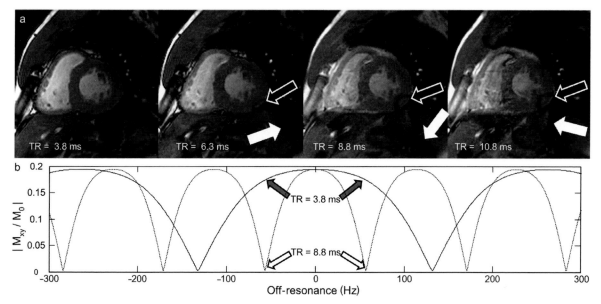

Figure 4.3 Effect of TR on bSSFP signal behavior. (a) Cine bSSFP images were acquired at 1.5T with variable TR. With longer TR, the images have greater banding artifacts, most notably along the inferolateral left ventricular wall (open arrows). Similar effects are observed at 3T. (b) This is due to narrower passbands with longer TR, which causes a drop in signal at lower off resonances as shown in the magnitude plot of the steady-state magnetization based on typical acquisition parameters at 1.5T – T1 = 1200 ms and T2 = 200 ms (blood), TE = TR/2, flip angle = 45°, and TR = 3.8 ms (solid line) and 8.8 ms (dotted line).

relatively robust in respect to B1 inhomogeneities that cause inconsistent flip angles.

One limitation of using bSSFP sequences is their sensitivity to severe imaging artifacts for off-resonances due to a complex signal behavior. The magnitude and the phase of the bSSFP signal depends not only on the T1 and T2 of the imaged species and the TR and TE of the acquistion but also on the phase (β) that accumulates during a TR as a result of magnetic field inhomogeneities or chemical shift. The presence of magnetic field inhomogeneities (ΔB0) leads to a phase shift between each RF pulse (Eq. 4.3),

$$\beta = \gamma \times \Delta B0 \times TR, \qquad (4.3)$$

where γ is the gyromagnetic ratio.

An off-resonance phase of β = 180° (π radians) corresponds to an isochromate that is off-resonance by 1/(2 × TR) so that Figure 4.3 can also be interpreted as a spectral response. At this phase offset, the signal in the magnitude response drops precipitously, corresponding to severe signal loss at locations in the image where the field inhomogeneity causes a 180° (π) phase shift between RF pulses. Since the off-resonances from susceptibilities are directly proportional to the field strength, bSSFP imaging at 3T is

equivalent to imaging at 1.5T at twice the TR with respect to these "banding" artifacts.

To reduce banding artifacts, two strategies are used. The first is to reduce the TR. Figure 4.3 demonstrates the significance of short TRs at 1.5T (similar findings are observed at 3T) where a banding artifact is apparent in the inferolateral wall of the left ventricle when longer TRs are used. As the TR is shortened, the band is pushed out of the myocardium and it completely disappears at a TR of 3.8 ms. The magnitude response in Figure 4.3 shows that an image is free of banding artifacts for all voxels with off-resonances less than ±40 Hz when acquired with a TR of 8.8 ms. If the TR is reduced to 3.8 ms, the passband widens and voxels with up to ±100 Hz are properly represented without significant signal drops.

To reduce the TR of the bSSFP acquisition we frequently use partial readout acquisitions. By acquiring an asymmetric readout, it is possible to reduce the TR by 20–30%, which is a significant decrease in TR, reducing banding artifacts substantially. This approach has the added benefits of improving the speed performance of the acquisition and reducing velocity artifacts by reducing the first moment of the readout gradient. This approach requires the use of homodyne reconstruction to reconstruct full

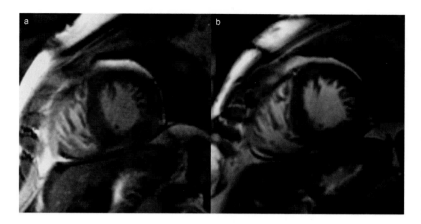

Figure 4.4 Short-axis bSSFP images acquired at (a) 1.5T and (b) 3T in a 58-year-old male with cardiac amyloidosis. The image at 1.5T was acquired with an 8-channel cardiac coil, TR = 2.89 ms, TE = 0.9 ms, flip angle = 45°, slice thickness = 8 mm, matrix = 256 × 256, and field of view 350 mm. The image at 3T was acquired with a 16-channel cardiac coil, TR = 3.41 ms, TE = 1.3 ms, flip angle = 45°, slice thickness = 7 mm, matrix = 256 × 256, and field of view 350 mm. The SNR and CNR are visibly greater at 3T (b) than at 1.5T (a), even with a slightly thinner slice thickness. Also note that with the relatively low TR used at 3T (TR = 3.41 ms), banding artifacts are not present over the heart.

resolution images, although this is a standard feature on most scanners. Partial readouts also affect the relative phase behavior of water and fat signals as discussed below.

The second approach to reduce banding artifacts is to reduce the field inhomogeneity across the heart by using local shimming and second order shimming of the static field to minimize these artifacts by reducing the variations of the off-resonance phase across the selected region to less than 180°. Schar *et al.* [7] suggested higher order local shimming procedures to avoid banding artifacts. An interesting alternative is the use of scout scans acquired with varying center frequencies to identify the center frequency that minimizes the presence of the dark band in the cardiac structures of interest. Short TRs and an improved B0 homogeneity are also essential to reduce flow-induced artifacts in bSSFP imaging.

As mentioned previously, SAR limitations reduce the maximum achievable flip angle at 3T. Figure 4.4 shows a comparison of images acquired at 1.5T and at 3T with a flip angle of 45°, often the highest achievable flip angle on clinical scanners. At this flip angle, the difference in blood-to-myocardial contrast is readily apparent and greater at 3T than at 1.5T. Methods described previously can be used to partially overcome these issues.

Cardiac bSSFP images acquired at 1.5T often have a black line, or "India ink" artifact that occurs at the interfaces of tissues that are predominantly water and predominantly fat (Figure 4.5). In cardiac MR imaging, this is present at the interface between the pericardium and epicardial fat. This appearance is a result of the phase behavior of bSSFP and not a result of chemical shift artifact, which is very small with

bSSFP because of the high readout bandwidth that is typically used. As shown in Figure 4.5, the phase behavior of the bSSFP signal alternates from 0° to 180° (π) (i.e., positive to negative) between alternating passbands. This phase behavior always occurs with bSSFP, no matter what the local magnetic field inhomogeneity, so long as TE = TR/2. The chemical shift between water and fat at 1.5T and 37 °C is −210 Hz, which corresponds exactly to the width of one passband (2π) when TR = 4.6 ms. This means that water and fat signals are always separated by exactly one passband, and will always have a 180° (π) phase shift relative to each other. This leads to destructive interference in pixels that contain both water and fat, including those pixels at water–fat interfaces, through partial volume effects. This creates the India ink artifact, as is seen with "out-of-phase" images acquired as part of in/out-phase imaging used in abdominal imaging.

At 3T, the situation changes, however, because the chemical shift between water and fat doubles to −420 Hz, while the gradient performance is roughly the same, and the passband profiles are identical for a given TR. In this situation, however, the water and fat resonances may be separated by two passbands. If the frequency of the passbands is separated by two passbands, the phase of water and fat are identical and signal from water and fat add constructively, and the India ink artifact disappears. Moreover, the presence of field inhomogeneities will cause the resonant peaks of water and fat to shift. Depending on the TR, this may push the resonant peak of fat, for example, into a new passband, before the water moves into a different passband. This complex behavior of the phase can result in changes in the appearance of the water–fat

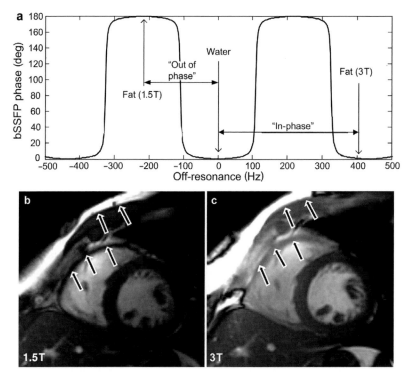

Figure 4.5 Demonstration of "India ink" artifact in a volunteer imaged at 1.5T and 3T with a TR of 4.6 ms. The phase of the bSSFP signal alternates from 0° to 180° between alternating passbands (a). The chemical shift between water and fat at 1.5T can lead to destructive interference (arrows) in pixels that contain both water and fat (b). The chemical shift doubles at 3T and leads to changes in the appearance of the water–fat interface. In the absence of field inhomogeneities, the phase of water and fat are identical and signal from water and fat add constructively and the "India ink" artifact disappears (c) at 3T when using the same TR.

interface, even within the same image (Figure 4.5c). Although this effect can also occur at 1.5T (unless the passbands are exactly spaced by 2π, when TR = 4.6 ms), it rarely occurs, because the passbands are relatively wide and the field inhomogeneities are smaller. At 3T, however, the passbands are narrow relative to the chemical shift and field inhomogeneities, and transitions of the water and fat peaks between different passbands frequently occur, as shown in Figure 4.5a. The importance of understanding this artifact is to understand differences in appearance between 1.5T and 3T, and to avoid pitfalls that can result from relying on the presence of this artifact (e.g., using the India ink artifact to identify fatty masses such as lipomas).

Finally, it is important to note that the phase behavior shown in Figure 4.5 occurs only when TE = TR/2, the most commonly used TE for symmetric echo acquisitions in SSFP. However, as we have suggested above, the use of partial readout (k_x) acquisitions is a useful way to shorten the TR at 3T to reduce banding and flow artifacts. For TEs not equal to TR/2, the phase behavior is more complex and will lead to more complex interference of water and fat at tissue interfaces. While the appearance is not disruptive to image interpretation, it is important to note this phase behavior to avoid diagnostic pitfalls regarding fatty tissue at tissue interface, i.e., the interpreting physician should not rely on the presence of the India ink artifact, particularly at 3T.

Parallel imaging

Combining the spatial sensitivities of multiple receiver coils in a phased array decreases the number of phase-encoding steps required, typically reducing the scan time by a factor, R, of 2–6 with multichannel cardiac coils [9, 10]. This acceleration in scan time can be taken advantage of to improve the spatial coverage for breath-hold CMR applications. However, the acceleration achievable is limited by the decrease in SNR, which is given by the following equation (Eq. 4.4):

$$SNR_R = \frac{SNR_o}{g\sqrt{R}}, \tag{4.4}$$

where SNR_o is the SNR of an unaccelerated image, R is the acceleration factor, and g, the "geometry factor" and which is equal to or greater than one, reflects the ill-conditioning of image unwrapping and is a measure of coil and imaging algorithm performance. The g-factor increases at higher reduction factors, limiting achievable accelerations. Fortunately, the performance of parallel imaging techniques improves at 3.0 T compared with 1.5T. This is a result of the smaller wavelengths of the RF signals at 3T. The smaller wavelengths lead to improved effective coil separation and help keep g close to one, even at higher R values.

For CMR at 3T, parallel imaging offers an opportunity to take advantage of the increased SNR to reduce the scan time or increase coverage within the same breath-hold [11]. For example, a fourfold increase in scan coverage is possible at 3T, using parallel imaging with an $R = 4$, in the same scan time, with the same SNR performance and image quality as 1.5T, assuming $g = 1$. In reality, this tremendous improvement may be tempered by other factors discussed previously in this chapter (i.e., T1, SAR, and B1 inhomogeneities).

Specific CMR sequences
Cardiac function

Cardiac MR imaging is the gold standard for the assessment of ventricular wall motion and function. Rapid gradient echo or bSSFP sequences, which provide images with high spatial and temporal resolution, as well as high contrast between blood pool and myocardium, are used to obtain CINE images of the beating heart. Typically multiple two-dimensional (2D) slices are obtained through the heart during multiple breath-holds. These images are then used to calculate multiple parameters of cardiac function, including cardiac output, ejection fraction, ventricular mass, etc. In addition, these image series allow for the assessment of regional wall thickness and motion abnormalities throughout the cardiac cycle.

Initially, CINE cardiac imaging was performed with spoiled gradient echo sequences, also known as fast low-angle shot (FLASH), SPGR, or fast field echo (FFE), an acquisition technique that uses RF spoiling and gradient spoiling to achieve a steady-state condition for the longitudinal magnetization. With bSSFP imaging, no spoiling is used and both the transverse and the longitudinal magnetizations reach a steady state and contribute to the MR signal [12]. This approach, also known as true fast imaging with steady-state free precession (trueFISP), fast imaging employing steady-state acquisition (FIESTA), and balanced fast field echo (bFFE), has become practical for clinical cardiac imaging [2] due to improvements in gradient performance and field shimming to avoid

artifacts described below. EKG-gated CINE bSSFP has become the sequence of choice for functional cardiac imaging, as a result of its high SNR performance and excellent blood–myocardial contrast. While the image contrast in the rapid SPGR sequence depends mostly on T1-dependent and inflow effects for a high blood signal, bSSFP provides an inherently high steady-state signal, particularly for blood, which has a large T2-to-T1 ratio.

Reports in the literature that compare CINE imaging between field strengths with SPGR and bSSFP sequences vary significantly in the reported gains of SNR and CNR [13, 14]. This might be partly explained by the variability in experimental setup (e.g., coils and sequence parameters such as TR and maximum flip angle). However, in general there is a gain in SNR and CNR with bSSFP compared to SPGR and with imaging at 3T compared with 1.5T. Several studies document the use of parallel MR imaging in cardiac CINE imaging with good correlation of volume measurements when using reduction factors of 2 for a 4-channel phased-array receiver coil and reduction factors of 4–6 for 32-element coils. It has been shown that parallel imaging at 3T introduces less SNR degradations than at 1.5T, that the increase in baseline SNR for 3T imaging overcompensated for the SNR reduction from parallel imaging, and that there is good agreement for the measurement of ejection fraction. These gains in acquisition speed can not only be used to improve spatial or temporal resolution or coverage or reduce a breath-hold duration, they can also decrease the SAR because of a reduced imaging time.

Myocardial tagging

MR tagging allows for the evaluation of complex intramyocardial contractile patterns and quantitative motion analysis of the cardiac walls [15]. With this method, intrinsic markers in the myocardial wall are created by the application of inversion bands across the imaging plane. This pattern is accomplished by the use of RF pulses in combination with gradient pulses that invert spins in thin parallel planes perpendicular to the imaging plane just prior to the application of the RF pulse used for the excitation of the imaging plane. Radial, line, and grid-shaped patterns have been applied to track the evolution of these bands throughout the cardiac cycle for the assessment of the deformation of the myocardium and

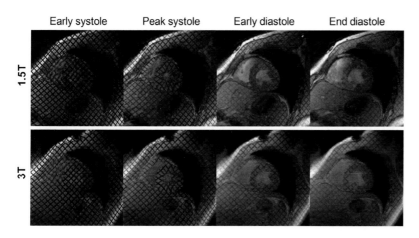

Early systole   Peak systole   Early diastole   End diastole

Figure 4.6 MR tagging images in a healthy volunteer acquired at 1.5T (upper row) and 3T (bottom row). The myocardial tags persist longer into diastole at 3T (bottom right image) due to the prolonged T1 relaxation time of the myocardium at 3T relative to 1.5T. The persistence of the tags throughout the cardiac cycles facilitates the identification of wall motion abnormalities during systole and diastole.

e.g. identify regions of impaired contractility. Spoiled gradient echo CINE sequences as described above for functional imaging are usually used for MR tagging with the simple addition of the saturation pulses. One challenge encountered with tagging at 1.5T is the fading of tags at end-diastole, greatly limiting the evaluation of myocardial function during diastole. Although MR tagging at 3T benefits from the increased SNR and CNR, the most important benefit is the prolonged T1 of myocardium. This leads to a slower recovery of the longitudinal magnetization and, therefore, improved tag persistence, particularly in mid- and end-diastole, where tags have typically faded when imaging at 1.5T (Figures 4.6 and 4.7). A recent study [16] showed SNR improvements of 35% and CNR improvements of 80% for myocardial tags at 3T as compared with 1.5T. Gutberlet *et al.* [9] measured gains in SNR and CNR during systole as 54% and 174% respectively.

First-pass perfusion

Most MR myocardial perfusion acquisitions measure myocardial signal changes during the first pass following the intravenous administration of a gadolinium-based contrast agent. As the extracellular contrast agent passes from the vascular space into the extravascular space of the myocardium, it shortens the T1 of myocardium. With rapid, dynamic T1-weighted imaging sequences it is possible to detect relative differences in the degree of enhancement, or T1 shortening. Areas with relatively less enhancement, which appear hypointense to normally perfused regions, correspond to areas of hypoperfusion, or less coronary artery blood flow. Typically first-pass

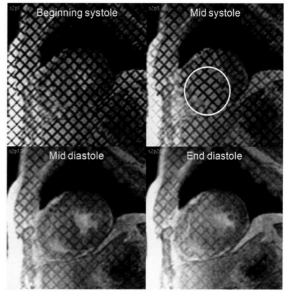

Beginning systole   Mid systole

Mid diastole   End diastole

Figure 4.7 MR tagging images obtained at 3T in a 45-year-old male with hypertrophic cardiomyopathy (HCM). The myocardial tags can be clearly seen throughout the cardiac cycle because of the prolonged T1 relaxation. In this patient, there is decreased deformation of the tags in the septum (circle) related to the abnormal myocytes and fibrosis in this area and related to HCM.

perfusion images are reviewed qualtitatively to identify areas of hypoperfusion. Because of the complex relationship between gadolinium concentration and measured signal, quantitative measurement of myocardial perfusion using first-pass perfusion MR imaging is still not yet routinely performed and is still under investigation. A reason for the strong interest in developing MR imaging-based myocardial perfusion imaging is that the in-plane resolution of MR perfusion imaging (2–3 mm) surpasses that of other imaging techniques, positron emission tomography

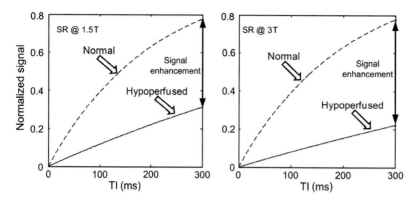

Figure 4.8 Signal intensity–saturation time (TI) curves for MR perfusion at 1.5T (left column) and 3T (right column) using a typical saturation recovery sequence. In normally perfused myocardium (dashed lines), extracellular gadolinium contrast agent leaves the vasculature and diffuses into the myocardium, shortening the T1 relaxation time. The T1 shortening for the normally enhancing areas of myocardium is similar at 1.5T and 3T. The abnormal, hypoperfused areas of myocardium (solid line) have a longer T1 relaxation time at 3T relative to 1.5T. As a result, the T1 relaxation takes longer at 3T and leads to greater contrast between normally perfused and underperfused areas.

(PET) and single-photon emission computed tomography (SPECT). As a result of the improved spatial resolution, MR imaging allows for greater delineation of small subendocardial perfusion defects. Despite marked improvements in scanner hardware and sequence design since its initial conception, there is still much room for improvement in the reproducibility and reliability of current myocardial perfusion MR imaging techniques. The development of accurate quantitative myocardial perfusion techniques should help increase the acceptance of MR imaging for the detection of myocardial ischemia. Ideally, the first-pass MR imaging acquisition should provide (1) high spatial (< 3 mm) and (2) high temporal (every heartbeat) resolution, (3) whole-heart coverage, (4) a quantifiable relationship between signal intensity and contrast agent concentration to allow for quantification, and (5) good image quality with sufficiently high contrast-to-noise ratio (CNR).

While various approaches for perfusion imaging exist, the most commonly used sequence is based on a 2D multislice, spoiled gradient echo sequence with saturation recovery (SR) preparation. The saturation pulse is applied prior to the readout for each acquired slice. The duration between the application of the saturation pulse and the acquisition of the contrast-defining central k-space lines, known as "TI," is similar to the inversion time in inversion recovery sequences. The signal difference between normal and hypoperfused myocardium is based on T1 and TI differences in the T1 (Figure 4.8). Myocardial perfusion at 3T is improved, relative to 1.5T by increases in SNR and CNR. In addition, there are greater differences in T1 times between normal and hypoperfused regions in the myocardium at 3T than

at 1.5T. In this way, an additional improvement in contrast between normal and hypoperfused myocardium can be achieved, beyond the factor of 2 increase from SNR improvements alone. The signal recovery of the normally perfused region is similar between 1.5T and 3T (Figure 4.8) because of the presence of the gadolinium-based contrast agent while the rate of signal recovery of underperfused areas is reduced at 3T, resulting in an increased contrast between normally perfused and hypoperfused myocardium. These theoretical predictions are supported by clinical results with significant image improvements and diagnostic performance at 3T (Figure 4.9). Gutberlet *et al.* measured an increase in SNR of 109% and in CNR between myocardium and the left ventricular cavity of 87% [9] while Araoz *et al.* measured an increase in contrast enhancement ratio of 70% and in myocardial enhancement ratio of 291% [17]. The increased CNR allows for an improved detection of small perfusion defects.

MR perfusion imaging at 3T can also benefit significantly from the use of parallel imaging with higher acceleration factors in order to improve temporal and spatial resolution of the acquisition, as well as increasing coverage over the entire heart. Optimal injection protocols should be determined for given sequences and modes of analysis to balance the optimization of contrast and minimization of contrast-induced susceptiblity artifacts.

Myocardial delayed enhancement

Evaluation of myocardial infarction using delayed imaging after intravenous injection of gadolinium-based contrast agents has become the gold standard

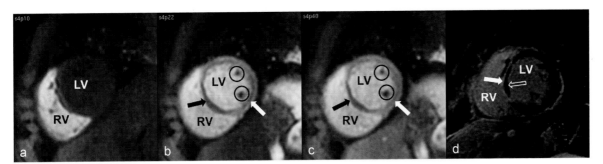

Figure 4.9 Cardiac MRI performed at 3T in a 29-year-old woman with Churg–Strauss syndrome (allergic angiitis and granulomatosis) and endomyocardial-biopsy-proven eosinophilic myocarditis. Short-axis, saturation-recovery, first-pass perfusion images first show (a) contrast arriving in the right ventricle (RV) and subsequently (b) in the left ventricle (LV). Areas of transmural hypoperfusion in the interventricular septum (black arrows), subendocardial hypoperfusion in the lateral wall (white arrows) and hypoperfusion of the papillary muscles (circles) persist on later perfusion images (c). Myocardial delayed contrast-enhanced images (d) show transmural enhancement in the interventricular septum (arrow) with an area of hypoenhancement (open arrow) indicating microvascular obstruction, or "no-reflow."

for the evaluation of myocardial viability [3]. Myocardial delayed enhancement (MDE) techniques allow for the differentiation between normal and abnormal myocardium because of differences in the extravascular concentration of gadolinium in normal and abnormal myocardium. At the time that MDE images are acquired, approximately 10–20 minutes after the intravenous injection of gadolinium-based contrast material, the concentration of gadolinium in normal myocardium has decreased due to normal wash-out kinetics while in infarcted myocardium the washout of gadolinium contrast is delayed. Similar washout kinetics are presumed to be responsible for the appearance of abnormal delayed contrast enhancement in a variety of nonischemic cardiomyopathies, such as inflammatory or infectious diseases of the myocardium, cardiomyopathy, cardiac neoplasms, and congenital or genetic cardiac pathologic conditions.

Although a variety of cardiac-gated T1-weighted MDE techniques can be used to visualize myocardial scar or infiltration, the inversion recovery SPGR (IR-SPGR) method first described by Simonetti *et al* [18] is the most widely used technique. In this approach, T1 weighting is achieved by applying a nonselective inversion pulse and waiting an inversion time (TI) until the normal myocardium has "nulled," i.e., zero longitudinal magnetization. Following the TI delay, a rapid, segmented SPGR acquisition acquires several lines of k-space. This is repeated over several heartbeats until the acquisition is complete. By choosing a TI that nulls the normal myocardium, areas of enhancing tissue appear very conspicuous and are easily visualized (Figure 4.10).

The correct TI, which depends on the T1 of the normal myocardium, is influenced by (1) the amount of gadolinium in the blood, which is determined by the initial dose given and (2) the time from that dose and the clearance of gadolinium from the blood. Clearance of contrast from blood depends on the patient's cardiac output and renal function. The T1 of the myocardium is also dependent on the field strength of the magnet. The maximum signal difference between normal and enhanced myocardium actually occurs later than the zero crossing of the signal intensity of the normal myocardium, but the conspicuity of lesions is the highest at this point. As discussed above, the T1 of myocardium increases considerably at 3T, meaning that the TI needed to null the myocardium will be longer than the values typically used at 1.5T. In our experience, the TI increases from 180–200 ms at 1.5T to approximately 220–250 ms at 3T. The patient-specific optimal TI is determined by trial and error or advanced scout scans that rapidly generate images with multiple TIs at a lower quality to identify the optimal timing. Alternatively, phase-sensitive inversion recovery (PSIR) provides MDE images with more stable contrast even if a suboptimal TI was chosen. This sequence has also been successfully applied on 3T systems.

MDE imaging benefits from a higher magnetic field in several ways [19]. In addition to the increase in SNR and CNR from the higher magnetization, the increase in T1 of the normal myocardium also leads to increased difference in the signal between normal and enhancing myocardium. This occurs because the normal myocardium recovers more slowly, requiring a long TI, which leads to an increase in the absolute signal difference between normal and enhancing myocardium. Recent studies have demonstrated

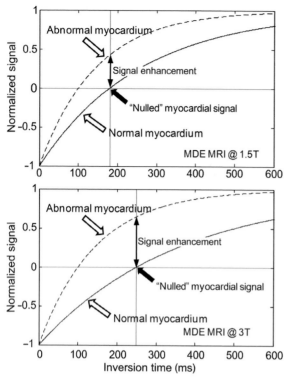

Figure 4.10 Signal intensity–inversion time (TI) curves for myocardial delayed enhancement MR imaging (MDE MRI) measurements at 1.5T (top row) and 3T (bottom row). The appropriate TI time for imaging is chosen such that the signal from normal myocardium (solid line) is "nulled." Because abnormal areas retain gadolinium contrast agent longer than normal myocardium, such as infarcted myocardium in patients with ischemic heart disease or fibrosis in patients with nonischemic heart disease, the T1 recovery will be shorter, resulting in areas of enhancement (dashed line). While the signal for enhancing myocardium (dashed line) is similar at 1.5T and 3T, the T1 lengthening of normal myocardium at 3T leads to greater contrast between normal and abnormal myocardium relative to 1.5T.

significant improvements in image quality, SNR, and CNR for MDE MR imaging at 3T over 1.5T. The improvement in CNR results in improved delineation of infarct extent. The improvements in SNR and CNR can also be used to acquire images with higher spatial resolution, including a smaller slice thickness (Figures 4.11–4.13).

Proper signal nulling with the inversion recovery sequence requires a homogeneous 180° flip angle across the imaging slice. The decreased B1 homogeneity at 3T causes larger deviations from the ideal flip angle and, therefore, signal nulling of the myocardium might not be achieved uniformly across the heart. The use of adiabatic pulses can provide a more homogeneous flip angle to avoid this undesired effect. These pulses are designed to sweep the resonant frequency and amplitude of the RF pulse to drive magnetization in a manner that is insensitive to the actual B1.

Conclusion

In conclusion, the most important benefits of cardiac imaging at 3T arise from the increased SNR and CNR and the longer longitudinal relaxation time T1. The latter leads to an improved background suppression and improved contrast and superior detection of small defects in first-pass perfusion imaging and an improved delineation of infarct extent in viability imaging. The increased SNR and benefits of 3T for parallel imaging can be used for accelerated imaging to provide more coverage or higher spatial or temporal resolution. The biggest challenges for cardiac imaging at a higher field strength are SAR limitations and the decreased B1 homogeneity and increased susceptibility effects. These issues can be partly

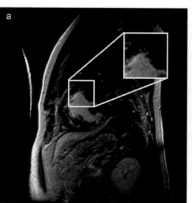

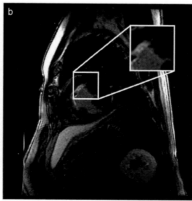

Figure 4.11 A 62-year-old male with prior subendocardial myocardial infarction. Myocardial delayed enhancement (MDE) images were acquired at 1.5T (a) with TR = 6.2 ms, TE = 1.5 ms, slice thickness = 8 mm, and matrix = 256. MDE images were also acquired in the same patient at 3T (b) with TR = 4.8 ms, TE = 1.3 ms, slice thickness = 8 mm, and matrix = 256. The infarct (inset images) is more conspicuous at 3T than at 1.5T.

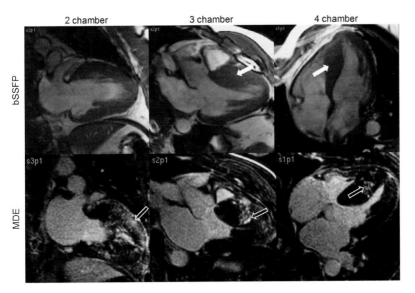

Figure 4.12 A 45-year-old male with prior hypertrophic cardiomyopathy (HCM; same as in Figure 4.6). Long-axis bSSFP (top row) and myocardial delayed enhancement (MDE) (bottom row) images were obtained at 3T. Asymmetric septal hypertrophy (arrows) and patchy, mid-myocardial areas of abnormal enhancement (open arrows) in the areas of hypertrophy on the MDE images are typical of HCM.

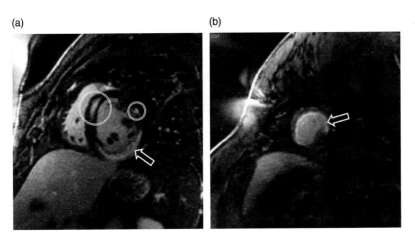

Figure 4.13 Short-axis myocardial delayed enhancement (MDE) images obtained through the mid (a) and apical (b) left ventricle in a 52-year-old female with cardiac sarcoidosis reveal mid-myocardial (circles) and subendocardial (open arrow) enhancement. The regions of subendocardial enhancement are due to myocardial infarcts, presumably as a result of granulomatous involvement of the coronary arteries while the areas of mid-myocardial enhancement correspond to cardiac granulomas, typical of cardiac sarcoidosis.

overcome by advanced sequence design, adiabatic pulses, and improved shimming techniques.

While the gains of a higher field strength are somewhat offset by the presence of more severe artifacts for CINE imaging with bSSFP, almost all other cardiac sequences including MR tagging, myocardial perfusion and delayed enhancement imaging clearly benefit from the higher field strength. With proper shimming, and attention to methods to maintain a short TR, it is relatively straightforward to acquire highly diagnostic bSSFP images in all patients.

Other important CMR applications not discussed in this chapter, including coronary artery imaging and phase contrast imaging, have also been successfully adopted to clinical 3T imaging. Particularly the combination of parallel MR imaging with multi-element coils and high acceleration factors offers unique opportunities for improved cardiovascular MR imaging.

In summary, cardiac imaging at 3T offers tremendous advantages beyond the increase in SNR performance, including improved contrast-enhanced perfusion and viability imaging, improved opportunities for aggressive parallel imaging techniques, and improved visualization of wall motion through myocardial tagging. Advancements in localized shimming methods and new RF pulses to reduce SAR to avoid pitfalls from B1 inhomogeneities will complete the transformation of 3T cardiac imaging from vision to a clinical reality in daily practice.

References

1. Pennell DJ. Cardiovascular magnetic resonance. *Circulation* 2010; **121**(5): 692–705.

2. Carr JC, Simonetti O, Bundy J, *et al.* Cine MR angiography of the heart with segmented true fast imaging with steady-state precession. *Radiology* 2001; **219**(3): 828–34.

3. Kim RJ, Wu E, Rafael A, *et al.* The use of contrast-enhanced magnetic resonance imaging to identify reversible myocardial dysfunction. *N Engl J Med* 2000; **343**(20): 1445–53.

4. Bottomley PA, Foster TH, Argersinger RE, Pfeifer LM. A review of normal tissue hydrogen NMR relaxation times and relaxation mechanisms from 1–100 MHz: dependence on tissue type, NMR frequency, temperature, species, excision, and age. *Med Phys* 1984; **11**(4): 425–48.

5. Pintaske J, Martirosian P, Graf H, *et al.* Relaxivity of Gadopentetate Dimeglumine (Magnevist), Gadobutrol (Gadovist), and Gadobenate Dimeglumine (MultiHance) in human blood plasma at 0.2, 1.5, and 3 Tesla. *Invest Radiol* 2006; **41**(3): 213–21.

6. Neubauer S. Cardiac magnetic resonance spectroscopy. *Curr Cardiol Rep* 2003; **5**(1): 75–82.

7. Schar M, Kozerke S, Fischer SE, Boesiger P. Cardiac SSFP imaging at 3 Tesla. *Magn Reson Med* 2004; **51**(4): 799–806.

8. Haacke EM, Brown RB, Thompson MR, Venekatesan R. *Magnetic Resonance Imaging – Principles and Sequence Design.* New York, NY, John Wiley & Sons, 1999.

9. Gutberlet M, Schwinge K, Freyhardt P, *et al.* Influence of high magnetic field strengths and parallel acquisition strategies on image quality in cardiac 2D CINE magnetic resonance imaging: comparison of 1.5T vs. 3T. *Eur Radiol* 2005; **15**(8): 1586–97.

10. Reeder SB, Wintersperger BJ, Dietrich O, *et al.* Practical approaches to the evaluation of signal-to-noise ratio performance with parallel imaging: application with cardiac imaging and a 32-channel cardiac coil. *Magn Reson Med* 2005; **54**(3): 748–54.

11. Niendorf T, Sodickson DK. Highly accelerated cardiovascular MR imaging using many channel technology: concepts and clinical applications. *Eur Radiol* 2008; **18**(1): 87–102.

12. Carr HY. Steady-state free precession in nuclear magnetic resonance. *Phys Rev* 1956; **112**: 1693–701.

13. Hudsmith LE, Petersen SE, Tyler DJ, *et al.* Determination of cardiac volumes and mass with FLASH and SSFP cine sequences at 1.5 vs. 3 Tesla: a validation study. *J Magn Reson Imaging* 2006; **24**(2): 312–18.

14. Tyler DJ, Hudsmith LE, Petersen SE, *et al.* Cardiac cine MR-imaging at 3T: FLASH vs SSFP. *J Cardiovasc Magn Reson* 2006; **8**(5): 709–15.

15. Zerhouni EA, Parish DM, Rogers WJ, Yang A, Shapiro EP. Human heart: tagging with MR imaging – a method for noninvasive assessment of myocardial motion. *Radiology* 1988; **169**(1): 59–63.

16. Kramer U, Deshpande V, Fenchel M, *et al.* Cardiac MR tagging: optimization of sequence parameters and comparison at 1.5 T and 3.0 T in a volunteer study. *Rofo* 2006; **178**(5): 515–24.

17. Araoz PA, Glockner JF, McGee KP, *et al.* 3 Tesla MR imaging provides improved contrast in first-pass myocardial perfusion imaging over a range of gadolinium doses. *J Cardiovasc Magn Reson* 2005; **7**(3): 559–64.

18. Simonetti OP, Kim RJ, Fieno DS, *et al.* An improved MR imaging technique for the visualization of myocardial infarction. *Radiology* 2001; **218**(1): 215–23.

19. Klumpp B, Fenchel M, Hoevelborn T, *et al.* Assessment of myocardial viability using delayed enhancement magnetic resonance imaging at 3.0 Tesla. *Invest Radiol* 2006; **41**(9): 661–7.

Chapter 5

Abdominal and pelvic MR angiography

Henrik J. Michaely

Introduction

Contrast-enhanced magnetic resonance angiography (CE-MRA) of the abdominal and pelvic vessels has evolved into the diagnostic modality of choice for various clinical indications ranging from suspected aortic dissection over portal-venous diseases to renovascular diseases and renal transplant surveillance [1–3]. Imaging of the renal arteries in hypertensive patients to rule out renal artery stenosis is by far the most common indication for abdominal MRA followed by diseases of the aorta such as aneurysms and aortitis as well as diseases of the mesenteric vessels. MRA of the abdominal vessels is also performed as part of peripheral run-off studies and part of whole-body MRA in patients with diabetes mellitus and/or generalized atherosclerosis [4].

The main attractiveness of MRA lies in the combination of three-dimensional (3D) noninvasive imaging with administration of only small amounts of well-tolerated contrast agents. Newer approaches even allow imaging of the renal arteries without contrast agent with good initial clinical results [5]. With current 1.5T MR scanners the achievable spatial resolution is about $1 \times 1 \times 1\,mm^3$ (depending on the equipment) with an acquisition time of about 25 to 30 seconds [4]. Even though this already represents a good spatial resolution it is still substantially inferior to the in-plane spatial resolution of $0.3\,mm^2$ of digital subtraction angiography (DSA) [6]. In addition, the longer acquisition time of MRA makes it prone to motion artifacts from breathing and nonvoluntary motion [7]. From previous theoretical calculations published by Hoogeveen et al., the required spatial resolution of MRA was requested to constitute at least three pixels within the cross-sectional lumen of the vessel in order to accurately measure the vessel and/or

stenotic segments [8]. For the renal arteries this implies an acquired spatial resolution of at least 1.5 mm for the proximal part, and an even better spatial resolution for the distal renal branches. While for the aorta itself a slightly lower spatial resolution may be sufficient, the aortic branches (which also need to be assessed) are the resolution-limiting structures. Equally important for the depiction of smaller vessels such as the distal renal arteries or the mesenteric vessels is to acquire the MRA data sufficiently fast to avoid motion artifacts and image blurring. Vasbinder and colleagues addressed the issue of distal renal artery motion during breath-hold MRA. They found that the distal parts of the renal vessels are always subject to random diaphragmatic motion even during breath-hold [7]. While this study only addressed the renal arteries one can assume that this holds equally true for the mesenteric arteries. The results from Vasbinder and colleagues are supported by several studies using two different factors of parallel imaging (PI) for renal MRA. The data group with the higher PI acceleration factor and hence with the faster MRA acquisition showed significantly better image quality of the distal renal arteries than the group with the longer-lasting MRA acquisition [9–11]. In addition, the use of isotropic voxels is a third requirement for high-quality MRA. Isotropic voxels allow for lossless reformations, which is an important prerequisite for successful post-processing particularly in assessing complex vascular anatomy such as aberrant vessels or postoperative changes. Isotropic voxels are also a prerequisite to assess the narrowed area in the cross-sectional view instead of assessing the degree of stenosis in the diameter view (Figure 5.1). This approach was found to be more accurate [12] and the results obtained with isotropic

Body MR Imaging at 3 Tesla, ed. Ihab R. Kamel and Elmar M. Merkle. Published by Cambridge University Press.
© Cambridge University Press 2011.

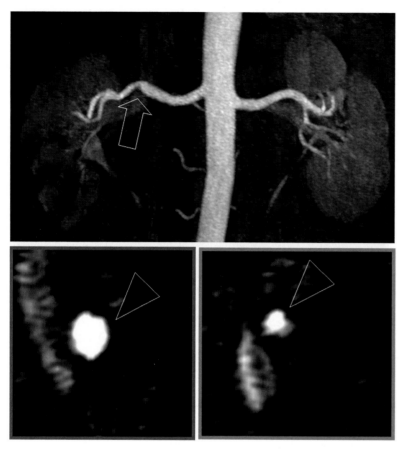

Figure 5.1 Coronal thin maximum-intensity-projection (MIP) view of a patient with 50% right-sided renal artery stenosis (arrow). In this view the stenosis is seen in the diameter view. In the two reformatted views perpendicular to the renal artery at the site of the stenosis (red frame) and in a normal segment (green frame) the normal vessel area as well as the stenotic vessel area (arrowheads) can be accurately measured to calculate the area of stenosis. See plate section for color version.

MRA showed a strong correlation with intravascular ultrasound. Lastly, the imaging volume of the MRA needs to be adequate to include the entire abdominal aorta and its major branches. If the pelvic arteries are to be imaged as well adaptation of the imaging volume is of utmost importance as the iliac arteries often demonstrate extensive elongation and kinking in elderly patients.

The image quality and contrast of an MRA with high spatial resolution, fast acquisition and sufficient volume coverage is ultimately dependent on the available signal-to-noise ratio (SNR). The achievable SNR of each sequence scales with the magnetic field strength. Thus, the SNR at 3T is theoretically twice as high as at 1.5T [13, 14]. Due to the lower SNR at 1.5T, abdominal and pelvic MRA is inherently confined to a lower spatial resolution. While the higher SNR at 3T is obviously the main reason for a shift towards 3T imaging, other factors also deserve being mentioned. What is often neglected but also beneficial for MRA is that the prolonged T1 relaxation times of all tissues

lead to a better background suppression [13, 15] and to an increased contrast agent effectiveness [16] (Table 5.1). Therefore 3T imaging is proclaimed the "field strength of choice" for MRA as it offers the best solution for most clinical requirements.

Imaging protocol for abdominal contrast-enhanced-MRA

Abdominal and pelvic MRA is typically embedded in a comprehensive imaging protocol consisting of a localizer, morphologic pulse sequences and dedicated MRA sequences. For the MRA fast gradient-recalled sequences (fast low-angle shot – FLASH, fast field echo – FFE, spoiled gradient recalled acquisition – SPGR) are commonly used. The MRA sequence should be acquired at least three times: once before the administration of the contrast agent bolus to serve as a mask for later image subtraction and to test the sequence parameters with regard to aliasing and noise. After contrast administration the MRA

Table 5.1 Typical sequence parameters for abdominal MRA at 1.5T and 3T (Siemens Avanto and TimTrio respectively)

	1.5T MRA	3T MRA
TR/TE (ms)	3.77/1.39	3.14/1.1
Flip angle (°)	25	23
Bandwidth (Hz/Px)	350	510
Matrix	512 × 80%	512 × 80%
FOV (mm²)	400 × 87%	400 × 81%
Phase oversampling [%]	0	8
Voxel size (mm³)	0.8	0.65
Spatial resolution (mm³)	1 × 0.8 × 1	0.9 × 0.8 × 0.9
Scan time (s)	19	18
Partitions	80	96
Parallel imaging	GRAPPA factor 3	GRAPPA factor 3

Michaely et al. [42].

sequence is typically acquired during the arterial peak contrast concentration in the area of interest for the actual MRA and a second time to allow for venous phase angiographic images. Some clinical sites acquire a third post-contrast phase routinely which can be of additional benefit in cases of venous pathology. Functional measurements such as phase-contrast flow sequences of the renal arteries [17] or dynamic contrast-enhanced renal perfusion measurements [18] increase the diagnostic accuracy and the level of confidence. These techniques are of particular value in patients with stents in whom an in-stent re-stenosis can not be excluded on morphologic images due to susceptibility artifacts and Eddy currents. This holds especially true for 3T as susceptibility artifacts increase with field strength [19]. For renal MRA the slab should cover the entire abdominal aorta from the diaphragm down to the external iliac arteries. This is clinically relevant as aberrant renal vessels may branch off from the entire abdominal aorta and from the iliac arteries. The slab thickness should include the vessels of interest ranging from 8 cm to 15 cm depending on the selected partition thickness and the number of partitions. A coronal slice orientation is usually preferred as the celiac axis and its branches, the superior and inferior mesenteric arteries, the renal arteries, the entire aorta and the iliac vessels can be imaged. If the mesenteric arteries represent the focus of the examination care should be taken to choose the slab large enough in anterior–posterior direction. The coronal field of view (FOV) should be minimized in left–right phase-encoding direction to minimize the acquisition time and to increase the spatial resolution [20]. If the patient's arms are positioned above the head a smaller FOV can be chosen – at the potential cost of motion artifacts when the elevated arms begin to hurt. A sagittal slab can be chosen if the examination is focused on the aorta only, e.g., dissecting aneurysms. Choosing a sagittal slab orientation allows for a smaller FOV with subsequent higher spatial resolution. However, the phase-encoding direction is usually swapped to anterior–posterior, which may lead to reconstruction artifacts when applying higher PI factors. With a coronal slab a phase (left → right phase-encoding) FOV between 380 mm and 500 mm should be chosen to avoid aliasing. Compared with 1.5T the specific parameters repetition time (TR), echo time (TE), flip angle, and receiver bandwidth (BW) need to be adopted specifically to optimize the image acquisition and quality at 3T. As the T1 relaxation times of blood are minimized during the first pass of the contrast agent the TR should be chosen as small as possible for a heavily T1-weighted image with minimal background signal. At 3T the readout BW can be increased by 40–100% (depending on the individual starting point) to minimize the TR without deteriorating image quality substantially [21]. Typically a TR of 3.0 ms to 3.5 ms can be achieved. However, short TRs may lead to a potential over-stimulation of peripheral nerves. The built-in stimulation monitor may automatically increase the TR to a noncritical level. A typical imaging protocol is given in Table 5.1. As susceptibility increases with the square of the field strength it is prudent to minimize the TE as well. At 3T fat and water protons are in-phase at 2.2 ms and 4.4 ms and out-of-phase at 1.1 ms and 3.3 ms. Therefore, with the typically utilized TE of 1 ms to 1.4 ms more chemical shift artifacts along the vessel border can be seen at 3T than at 1.5T. The increased chemical shift artifacts may additionally increase the background suppression. Fast gradient echo sequences as used for MRA will lead to a better background suppression at 3T as the longitudinal relaxation is slower due to the increased T1 times at higher field strengths [15]. The kidney and liver for example reveal 9–38% higher T1 relaxation times, while the T1 relaxation time of subcutaneous fat is

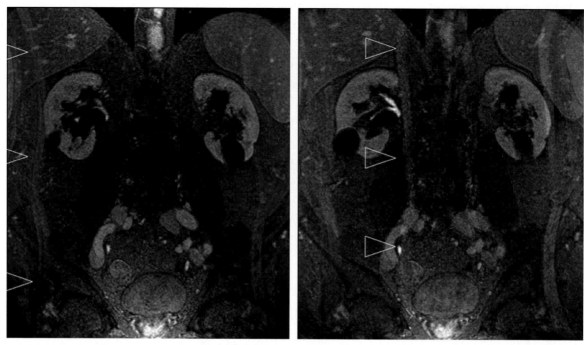

Figure 5.2 Coronal MRA source data demonstrating the influence of different parallel imaging reconstruction algorithms on aliasing. GRAPPA (left image) demonstrates aliasing more peripherally (arrowheads) than SENSE (right image) where the artifacts are propagated towards the image center (arrowheads).

increased by 11% [15]. Probably the most important parameter in MRA at 3T is the PI acceleration factor. PI techniques such as generalized autocalibrating partially parallel acquisitions (GRAPPA) [22] and sensitivity encoding (SENSE) [23] acquire fewer phase-encoding steps than conventional readout schemes. By using the inherent local information of multi-element coils the lacking data in k-space or in the image domain can be reconstructed and a full image can be reconstructed. PI can be used to either increase the spatial resolution or to shorten the scan time. Most institutions chose a combination of both. Currently at 1.5T, PI factors of 2 or rarely 3 are being used [4, 12]. Further increasing the PI factors – and hence increasing the spatial resolution – is ultimately limited by SNR as the SNR in PI is inversely proportional to the square root of the PI acceleration factor. At 3T, PI acceleration factors of 3 or higher are feasible [21] depending on the coil used. Parallel acquisition techniques (PAT) factors greater than 3 are particularly applicable when parallel acceleration is chosen in the phase-encoding and the partition-encoding direction [24]. In the case of two-dimensional (2D) PI, the acceleration factors in the phase-encoding and partition-encoding direction are multiplied to yield the overall acceleration factor.

Two-dimensional PI with higher PI factors is superior to PI in one direction as the coil sensitivity profiles can better be differentiated over an entire 3D volume leading at least theoretically to less reconstruction artifacts. Studies on the image quality of abdominal vessels report a better image quality with PI and with higher factors of PI [9, 25]. Artifacts that occur with PI are mainly noise bands in the center of the body that result from imperfect reconstruction due to a too small difference of the coil sensitivity profiles (Figure 5.2). Image noise is not a problem when the PI factors do not exceed 3 at 3T. Clinical MRA examinations with acceleration factors greater than 3 were first implemented by Fenchel *et al.* when acquiring renal MRA examinations with PI in phase-encoding and partition-encoding direction, the so called PAT²-algorithm in which GRAPPA and SENSE algorithms are combined (one being used in the phase-encoding, and the other in partition-encoding direction) [24]. This approach yielded high image quality but required an experimental 32-channel receiver coil. Depending on the reconstruction algorithm used aliasing might become visible in the image center with small FOV acquisitions. Image domain-based algorithms such as SENSE tend to propagate artifacts into the image center more than

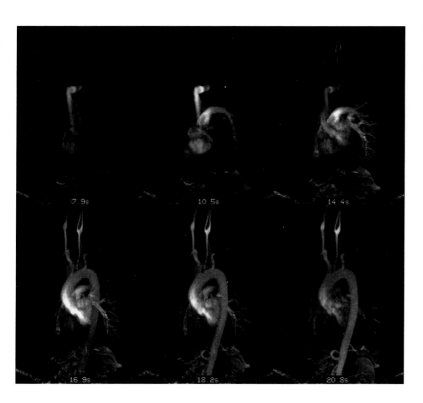

Figure 5.3 Time-resolved MRA at 3T using 1 mL of contrast (temporal resolution slightly above 1 second). This approach can be used for bolus timing and yields hemodynamic information of the target area at no extra cost.

auto-calibrating algorithms such as 2D-Arc [26] and GRAPPA [22] (Figure 5.2). Overall, abdominal MRA at 3T benefits greatly from PI with acceleration factors up to 3 while maintaining SNR and contrast-to-noise ratio (CNR).

PI is also a suitable technique for minimizing the energy deposition in the patient, which is strictly limited by governing bodies such as the US Food and Drug Administration (FDA). While the SNR is approximately doubled at 3T the specific absorption rate (SAR) is increased by a factor of 4 with the transition from 1.5T to 3T [13]. Therefore, there is a strong desire to reduce the number of applied radio-frequency (RF) pulses and to minimize the flip angle to stay within SAR limits. Theoretically, a PAT factor of 4 compensates for the increase in SAR at 3T. However, limiting factors such as imperfect coil design disprove the above equation. In addition, potentially faster TR times that could be achieved often exceed the critical threshold of the stimulation monitor, resulting in a net speed gain that sometimes may be smaller than expected.

Perfect bolus timing is crucial for high image quality. There are different approaches ranging from a conventional test-bolus technique over semiautomatic fluoroscopic approaches to fully automated techniques, e.g., SmartPrep® (GE Healthcare, Little Chalfont, UK). As they are basically independent of field strength in how they are applied they will not be further discussed apart from one recent development. Conventional test-bolus techniques acquire repeated single 10- to 20-mm images at the level of interest (e.g., the renal arteries) with a temporal resolution of 1 second per image. From the vessel of interest a signal–time curve can be derived. With the widespread use of view-sharing techniques time-resolved thick-slab MRAs can be acquired after the injection of 0.5 to 1.0 mL of contrast. Though the idea itself is not new [27], the combination of 3T and view-sharing now allows performance of timing-run MRAs with high-quality and minimal amount of contrast (Figure 5.3). By this means valuable additional information on altered hemodynamics or collaterals can be obtained at no additional cost.

Contrast agents for abdominal MRA

Despite its widespread use all over the world, CE-MRA might be considered an off-label use depending on the country of residence, the type of contrast agent used, and the target vessels studied.

Historically, MRA examinations were typically performed at 1.5T after the bolus injection of 0.2 mmol/kg body weight or even 0.3 mmol/kg body weight of standard extracellular contrast agents (Gd-DTPA, Magnevist®, Bayer Schering Pharma, Berlin, Germany; gadodiamide, Omniscan®, GE Healthcare, Little Chalfont, UK; Gd-DOTA, Dotarem®, Guerbet, Paris, France; gadoteridol, ProHance®, Bracco, Milan, Italy). Due to the longer acquisition times of MRA sequences at 1.5T, an injection rate of 1.5–2.0 ml/s is typically chosen. With a decreasing voxel size, higher factors of PI and hence a decreasing SNR the use of dedicated contrast agents for state-of-the-art MRA seems useful. At the time of this writing, three "high-end" contrast agents are commercially available, some in Europe only, some also in the USA. These contrast agents are either characterized by a 1-molar formulation (gadobutrol, Gadovist®, Bayer Schering Pharma, Berlin, Germany), a slight protein interaction with a 20–30% higher relaxivity than standard extracellular contrast agents (Gd-BOPTA, MultiHance®, Bracco, Milan, Italy), or a strong transient protein binding (gadofosveset [formerly MS-325], Vasovist®, Ablavar®, Lantheus Medical Imaging, N. Billerica, MA) which reveals an up to fourfold higher relaxivity than standard extracellular contrast agents [16] and has a markedly longer plasma half life. Despite their different pharmacokinetic properties, they are all suitable agents for MRA as they provide better enhancement than standard extracellular contrast agents [28–33].

In a recent clinical study comparing Gd-DTPA and gadobutrol for renal MRA at 1.5T, better image quality and particularly better depiction of small vessels was seen with gadobutrol [34]. Older studies demonstrated higher CNR with gadobutrol or Gd-BOPTA and an increased number of visualized small vessels [31, 35]. The increased CNR that can be seen with these substances is thought to be caused by the better bolus geometry in the case of the 1-molar agent and due to the higher relaxivity during the first pass in the case of the protein-binding agents. In addition, gadofosveset allows for an extended imaging window of up to one hour post-injection [36]. It can be used for first-pass MRA like a conventional extracellular contrast agent and allows for repetitive MRA examinations in the steady state [37–39]. One possible application is to acquire the first-pass MRA as a time-resolved study to display the blood flow hemodynamics and to measure the renal perfusion. In the

Table 5.2 The higher blood/fat ratio at 3T allows for a better background suppression and a higher vessel contrast

	1.5T	3T
T1 arterial blood (ms)	1250	1650
T1 fat (ms)	343	382
R1 Gd-DTPA (L/mmol/s)	4.1	3.7
T1 blood + Gd (5 mmol/L) (ms)	47	52
Ratio blood/fat	5.15	5.30

steady-state phase the renal arteries can be examined again with high spatial resolution. The injection speed of the first-pass MRA with gadofosveset can be chosen between 1 mL/s and 4 mL/s which allows for homogeneous good image quality [39]. Other potential applications comprise venous imaging with high SNR or extended anatomical coverage with MRA of other vascular territories during the steady state.

As the relaxivity of most contrast agents – i.e., those with no or slight protein interaction – is decreased by less than 20% with the transition from 1.5T to 3T (e.g., gadobutrol from R1 = 5.2 L/mmol/s at 1.5T to R1 = 5.0 L/mmol/s at 3T, Gd-DTPA from R1 = 4.1 L/mmol/s at 1.5T to R1 = 3.7 L/mmol/s at 3T) the relative contrast agent efficacy is increased at 3T (Table 5.2). For gadofosveset (Europe – Vasovist®, USA – Ablavar®), a strongly protein-binding contrast agent for vascular imaging, the decrease in relaxivity with the transition from 1.5T to 3T of 50% is seen. Yet, gadofosveset still reveals the highest R1 relaxivity at both field strength of 9.9 L/mmol/s at 3T compared with 19.0 L/mmol/s at 1.5T [16]. Recent studies therefore report an unchanged or even improved image quality of 3T MRA with reduced administered amounts of contrast agent [40–42] (Figure 5.4). Depending on the study design, the amount of contrast agent was reduced by 25% to 50% to an overall dose of 0.1 mmol/kg body weight. Reduction of the administered amount of contrast is economically desirable but of particular importance in patients with impaired renal function. Patients with severely decreased renal function (glomerular filtration rate [GFR] < 30 mL/min/1.72m²) are at particular risk for developing nephrogenic systemic fibrosis (NSF), a rare but potentially deadly disease which seems to be linked to the prior administration of certain gadolinium chelates (Gd-chelates) [43]. Particularly, higher doses (0.2 mmol/kg body weight and

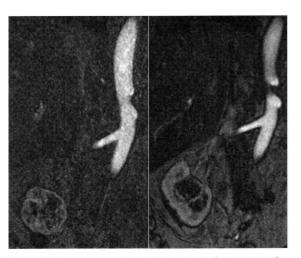

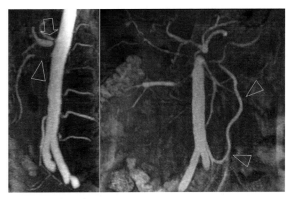

Figure 5.5 Focused thin-volume sagittal (left image) and coronal (right image) multiplanar reformation of a patient suffering from severe atherosclerosis. These images were acquired in a peripheral run-off study with continuous table movement after the injection of 0.07 mmol/kg gadobutrol. A high-grade stenosis of the celiac axis (arrow) as well as proximal occlusion of the superior mesenteric artery (arrowhead) is appreciated in the sagittal image. In the coronal image a large collateral vessel originating from the inferior mesenteric artery (Riolan's anastomosis) (arrowheads) is seen.

Figure 5.4 In comparison to an MRA acquired after injection of 20 mL gadobutrol at 1.5T (left), the 3T image of the same volunteer (right) acquired after injection of 15 mL Gd-BOPTA demonstrates higher SNR with a more homogeneous signal despite voxel volume and acquisition time being decreased at the same time.

higher) of gadodiamide in patients with chronic renal failure and with previous pro-inflammatory events seem to increase the relative risk for developing NSF significantly [44, 45]. Thus, MRA at 3T using a single dose (0.1 mmol/kg body weight) of one of the more suitable agents is currently considered the best clinical practice in these patients. Probably even lower doses of contrast agent up to 0.05 mmol/kg could be used. Many groups are currently investigating this scientifically. If a CE-MRA is clinically warranted in high-risk patients it seems appropriate to perform the examination with a minimal dose of a macrocyclic contrast agent (Gd-DOTA, gadoteridol, or gadobutrol) according to the latest guideline from the European Medicines Agency (EMA). Imaging at 3T with a 0.07 mmol/kg dose of contrast is one potential solution where a good spatial resolution and SNR can be achieved with a minimal amount of contrast only [42] (Figure 5.5). The relative risk of developing NSF after the injection of Gd-chelates is still markedly lower than the risk of contrast-induced nephropathy in cases of exposure to iodinated contrast agents, e.g., computed tomography (CT)-angiography or DSA.

Non-contrast-enhanced (NCE)-MRA

NCE-MRA has been available throughout the past 15 years. Unfortunately, the techniques available at the time, time-of-flight (TOF) and phase contrast (PC) MRA, were characterized by several disadvantages precluding widespread clinical application. Mainly driven by Japanese development – contrast agent is poorly reimbursed in Japan – and massively supported by the discussion about NSF, new NCE-MRA techniques have appeared. These techniques are typically based on steady-state free precession (SSFP) sequences with or without EKG-gating and venous background suppression. Typically the tissue in the imaging plane is inverted and the venous inflow caudally is suppressed by a saturation band. The blood flowing cranially into the imaging volume is not suppressed and hence demonstrates bright signal. In order to optimize the image quality imaging is performed with EKG-gating. In some applications selective excitation is performed, i.e., magnetic labeling, of the inflowing blood. NCE-MRA benefits from 3T with its inherent prolonged T1 times in two ways. First, the improved background suppression allows for a higher vessel-background contrast. Second, the prolonged T1 times also lead to a slower decay of the magnetically labeled inflowing blood.

While breath-hold examinations have been described, NCE-MRA is typically acquired over 2–4 minutes during free breathing. Clinical results of current studies conducted at 1.5T hold promise for a high accuracy [46, 47]. NCE-MRA based on SSFP sequences showed good correlation to DSA and to CE-MRA. NCE-MRA had the advantage over CE-MRA of demonstrating distal vessels better than CE-MRA as no

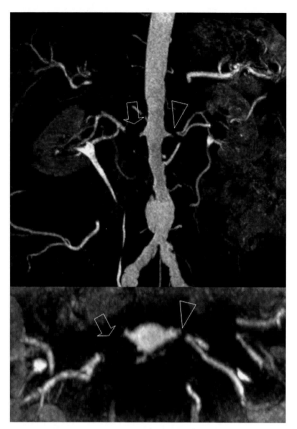

Figure 5.6 Coronal (upper image) and transversal (lower image) thin-volume MIP of a patient suffering from bilateral renal artery stenosis. The MRA was acquired after injection of 0.1 mmol/kg Gd-chelate and reveals severe and diffuse atherosclerotic changes including an infrarenal aortic aneurysm. The left renal artery shows a high-grade focal stenosis (arrowhead). The right renal artery was stented (arrow) prior to this MRA examination and demonstrates a signal void.

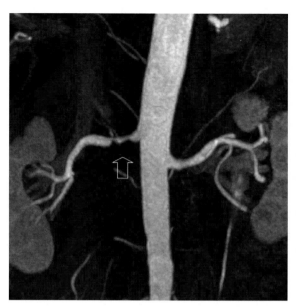

Figure 5.7 Thin-volume MIP of a 3T MRA of the renal arteries (0.1 mmol/kg Gd-chelate) demonstrating a normal aorta and left renal artery. The right renal artery demonstrates a proximal tandem-stenosis (arrow).

superimposed enhancement of the renal cortex was seen. A single study currently compares SSFP-MRA of the renal arteries at 1.5T intraindividually with SSFP-MRA of the renal arteries at 3T [48]. In this study the authors demonstrated a higher image quality scoring for the 3T SSFP-MRA which also allowed better depiction of the most distally located renal arteries.

Clinical application

Renal artery imaging: renal artery stenosis and more

Renal artery stenosis (RAS) is the most common cause of secondary hypertension [49, 50], with a prevalence of approximately 4% in Western countries [51].

The prevalence of atherosclerotic RAS increases with age and concomitant diseases such as hypertension, diabetes mellitus, or coronary artery disease to up to 47% [52–56] (Figures 5.6 and 5.7). RAS will lead to ischemic nephropathy with subsequent end-stage renal disease (ESRD) [49] if not detected and treated properly. RAS is estimated to account for 10–40% of ESRD [57] in patients without identified primary renal disease such as glomerulonephritis or autosomal dominant polycystic kidney disease. Among all patients with RAS, atherosclerotic RAS can be found in 90% of patients with RAS while fibromuscular dysplasia (FMD) accounts for the remaining 10% of cases [49, 56, 58] (Figure 5.8). FMD mainly affects younger female patients whereas atherosclerotic RAS is a disease of elderly patients.

Detection and characterization of RAS is problematic in two ways. First, there is a considerable overlap of different renal disease complexes including atherosclerotic vascular disease, primary hypertension, and renal parenchymal disease [49]. Secondary hypertension may be the consequence of RAS but in a patient with concomitant renoparenchymal disease the initial reason for the hypertension often cannot be determined based on morphologic imaging only. Second, the accuracy of the currently utilized diagnostic tests varies significantly. While ultrasound is

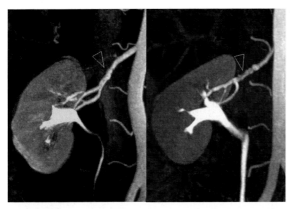

Figure 5.8 Fibromuscular dysplasia in two different patients. At 3T high spatial resolution (0.9 × 0.8 × 0.9 mm³) and fast acquisition allow for robust depiction of the classic string-of-beads appearance (arrowhead) in the distal renal arteries following single-dose Gd-chelate administration.

heavily user-dependent, the reported studies on MRA are quite nonconclusive. Initial studies and meta-studies on the accuracy of detecting and grading RAS with MRA were extremely promising [59–62] while a more recent meta-study found a sensitivity/specificity of only 62%/84% for the correct grading of RAS with MRA [63]. The poor results of this meta-study can be contributed to several factors. In contrast to the positive initial studies a retrospective approach was chosen and also patients suffering from FMD were included. Due to the subtle changes and the oftentimes distal location of FMD, there may have been lesions missed on the 1.5T and 1T MRA examinations due to their inherent lower spatial resolution.

MRA at 3T offers several advantages that are very beneficial for imaging the renal arteries and for differentiating between renovascular and renoparenchymal disease. As explained above, the higher SNR at 3T can be directly translated into a higher spatial resolution and shorter acquisition times, which are two prerequisites for successful depiction of FMD and distal RAS [21] (Figure 5.8). The high accuracy has also been confirmed by initial clinical studies with correlation to invasive angiography [64]. However, studies with a larger number of patients have not been published at this time. Functional imaging studies such as first-pass renal perfusion studies and blood oxygen level-dependent (BOLD) imaging, which can be helpful in differentiating renovascular disease from renoparenchymal disease, also directly benefit from higher field strength [65, 66].

Imaging with high spatial resolution and isotropic voxels which is facilitated by the higher SNR at 3T is a prerequisite for lossless post-processing including the generation of curved multiplanar reformats and double oblique cross-sectional views. This is of importance as the *"area stenosis"* correlates better with DSA than the *"diameter stenosis"* [12] with subsequently improved interobserver agreement, in particular for intermediate-grade RAS. In previous studies high-grade stenoses and occlusions were almost always correctly graded while intermediate-grade stenoses were always a source of error. Apart from the detection of FMD and the correct grading of RAS high spatial resolution is also mandatory in the evaluation of potential living kidney donors. To avoid transplant dysfunction all renal arteries – including small accessory arteries often supplying the uretero-pelvic junction – have to be displayed on preoperative imaging to be successfully included in the transplantation. As accessory arteries may originate from the entire aorta or the iliac arteries a large FOV is indicated in patients who are evaluated as potential living kidney donors (Figure 5.9). In these patients multiphasic examinations are of particular interest as the venous anatomy has to be reported as well. Intravascular contrast agents or those with a slight protein interaction are particularly well suited for this purpose. In renal transplant patients with suspected graft dysfunction, multiphasic MRA examinations are indicated to rule out RAS, renal vein thrombosis, iliac artery dissection, or aneurysm, all common complications during the peri-operative time [67]. The clinical accuracy of CE-MRA in native kidneys but also in renal transplants is significantly increased if functional perfusion measurements are acquired during the same examination [68] (Figure 5.10).

Aneurysms of the renal arteries are rare and occur mainly in patients with FMD or with long-standing atherosclerosis. They can lead to hypertension and renal infarction, but are generally not likely to rupture. Imaging of aneurysms of the main renal arteries can be easily achieved with standard CE-MRA. Distal renal artery aneurysms that may occur in patients with panarteritis nodosa or neurofibromatosis can only be seen with CE-MRA when timing and enhancement are optimal as enhancement of the renal parenchyma may easily obscure these findings. Other manifestations of vasculitis of the renal arteries are concentric long-segment high-grade stenoses, which can be encountered in patients with Takayasu disease.

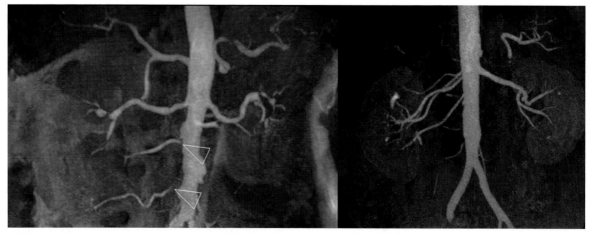

Figure 5.9 Thin-volume 3T coronal MIPs of two patients with multiple renal arteries on the right side. The left patient additionally demonstrates renal artery stenoses of the lower two renal arteries (arrowheads). Please note that the origin of the renal arteries of the left patient almost reaches the aortic bifurcation. Particularly in patients with variant renal anatomy (malrotation or horseshoe kidney) renal arteries coming off the iliac arteries are not uncommon.

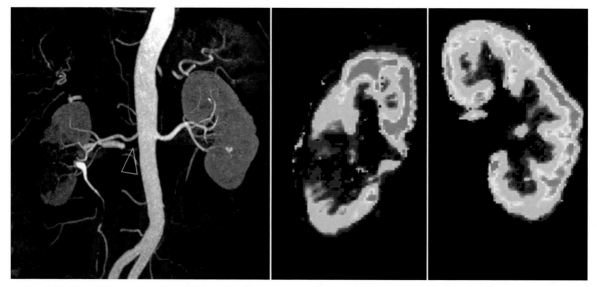

Figure 5.10 In the coronal thin-volume MIP of the renal arteries (left image) two renal arteries on the patient's right side can be seen. The upper vessel appears slender and normal while the lower renal artery cannot be visualized proximally (arrowhead) with post-stenotic dilation. The color-perfusion maps demonstrate normal perfusion on the left side while the right kidney demonstrates a reduced (lower pole) and almost absent (mid portion) plasma flow in the lower half of the organ. See plate section for color version.

Imaging of the aorta and iliac vessels: from aneurysms to aortitis

Imaging of the aorta can be performed with similar sequences as renal imaging apart from a sagittal orientation of the imaging volume rather than coronal. The best image quality of the high-resolution MRA can be achieved if a homogeneous enhancement is present throughout the aorta. This is best achieved with slow injection rates of 0.5–1.0 mL/s. In patients with abdominal aortic aneurysm the enhancement of the aneurysmal sac demonstrates large interindividual differences and might be due to the turbulent flow in the aneurysm. Therefore a homogeneous enhancement of the aneurysm will often be appreciated in the venous phase only. MRA allows for reliable differentiation of

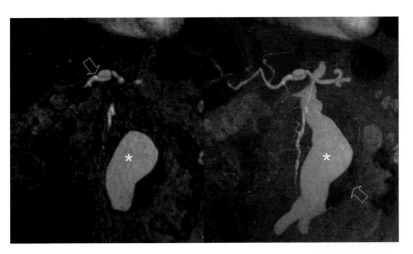

Figure 5.11 Source data (left) and thin-volume MIP (right) image of a patient suffering from severe atherosclerosis. The high spatial resolution MRA at 3T clearly demonstrates an elongated aorta with infrarenal aortic aneurysm (asterisk) and lateral thrombus formation (arrow on right image). In addition, a focal dissection of the hepatic artery is seen (arrow on left image).

thrombus and flowing blood in the aneurysmal sac – yet the exact extent of calcifications cannot be estimated with MRA (Figure 5.11).

In cases of severe atherosclerosis the assessment of the aorta and of the iliac arteries is typically included in a run-off MRA study that starts at the diaphragm and extends to cover the pedal arteries as well. With current MR scanners the large FOV can be easily covered with several MRA steps [69] or with a single continuous FOV [70]. Both approaches yield comparable high image quality as seen in single-station high-resolution MRA in the abdomen (Figure 5.12). At 3T the entire FOV can be acquired with a minimal dose (0.07 mmol/kg) of contrast agent only [71].

In patients with suspected dissection or occlusion of the abdominal aorta multiphasic or time-resolved MRA examinations should be added to the examination protocol [72] (Figure 5.13). This allows characterization of the blood flow in the true and false lumen and to assess the perfusion of the kidneys [73]. State-of-the-art sequences for this purpose comprise time-resolved view-sharing techniques such as TWSIT (time-resolved MRA with stochastic interleaved trajectories) [74] or TRICKS (time-resolved imaging of contrast-kinetics) [75]. The advantage of view-sharing is that a higher temporal resolution can be achieved with no SNR-penalty. In combination with parallel imaging a temporal resolution of 2–3 seconds per full 3D volume with a spatial resolution of $1.2 \times 1.2 \times 2$ mm^3 can be achieved. At 3T, time-resolved studies of the aorta can be successfully acquired with small amounts of contrast agent (3–6 mL) only. When the high spatial resolution is

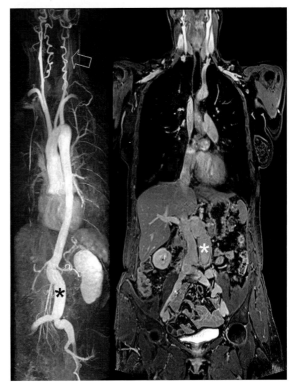

Figure 5.12 Full-thickness composed coronal MIP (left) of a 3T MRA of the chest and abdomen in a patient with Marfan's syndrome. There are bilateral elongated vertebral arteries (arrow) as well as a treated abdominal aortic aneurysm (asterisk). The metal artifact from the MR-compatible endovascular aortic stent is better depicted on the coronal 3D fat-suppressed T1-weighted gradient echo (GRE) sequence (right image) acquired immediately after the MRA.

traded for a higher temporal resolution, time-resolved techniques can also be used as an improved timing-run after the injection of just 1 mL of contrast

(a)

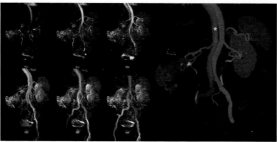

(b)

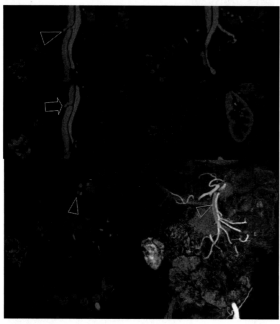

Figure 5.13 (a) Full-thickness coronal MIP (left) of a time-resolved MRA of the abdomen acquired after injection of 4 ml of a Gd-chelate. A complete dissection of the aorta can be seen with the false lumen supplying the right common iliac artery and the true lumen the left common iliac artery. A full-thickness MIP of a high-spatial-resolution MRA of the same patient (right) demonstrates a weaker enhancement in the false lumen (asterisk) and the right kidney (arrowhead). (b) Selected coronal source images of the origin of the right renal artery (upper two rows) as well as of the superior mesenteric artery (lower row) of the same patient. The right renal artery obtains its flow mainly from the false lumen with only a minor contribution from the true lumen. This results in a marked side-different perfusion of the kidney. The dissection membrane extends into the superior mesenteric artery, which is well visualized on the thin coronal MIP view. The celiac axis originates from the true lumen only.

(Figure 5.3). This kind of timing-run allows for a rough assessment of the aorta: dissecting aneurysms or larger collaterals can already be visualized with the timing-run, which allows for a better planning of the

subsequent high-resolution MRA. In patients in whom contrast agent administration is contraindicated, nonenhanced SSFP sequences are the default option for the depiction of the aorta [76]. SSFP sequences are well suited to measure the diameter of the aorta and can also demonstrate a dissection membrane – particularly if EKG-gating is used – but are not suitable for assessing the abdominal branches of the aorta at this time.

Time-resolved images or arterial and venous CE-MRA often fail to demonstrate endoleaks as the flow into the endoleaks can be rather slow. A study on the detection of endoleaks favored the application of intravascular contrast agents with delayed images after 30 minutes on which a slow blood flow into the aneurysm could be demonstrated [77]. Therefore delayed T1-weighted axial images seem to be most useful for the detection of endoleaks (Figure 5.14).

With the introduction of the new intravascular contrast agent gadofosveset venous imaging has been largely facilitated. Venous studies can now be easily acquired in the steady state after the injection of gadofosveset without sacrificing image quality [78]. If this intravascular contrast agent is not available, contrast agents with slight protein interaction such as Gd-BOPTA or higher concentrated agents such as gadobutrol can serve as a suitable alternative. The imaging window however is limited requiring the acquisition of the venous MRA immediately after the arterial data set. Immediate post-contrast 3D VIBE (volume-interpolated breath-hold sequence), LAVA (liver acquisition with volume acceleration), or THRIVE (T1-weighted high-resolution isotropic volume examination) sequences in two orientations (axial and coronal) allow for an excellent depiction of the vessel lumen as well as the para-aortic soft tissue, e.g., thrombotic material of aortic aneurysms or endoleaks (Figure 5.15). In some cases wall enhancement of the aortic wall can be seen in cases of vasculitis even though these cases are rare. Better sequences to specifically investigate vessel wall involvement in inflammatory diseases comprise single-slice EKG-gated dark-blood T1-weighted-fat saturated turbo spin echo sequences and single-slice EKG-gated dark-blood T2-weighted-fat saturated sequences. Typical inflammatory diseases affecting the abdominal aorta are Ormond's disease – also known as periaortitis or retroperitoneal fibrosis – and Takayasu disease. In Ormond's disease uni- or

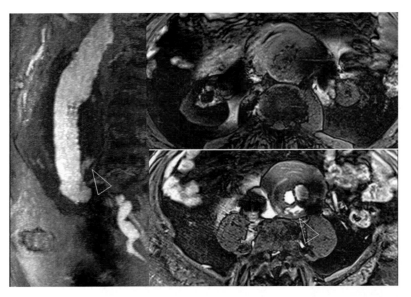

Figure 5.14 Thin sagittal MIP of the high-spatial-resolution MRA (left column), pre-contrast (top right), and 5 minutes post-contrast (bottom right) axial fat-suppressed 3D T1-weighted GRE images in a patient post endovascular abdominal aortic repair. A single dose of 0.5 M Gd-chelate was administered. A type II endoleak can be seen in the MRA (arrowhead) but is more conspicuous on the fat-suppressed 2-mm 3D T1-weighted GRE images acquired at 3T.

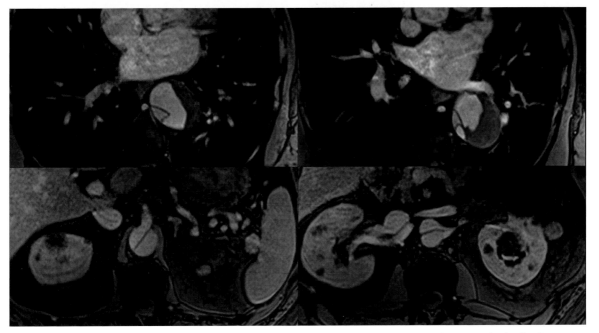

Figure 5.15 Multiple axial fat-suppressed 2-mm 3D T1-weighted GRE images acquired in the venous phase immediately after the high-spatial-resolution MRA. At 3T the spatial resolution of volumetric sequences such as VIBE, LAVA, or THRIVE allows for the exact depiction of the dissection membrane, and the visualization of slow/delayed flow into the aneurysm sac. In this case multiple different lumina are seen in the thoracic aorta (top row). The split blood supply to the left renal artery and the well-preserved origin of the superior mesenteric artery are also well appreciated on these images (bottom row).

bilateral hydronephrosis is the main reason for presentation. Even though the inflammatory tissue is located around the aorta, a relevant luminal narrowing of the aorta is rare. Dedicated imaging with specific sequences as above is rarely indicated.

On the contrary, in Takayasu disease high-grade aortic narrowing and concentric stenoses of the abdominal branches can be seen [79]. In the current classification of Takayasu the forms III–V affect the abdominal aorta and its branches (Table 5.3). CE-MRA

Table 5.3 Classification of Takayasu disease

Type	Localization
Type I	Branches of aortic arch
Type IIa	Ascending aorta, aortic arch, and branches of the aortic arch
Type IIb	Ascending aorta, aortic arch and its branches, and thoracic descending aorta
Type III	Thoracic descending aorta, abdominal aorta, and/or renal arteries
Type IV	Abdominal aorta and/or renal arteries
Type V	Features of types IIb and IV

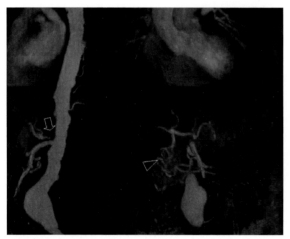

Figure 5.16 Thin sagittal (left) and coronal (right) MIP view of a patient suffering from severe atherosclerosis. The entire aorta exhibits an irregular wall and an additional infrarenal abdominal aortic aneurysm. In the sagittal view a proximal occlusion of the celiac axis is seen (arrow). No relevant post-stenotic dilation is seen. The blood supply to the liver and spleen is maintained via collateral gastroduodenal arteries (arrowhead).

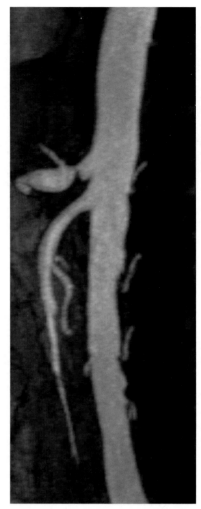

Figure 5.17
Sagittal thin MIP view of a high-spatial MRA acquired at 3T after injection of 0.1 mmol/kg Gd-chelate. A proximal high-grade stenosis of the celiac axis can be appreciated. The hemodynamic relevance of this finding is underlined by the post-stenotic dilation seen in this patient.

will show concentric long-segment stenoses with thick edematous and enhancing vessel wall.

Imaging of the mesenteric arteries

Imaging of acute mesenteric ischemia is rarely performed with MRA as most patients are being examined with CT-angiography. Due to the longer examination times MRA is not suited for emergency examinations but well suited to demonstrate the status of the visceral arteries in a nonemergency situation. Typical indications comprise the depiction of the origin of the celiac axis, the superior mesenteric artery and the inferior mesenteric artery in patients with atherosclerosis to

rule out chronic mesenteric ischemia (Figures 5.16 and 5.17). MRA at 3T allows pathologic changes such as proximal stenoses, focal or long-segment dissections, and collateral vessels to be safely demonstrated. From a technical point of view optimization of the sequence can be done according to what has been stated for the renal arteries above. PI is mandatory as it improves image quality due to less artifacts and even showed an increase in CNR in a single study of the hepatic artery and aorta [25]. Stenoses of the mesenteric vessels are common in patients with systemic atherosclerosis. In this case MRA clearly demonstrates the luminal narrowing which is almost always located at the origin of the vessel. If clinically relevant a post-stenotic dilation and/or collateral vessels can be

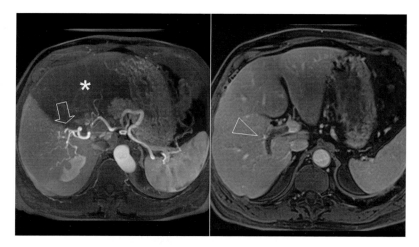

Figure 5.18 10-mm-thin axial MIPs based on fat-suppressed 3D T1-weighted GRE sequences acquired during the arterial (left) and venous (right) phase. A large caliber hepatic artery can be seen (arrow) as well as a perfusion difference between the right and left (asterisk) hepatic lobe. In the venous phase a bland thrombus (arrowhead) in the right portal vein is seen. These imaging findings are consistent with a hepatic artery buffer response syndrome.

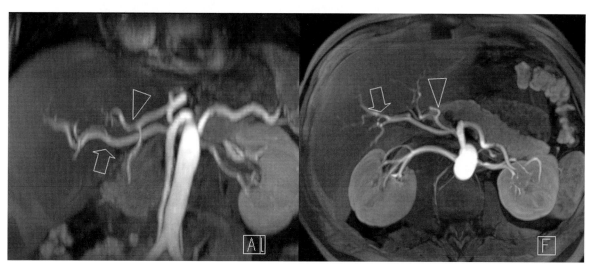

Figure 5.19 Coronal (left) and axial (right) thin MIP views of a 3T abdominal fat-suppressed 3D T1-weighted GRE examination. The high and almost isotropic spatial resolution of the fat-suppressed 3D T1-weighted GRE sequence at 3T (1.4 × 1.1 × 2.0 mm³) allows near lossless multiplanar reformats. In this patient a variant blood supply to the liver is seen. The right hepatic artery originates from the superior mesenteric artery (arrow) while the left hepatic artery originates from the celiac axis (arrowhead). A = anterior, L = left, F = feet.

appreciated (Figures 5.16 and 5.17). However, if a narrowing of the celiac axis is seen in young and slender patients close attention has to be paid to this finding. Most stenoses of the celiac axis are caused by the diaphragm crus and do not cause clinical symptoms. Only in a minority of patients with clinical symptoms such as postprandial upper abdominal pain can a relevant functional narrowing of the celiac axis be found. In these patients repeated CE-MRA measurements in inspiration and expiration demonstrate diaphragm position-dependent luminal narrowing.

Imaging of the hepatic vessels is rarely done to detect and grade luminal narrowing as in the case of the renal arteries. In most cases, the number and origin of the hepatic arteries is of interest in patients before intervention or surgery. CE-MRA can be used for this purpose but contrast-enhanced 3D sequences such as VIBE, LAVA, or THRIVE are equally well suited at 3T. These sequences are basically less "aggressive" MRA sequences, and can be acquired with 2-mm-thin slices yielding MRA-like images during the arterial phase. At the same time they yield additional information about the hepatic perfusion and about the portal vein when acquired several times (Figures 5.18 and 5.19).

Future developments

MRA has always been a driving force behind the development of MR techniques. New technical innovations on the horizon of MRA are already in sight and have been used in initial studies. Among the very promising techniques are developments of PI with acceleration in phase-encoding and partition-encoding direction, further optimizing temporal resolution [24]. Combined with improvements of the RF coil systems and with more stable PI reconstruction algorithms, this technique is likely to become clinical routine in the near future. Still far away from clinical applications is the so-called off-resonance contrast angiography (ORCA) [80]. ORCA contrast depends not on T1 shortening of the blood but on gadolinium-induced shifts in intravascular resonance frequency due to the bulk magnetic susceptibility effects of gadolinium and seems to provide very good background suppression without image subtraction. Edelman and colleagues also presented the idea of a scoutless abdominal MRA examination based on nonselective RF excitation with 2D acceleration that yielded a 30% decrease in imaging time without a significant loss in SNR [80]. Other very promising and commercially already available techniques are the Dixon-based fat saturation techniques which allow for the reconstruction of fat-only and water-only images at the expense of imaging time [82, 83]. The potential of the intravascular contrast agent gadofosveset, which has been commercially available in Europe since April 2006 and in the USA since the beginning of 2010, has not been fully explored yet. Dedicated MRA sequences with respiratory-gating and EKG-gating seem very promising for imaging in the steady state as they allow extended imaging times and hence higher SNR and a higher spatial resolution. Proof-of-concept studies have already been performed in animals but no clinical studies have been published at the time of this writing [84]. Similarly, proof-of-concept animal studies for the detection of gastrointestinal bleeding with intravascular contrast agents have been published [85] without any clinical follow-up studies in humans.

Conclusion

MRA of the abdominal and pelvic vessels greatly profits from the higher SNR at 3T. MRA sequences which are adapted to 3T allow for higher spatial resolution of less than 1 mm isotropic, shorter acquisition times, and reduced amount of administered contrast agent. Particularly, the combination of PI

Table 5.4 Requirements for state-of-the-art CE-MRA with focus on the renal arteries

Criterion	Comments
High spatial isotropic resolution	At most 1-mm voxel edge length to depict subtle changes and allow for lossless reformats
	With current 3T equipment 0.9 mm isotropic can be achieved
Minimized acquisition time	At most 20 s acquisition time to minimize motion artifacts
Sufficient slab volume	Particularly in mesenterial MRA make sure to have enough coverage in anterior–posterior direction
Sufficient z-axis field of view (FOV)	Inclusion of the entire abdominal aorta and of the iliac arteries to depict all aberrant renal artery origins
Homogeneous, good enhancement	Correct bolus timing to provide high CNR to depict also smaller vessels. Use automated power injector. Consider using improved contrast agents (higher relaxivity, higher concentration)
Multiphasic examination	Acquire one arterial phase and at least one venous phase. Mask sequence should be acquired for later image subtraction
Functional imaging	Add functional sequences such as MR PC-flow measurements and MR perfusion measurements
Standardized reading criteria	Area stenosis more accurate than diameter stenosis, use source data and 3D post-processing

and 3T is beneficial in increasing image quality and minimizing 3T-specific problems such as the increased SAR. Optimal protocol settings are depicted in Table 5.4. Initial clinical studies which were performed on a small level show promising results for the accuracy of the detection of vascular disease. The advent of new intravascular contrast agents such as gadofosveset will additionally broaden the spectrum of potential MRA applications towards more comprehensive examinations. Overall, the benefits of 3T can be translated into an improved MRA examination.

References

1. Leiner T. Magnetic resonance angiography of abdominal and lower extremity vasculature. *Top Magn Reson Imaging* 2005; **16**: 21–66.

2. Schoenberg SO, Rieger J, Nittka M, *et al.* Renal MR angiography: current debates and developments in imaging of renal artery stenosis. *Semin Ultrasound CT MR* 2003; **24**: 255–67.

3. Gufler H, Weimer W, Neu K, *et al.* Contrast enhanced MR angiography with parallel imaging in the early period after renal transplantation. *J Magn Reson Imaging* 2009; **29**: 909–16.

4. Michaely HJ, Dietrich O, Nael K, *et al.* MRA of abdominal vessels: technical advances. *Eur Radiol* 2006; **16**: 1637–50.

5. Wyttenbach R, Braghetti A, Wyss M, *et al.* Renal artery assessment with nonenhanced steady-state free precession versus contrast-enhanced MR angiography. *Radiology* 2007; **245**: 186–95.

6. Vosshenrich R, Fischer U. Contrast-enhanced MR angiography of abdominal vessels: is there still a role for angiography? *Eur Radiol* 2002; **12**: 218–30.

7. Vasbinder G, Maki J, Nijenhuis R, *et al.* Motion of the distal renal artery during 3D contrast-enhanced breath-hold MRA. *J Magn Reson Imaging* 2002; **16**: 685–96.

8. Hoogeveen RM, Bakker CJ, Viergever MA. Limits to the accuracy of vessel diameter measurement in MR angiography. *J Magn Reson Imaging* 1998; **8**: 1228–35.

9. Michaely HJ, Herrmann KA, Kramer H, *et al.* High-resolution renal MRA: Comparison of image quality and vessel depiction with different parallel imaging acceleration factors. *J Magn Reson Imaging* 2006; **24**: 95–100.

10. Wilson GJ, Eubank WB, Vasbinder GB, *et al.* Utilizing SENSE to reduce scan duration in high-resolution contrast-enhanced renal MR angiography. *J Magn Reson Imaging* 2006; **24**(4): 873–9.

11. Born M, Willinek WA, Gieseke J, *et al.* Sensitivity encoding (SENSE) for contrast-enhanced 3D MR angiography of the abdominal arteries. *J Magn Reson Imaging* 2005; **22**: 559–65.

12. Schoenberg SO, Rieger J, Weber CH, *et al.* High-spatial-resolution MR angiography of renal arteries with integrated parallel acquisitions: comparison with digital subtraction angiography and US. *Radiology* 2005; **235**: 687–98.

13. Campeau NG, Huston J, 3rd, Bernstein MA, *et al.* Magnetic resonance angiography at 3.0 Tesla: initial clinical experience. *Top Magn Reson Imaging* 2001; **12**: 183–204.

14. Merkle EM, Dale BM, Paulson EK. Abdominal MR imaging at 3T. *Magn Reson Imaging Clin N Am* 2006; **14**: 17–26.

15. de Bazelaire CM, Duhamel GD, Rofsky NM, *et al.* MR imaging relaxation times of abdominal and pelvic tissues measured in vivo at 3.0 T: preliminary results. *Radiology* 2004; **230**: 652–9.

16. Rohrer M, Bauer H, Mintorovitch J, *et al.* Comparison of magnetic properties of MRI contrast media solutions at different magnetic field strengths. *Invest Radiol* 2005; **40**: 715–24.

17. Schoenberg SO, Knopp MV, Londy F, *et al.* Morphologic and functional magnetic resonance imaging of renal artery stenosis: a multireader tricenter study. *J Am Soc Nephrol* 2002; **13**: 158–69.

18. Michaely HJ, Schoenberg SO, Oesingmann N, *et al.* Renal artery stenosis: functional assessment with dynamic MR perfusion measurements – feasibility study. *Radiology* 2006; **238**: 586–96.

19. Merkle EM, Dale BM. Abdominal MR imaging at 3T: the basics revisited. *AJR Am J Roentgenol* 2006; **186**: 1524–32.

20. Fain SB, King BF, Breen JF, *et al.* High-spatial-resolution contrast-enhanced MR angiography of the renal arteries: a prospective comparison with digital subtraction angiography. *Radiology* 2001; **218**: 481–90.

21. Michaely HJ, Nael K, Schoenberg SO, *et al.* The feasibility of spatial high-resolution magnetic resonance angiography (MRA) of the renal arteries at 3T. *Rofo* 2005; **177**: 800–4.

22. Griswold MA, Jakob PM, Heidemann RM, *et al.* Generalized autocalibrating partially parallel acquisitions (GRAPPA). *Magn Reson Med* 2002; **47**: 1202–10.

23. Pruessmann KP, Weiger M, Scheidegger MB, *et al.* SENSE: sensitivity encoding for fast MRI. *Magn Reson Med* 1999; **42**: 952–62.

24. Fenchel M, Nael K, Deshpande VS, *et al.* Renal magnetic resonance angiography at 3.0 Tesla using a 32-element phased-array coil system and parallel imaging in 2 directions. *Invest Radiol* 2006; **41**: 697–703.

25. Ho LM, Merkle EM, Paulson EK, *et al.* Contrast-enhanced hepatic magnetic resonance angiography at 3T: does parallel imaging improve image quality? *J Comput Assist Tomogr* 2007; **31**: 177–80.

26. Lum DP, Busse RF, Francois CJ, *et al.* Increased volume of coverage for abdominal contrast-enhanced MR angiography with two-dimensional autocalibrating parallel imaging: initial experience at 3.0 Tesla. *J Magn Reson Imaging* 2009; **30**: 1093–100.

27. Finn JP, Baskaran V, Carr JC, *et al.* Thorax: low-dose contrast-enhanced three-dimensional MR angiography

with subsecond temporal resolution – initial results. *Radiology* 2002; **224**: 896–904.

28. Huppertz A, Rohrer M. Gadobutrol, a highly concentrated MR-imaging contrast agent: its physicochemical characteristics and the basis for its use in contrast-enhanced MR angiography and perfusion imaging. *Eur Radiol* 2004; **14** Suppl 5: M12–18.

29. Tombach B, Heindel W. Value of 1.0-M gadolinium chelates: review of preclinical and clinical data on gadobutrol. *Eur Radiol* 2002; **12**: 1550–6.

30. Goyen M, Herborn CU, Vogt FM, *et al.* Using a 1 M Gd-chelate (gadobutrol) for total-body three-dimensional MR angiography: preliminary experience. *J Magn Reson Imaging* 2003; **17**: 565–71.

31. Herborn CU, Lauenstein TC, Ruehm SG, *et al.* Intraindividual comparison of gadopentetate dimeglumine, gadobenate dimeglumine, and gadobutrol for pelvic 3D magnetic resonance angiography. *Invest Radiol* 2003; **38**: 27–33.

32. Wikstrom J, Wasser MN, Pattynama PM, *et al.* Gadobenate dimeglumine-enhanced magnetic resonance angiography of the pelvic arteries. *Invest Radiol* 2003; **38**: 504–15.

33. Goyen M, Debatin JF. Gadobenate dimeglumine (MultiHance) for magnetic resonance angiography: review of the literature. *Eur Radiol* 2003; **13** Suppl 3: N19–27.

34. Hadizadeh DR, Von Falkenhausen M, Kukuk GM, *et al.* Contrast material for abdominal dynamic contrast-enhanced 3D MR angiography with parallel imaging: intraindividual equimolar comparison of a macrocyclic 1.0 M gadolinium chelate and a linear ionic 0.5 M gadolinium chelate. *AJR Am J Roentgenol* 2010; **194**: 821–9.

35. Goyen M, Lauenstein TC, Herborn CU, *et al.* 0.5 M Gd chelate (Magnevist) versus 1.0 M Gd chelate (Gadovist): dose-independent effect on image quality of pelvic three-dimensional MR-angiography. *J Magn Reson Imaging* 2001; **14**: 602–7.

36. Goyen M, Edelman M, Perreault P, *et al.* MR angiography of aortoiliac occlusive disease: a phase III study of the safety and effectiveness of the blood-pool contrast agent MS-325. *Radiology* 2005; **236**: 825–33.

37. Huppertz A, Kroll H, Klessen C, *et al.* Biphasic blood pool contrast agent-enhanced whole-body MR angiography for treatment planning in patients with significant arterial stenosis. *Invest Radiol* 2009; **44**: 422–32.

38. Nikolaou K, Kramer H, Grosse C, *et al.* High-spatial-resolution multistation MR angiography with parallel imaging and blood pool contrast agent: initial experience. *Radiology* 2006; **241**: 861–72.

39. Nissen JC, Attenberger UI, Fink C, *et al.* Thoracic and abdominal MRA with gadofosveset: influence of injection rate on vessel signal and image quality. *Eur Radiol* 2009; **19**(8): 1932–8.

40. Herborn CU, Runge VM, Watkins DM, Gendron JM, Naul LG. MR angiography of the renal arteries: intraindividual comparison of double-dose contrast enhancement at 1.5T with standard dose at 3T. *AJR Am J Roentgenol* 2008; **190**: 173–7.

41. Michaely HJ, Herrmann KA, Nael K, *et al.* Functional renal imaging: nonvascular renal disease. *Abdom Imaging* 2007; **32**: 1–16.

42. Michaely HJ, Kramer H, Dietrich O, *et al.* Intraindividual comparison of high-spatial-resolution abdominal MR angiography at 1.5T and 3T: initial experience. *Radiology* 2007; **244**: 907–13.

43. Grobner T. Gadolinium – a specific trigger for the development of nephrogenic fibrosing dermopathy and nephrogenic systemic fibrosis? *Nephrol Dial Transplant* 2006; **21**: 1104–8.

44. Sadowski EA, Bennett LK, Chan MR, *et al.* Nephrogenic systemic fibrosis: risk factors and incidence estimation. *Radiology* 2007; **243**: 148–57.

45. Broome DR, Girguis MS, Baron PW, *et al.* Gadodiamide-associated nephrogenic systemic fibrosis: why radiologists should be concerned. *AJR Am J Roentgenol* 2007; **188**: 586–92.

46. Liu X, Berg N, Sheehan J, *et al.* Renal transplant: nonenhanced renal MR angiography with magnetization-prepared steady-state free precession. *Radiology* 2009; **251**: 535–42.

47. Lanzman RS, Voiculescu A, Walther C, *et al.* ECG-gated nonenhanced 3D steady-state free precession MR angiography in assessment of transplant renal arteries: comparison with DSA. *Radiology* 2009; **252**: 914–21.

48. Lanzman RS, Kropil P, Schmitt P, *et al.* Nonenhanced free-breathing ECG-gated steady-state free precession 3D MR angiography of the renal arteries: comparison between 1.5T and 3T. *AJR Am J Roentgenol* 2010; **194**: 794–8.

49. Safian RD, Textor SC. Renal-artery stenosis. *N Engl J Med* 2001; **344**: 431–42.

50. Klatte EC, Worrell JA, Forster JH, *et al.* Diagnostic criteria of bilateral renovascular hypertension. *Radiology* 1971; **101**: 301–4.

51. Sawicki PT, Kaiser S, Heinemann L, *et al.* Prevalence of renal artery stenosis in diabetes mellitus – an autopsy study. *J Intern Med* 1991; **229**: 489–92.

52. Rihal CS, Textor SC, Breen JF, *et al.* Incidental renal artery stenosis among a prospective cohort of hypertensive patients undergoing coronary angiography. *Mayo Clin Proc* 2002; **77**: 309–16.

53. Harding MB, Smith LR, Himmelstein SI, *et al.* Renal artery stenosis: prevalence and associated risk factors

in patients undergoing routine cardiac catheterization. *J Am Soc Nephrol* 1992; **2**: 1608–16.

54. Olin JW, Melia M, Young JR, *et al.* Prevalence of atherosclerotic renal artery stenosis in patients with atherosclerosis elsewhere. *Am J Med* 1990; **88**: 46N–51N.

55. Wachtell K, Ibsen H, Olsen MH, *et al.* Prevalence of renal artery stenosis in patients with peripheral vascular disease and hypertension. *J Hum Hypertens* 1996; **10**: 83–5.

56. Textor SC. Epidemiology and clinical presentation. *Semin Nephrol* 2000; **20**: 426–31.

57. Scoble JE, Hamilton G. Atherosclerotic renovascular disease. *BMJ* 1990; **300**: 1670–1.

58. Slovut DP, Olin JW. Fibromuscular dysplasia. *N Engl J Med* 2004; **350**: 1862–71.

59. Thornton J, O'Callaghan J, Walshe J, *et al.* Comparison of digital subtraction angiography with gadolinium-enhanced magnetic resonance angiography in the diagnosis of renal artery stenosis. *Eur Radiol* 1999; **9**: 930–4.

60. Leung DA, Hoffmann U, Pfammatter T, *et al.* Magnetic resonance angiography versus duplex sonography for diagnosing renovascular disease. *Hypertension* 1999; **33**: 726–31.

61. Wasser MN, Westenberg J, van der Hulst VP, *et al.* Hemodynamic significance of renal artery stenosis: digital subtraction angiography versus systolically gated three-dimensional phase-contrast MR angiography. *Radiology* 1997; **202**: 333–8.

62. Tan KT, van Beek EJ, Brown PW, *et al.* Magnetic resonance angiography for the diagnosis of renal artery stenosis: a meta-analysis. *Clin Radiol* 2002; **57**: 617–24.

63. Vasbinder GB, Nelemans PJ, Kessels AG, *et al.* Accuracy of computed tomographic angiography and magnetic resonance angiography for diagnosing renal artery stenosis. *Ann Intern Med* 2004; **141**: 674–82.

64. Kramer U, Nael K, Laub G, *et al.* High-resolution magnetic resonance angiography of the renal arteries using parallel imaging acquisition techniques at 3T: initial experience. *Invest Radiol* 2006; **41**: 125–32.

65. Li LP, Vu AT, Li BS, *et al.* Evaluation of intrarenal oxygenation by BOLD MRI at 3.0 T. *J Magn Reson Imaging* 2004; **20**: 901–4.

66. Michaely HJ, Kramer H, Oesingmann N, *et al.* Intraindividual comparison of MR-renal perfusion imaging at 1.5 T and 3.0 T. *Invest Radiol* 2007; **42**: 406–11.

67. Michaely HJ, Schoenberg SO, Rieger JR, *et al.* MR angiography in patients with renal disease. *Magn Reson Imaging Clin N Am* 2005; **13**: 131–51.

68. Attenberger UI, Sourbron SP, Schoenberg SO, *et al.* Comprehensive MR evaluation of renal disease: added

clinical value of quantified renal perfusion values over single MR angiography. *J Magn Reson Imaging* 2010; **31**: 125–33.

69. Meaney J, Ridgway J, Chakraverty S, *et al.* Stepping-table gadolinium-enhanced digital subtraction MR angiography of the aorta and lower extremity arteries: preliminary experience. *Radiology* 1999; **211**: 59–67.

70. Vogt FM, Zenge MO, Ladd ME, *et al.* Peripheral vascular disease: comparison of continuous MR angiography and conventional MR angiography – pilot study. *Radiology* 2007; **243**: 229–38.

71. Voth M, Haneder S, Huck K, *et al.* Peripheral magnetic resonance angiography with continuous table movement in combination with high spatial and temporal resolution time-resolved MRA with a total single dose (0.1 mmol/kg) of gadobutrol at 3T. *Invest Radiol* 2009; **44**: 627–33.

72. Schoenberg SO, Wunsch C, Knopp MV, *et al.* Abdominal aortic aneurysm. Detection of multilevel vascular pathology by time-resolved multiphase 3D gadolinium MR angiography: initial report. *Invest Radiol* 1999; **34**: 648–59.

73. Michaely HJ, Nael K, Schoenberg SO *et al.* Renal perfusion: comparison of saturation-recovery TurboFLASH measurements at 1.5T with saturation-recovery Turbo FLASH and time-resolved echo-shared angiographic technique (TREAT) at 3.0 T. *J Magn Reson Imaging* 2006; **24**: 1413–19.

74. Nael K, Krishnam M, Ruehm SG, *et al.* Time-resolved MR angiography in the evaluation of central thoracic venous occlusive disease. *AJR Am J Roentgenol* 2009; **192**: 1731–8.

75. Korosec FR, Frayne R, Grist TM, *et al.* Time-resolved contrast-enhanced 3D MR angiography. *Magn Reson Med* 1996; **36**: 345–51.

76. von Tengg-Kobligk H, Ley-Zaporozhan J, Henninger V, *et al.* Intraindividual assessment of the thoracic aorta using contrast and non-contrast-enhanced MR angiography. *Rofo* 2009; **181**: 230–6.

77. Cornelissen SA, Prokop M, Verhagen HJ, *et al.* Detection of occult endoleaks after endovascular treatment of abdominal aortic aneurysm using magnetic resonance imaging with a blood pool contrast agent: preliminary observations. *Invest Radiol* 2010; **45**: 548–53.

78. Ruehm SG. MR venography. *Eur Radiol* 2003; **13**: 229–30.

79. Nastri MV, Baptista LP, Baroni RH, *et al.* Gadolinium-enhanced three-dimensional MR angiography of Takayasu arteritis. *Radiographics* 2004; **24**: 773–86.

80. Edelman RR, Storey P, Dunkle E, *et al.* Gadolinium-enhanced off-resonance contrast angiography. *Magn Reson Med* 2007; **57**: 475–84.

81. Carrillo A, Shankaranarayanan A, Gurr D *et al.* Scoutless abdominal angiography at 3 Tesla with two-dimensional acceleration. *Proceedings 13th Scientific Meeting, International Society for Magnetic Resonance in Medicine*, Seattle, 2006. p. 1930.

82. Reeder SB, Hargreaves BA, Yu H, *et al.* Homodyne reconstruction and IDEAL water-fat decomposition. *Magn Reson Med* 2005; **54**: 586–93.

83. Reeder SB, McKenzie CA, Pineda AR, *et al.* Water-fat separation with IDEAL gradient echo imaging. *J Magn Reson Imaging* 2007; **25**: 644–52.

84. Spuentrup E, Buecker A, Meyer J, *et al.* Navigator-gated free-breathing 3D balanced FFE projection renal MRA: comparison with contrast-enhanced breath-hold 3D MRA in a swine model. *Magn Reson Med* 2002; **48**: 739–43.

85. Hilfiker PR, Weishaupt D, Kacl GM, *et al.* Comparison of three dimensional magnetic resonance imaging in conjunction with a blood pool contrast agent and nuclear scintigraphy for the detection of experimentally induced gastrointestinal bleeding. *Gut* 1999; **45**: 581–7.

Chapter 6

Liver MR imaging at 3T: challenges and opportunities

Elizabeth M. Hecht and Bachir Taouli

Introduction

Increasing the main magnetic field strength for magnetic resonance (MR) imaging offers several theoretical advantages including higher signal to background noise, increased spectral separation, and better tissue contrast. The questions remain as to whether these theoretical advantages can be realized in the clinical setting and whether this implementation will lead to better lesion detection and characterization, more accurate diagnoses, and ultimately better patient outcome compared with 1.5T systems. While clinical 3T liver imaging is now more widely available, these questions still remain unanswered, as published scientific data are small. The answers will not only depend on the optimization of field strength-specific parameters but also on concomitant improvements in software and hardware.

The purpose of this chapter is to introduce the reader to the challenges and opportunities of 3T liver imaging as compared with 1.5T. Sequence optimization will be discussed in the context of focal and diffuse liver diseases and an optimized clinical protocol will be presented. Advanced functional liver imaging will also be discussed in the context of 3T and its potential clinical applications. This chapter serves as an introduction to high-field liver imaging and should be used as a foundation on which to build as future improvements in imaging sequences and high field coil and magnet design are ongoing.

Opportunities and challenges of liver imaging at 3T: the fundamentals

B0 field homogeneity

B0 defines the main effective static field of the scanner. In the abdomen, susceptibility artifacts occur mostly at the air–tissue interfaces, and can also be caused by bowel air, surgical clips, and metallic objects. These susceptibility effects are generally larger at 3T than 1.5T, because of a linear dependence of the magnetization on the field strength [1] (Figure 6.1). The shortened T2* relaxation times that result from local field distortions cause greater signal loss at a given echo time (TE) at 3T than at 1.5T (Figure 6.2). Given that spatial localization relies on gradient-induced frequency and phase-encoding, susceptibility-induced field alterations also lead to image distortions. Susceptibility-weighted imaging of the brain, and even some abdominal imaging applications, may benefit from greater susceptibility. For example, improved sensitivity to iron deposition in the liver and other organs may be useful in the detection of hemosiderosis and hemochromatosis [2]. Greater sensitivity to iron-containing contrast agents may also prove advantageous by reducing the required amount of administered iron contrast, although a study on volunteers failed to show stronger signal attenuation of SPIO (superparamagnetic iron oxide)-enhanced liver parenchyma at 3T compared with 1.5T [3].

Strategies to minimize susceptibility effects include improved localized shimming, reduced voxel size, and shortening of TE and echo train lengths (ETL). Improvements in shimming aim to reduce the magnetic field inhomogeneity directly. Smaller voxel size minimizes intravoxel dephasing. Additionally, gradient echo sequences using short TE will have less signal loss due to T2* shortening. Unfortunately, higher receiver bandwidths are usually necessary to shorten TE, in turn, reducing the gain in signal-to-noise ratio (SNR). As will be discussed below, parallel imaging strategies can be beneficially applied to echo planar imaging (EPI), whereby the center of k-space is traversed earlier and at shorter

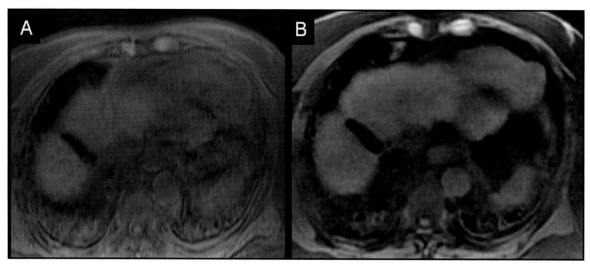

Figure 6.1 Susceptibility artifacts demonstrated in the same patient at 1.5T and 3T. Unenhanced gradient echo (GRE) images at 1.5T (A) and 3T (B). Patient is status post partial hepatectomy for hepatocellular carcinoma (HCC), with hepatic dome clips creating susceptibility artifacts worse at 3T compared with 1.5T, the TEs being approximately equivalent (1.14 ms at 1.5T vs. 1.34 ms at 3T).

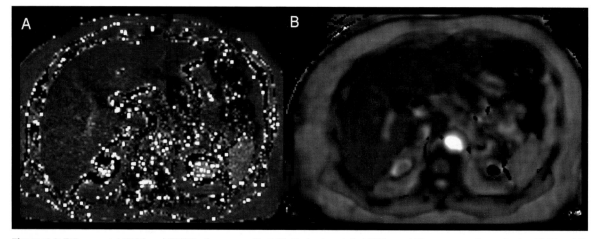

Figure 6.2 T2* maps at 1.5T (A) and 3T (B) in the same patient. Multiecho breath-hold T2* acquisitions were performed using TR 80 ms/TEs 0.94–17.26 ms at 3T, and TR 169 ms/TEs 2.38–23.82 ms at 1.5T. Liver T2* values were shorter at 3T than at 1.5T (14 vs. 32 ms).

effective TE compared with an EPI sequence without parallel imaging. In addition, the undersampling of k-space with parallel imaging allows the reduction of acquisition time. In theory, a well-shimmed 3T whole-body MR system can provide field homogeneity specifications that are comparable with or even improved over 1.5T systems.

With the increase in precessional frequency at 3T (the Larmor frequency at 3T is twice as long as that at 1.5T), the chemical shift between compounds, similarly proportional to the magnetic field strength, also increases. This greater spectral separation of fat and water and other compounds, combined with greater SNR, provides great promise for MR spectroscopy at high fields [4, 5]. For imaging applications, the greater chemical shift between fat and water, equaling about 440 Hz at 3T, compared with 220 Hz at 1.5T, has several practical consequences. First, the TEs at which fat and water protons are in-phase and opposed-phase (or out-of-phase) become much more closely spaced at 3T. The protons are in-phase at TEs of 2.28 ms and multiples thereafter (4.56 ms, 6.84 ms, etc.), while fat and water protons are opposed phase at TE of 1.14 ms, 3.42 ms, 5.7 ms, and so on (Figure 6.3).

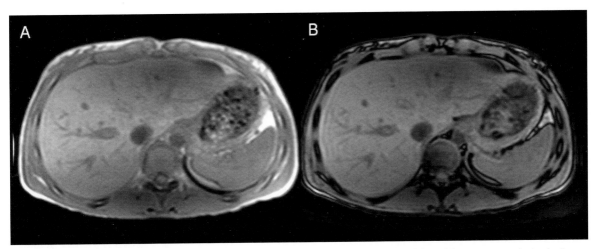

Figure 6.3 2D in- and out-of-phase images at 3T in a healthy volunteer. In-phase (A) and out-of-phase (B) images were obtained using TR/TE of 179 ms/1.14 ms (out-of-phase) and 2.3 (in-phase), slice thickness 6 mm, flip angle 50°.

Second, given the greater separation of fat and water at 3T, chemical shift artifact of the first kind, due to mismapping of the frequency-encoded signal of fat into water voxels, can be seen at higher receiver bandwidths than at 1.5T. Last, for applications that depend on frequency-selective fat suppression pulses, the greater spectral separation lends itself to more successful suppression, provided reasonable B0 field homogeneity is maintained.

B1 field homogeneity

B1 refers to the radiofrequency (RF) field strength. Inhomogeneity in the B1 field results in imperfect excitation and may manifest as regions of signal loss or, less commonly, signal brightening. At increasing field strength, RF homogeneity becomes more challenging to maintain. The human body is composed predominantly of water and thereby amenable to proton MR imaging. However, water is a very conductive medium with high electrical permittivity and these properties in human tissue can inhibit the generation of a uniform B1 field. At higher field strengths, the interaction between the human body and the coil becomes more pronounced in part because the size of the body becomes comparable to the operating RF wavelength. Compared with 1.5T, at 3T unwanted RF behavior in the body becomes more apparent. Although the distribution of these effects can be unpredictable, in abdominal imaging they commonly manifest as regions of signal loss over vital structures such as the left lobe of the liver (Figure 6.4).

In addition, excitation field variations can result in nonuniformities of flip angle across the image and may manifest as spatial variations of contrast.

The B1 field shaping effects of the human body are commonly grouped under the general term "dielectric effects" but are a result of both standing wave and dielectric effects. At sufficiently high frequency, several complex influences come into play including construction and destructive interferences due to wave propagation effects at the shortened wavelength associated with high internal permittivities; shielding effects of the RF eddy currents induced by the coil fields in electrically conductive tissues; and distortion of electromagnetic fields at tissue boundaries. The net effect of these dynamic phenomena depends on the geometry and composition of the patient's body, e.g., in obese patients and in the presence of ascites or amniotic fluid, these effects are more pronounced [6].

The most straightforward and pragmatic solution to alleviate these types of artifacts is by using an RF cushion. An RF cushion (or dielectric pad) is simply a pad filled with a conductive medium (e.g., dilute manganese chloride solution) that has a very high dielectric constant and low conductivity (Figure 6.4). The cushion is designed to alter the geometry of the object being imaged and changes the phase of the RF standing waves. While this does not serve to eliminate the artifact, it displaces out of the imaging field of view. In a study of Franklin *et al.*, the RF cushion was found to reduce the B1 inhomogeneity artifact in the liver on single-shot fast spin echo (FSE) T2-weighted

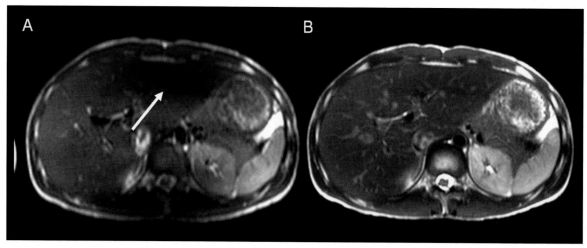

Figure 6.4 Dielectric effect at 3T. Single-shot T2 fast spin echo (FSE) images obtained without (A) and with a dielectric pad (B). A dielectric effect (shading) is seen over the left hepatic lobe (arrow) on the image without the pad. The effect is suppressed with the use of a dielectric pad.

images [7]. Compared with T1-weighted gradient echo sequences, T2-weighted turbo spin echo (TSE) type sequences can suffer more from B1 inhomogeneity artifacts possibly due to the higher number of refocusing pulses required for the T2-weighted sequences. Of note, based on initial observations two-dimensional (2D) T1-weighted gradient echo sequences appear to be slightly more vulnerable to these artifacts compared with three-dimensional (3D) gradient echo sequences [8].

Post-processing filters have been introduced on some systems and serve to equalize signal throughout an image and can alleviate the effects of the artifact. However, the filters do not address the source of the problem and cannot regain lost SNR. Other approaches may offer more enduring and systematic solutions. These include alternative pulse sequences that utilize innovative RF excitation pulses that aim to generate more uniform excitation [9] and new phased-array transmit coil designs that permit customized excitation pulses for uniformity [10, 11]. In a preliminary study by Vaughan *et al.*, 9.4 T imaging of the human brain was achieved and image quality optimized by using interactive, multichannel RF field magnitude and phase shimming to compensate for field inhomogeneity as encountered [12]. Parallel excitation with transmit coil arrays would also permit additional control over field homogeneity. This technique could be used to accelerate complex RF pulses, and may also improve signal homogeneity and reduce specific absorption rate (SAR) [11, 13].

Specific absorption rate (SAR)

In theory, the SAR increases proportionally to the main magnetic field, and should be increased by a factor of 4 at 3T compared with 1.5T. As baseline SAR increases, the local distribution of SAR becomes more heterogeneous and subject-specific for similar reasons discussed above related to human tissue conductivity and permittivity.

Limiting SAR becomes technically challenging for body imaging at 3T as many RF-intensive pulse sequences are utilized, e.g., frequency-selective fat-suppressed T2-weighted TSE. Acceleration of data reception using parallel imaging may be used to reduce SAR for individual data sets because it reduces the number of RF excitations required to generate a given data set. However, to have a significant impact on SAR, much higher order parallel imaging would be required than is currently feasible in routine practice.

At 3T in general practice, imaging parameters are significantly constrained by the SAR limits imposed by the US Food and Drug Administration (FDA) and implemented by manufacturers. Straightforward parameter adjustments such as decreasing slices per repetition time (TR), decreasing flip angle, lengthening TR, increasing inter-echo spacing, and prolonging the RF pulse duration can reduce SAR; however, adjusting these parameters leads to reduced coverage, alteration of tissue contrast, and diminished SNR.

There are several new sequence designs that can reduce SAR and have been successfully implemented at 3T. Variable-rate selective excitation (VERSE) uses a time-varying gradient which modifies the shape of the RF pulse to reduce the amplitude of the RF signal without significantly affecting other parameters that may affect tissue contrast [14]. In a study of 12 volunteers, van den Bos *et al.* found that fat-suppressed T2-weighted breath-hold imaging of the liver was facilitated by using VERSE RF pulses [15]. Using the lower RF power, VERSE pulse enables more image slices within a given time period and thus could be used to scan a larger volume or for thin-slice volumetric imaging. In addition, better blood vessel suppression was noted with the VERSE pulse which in addition to thinner slice could potentially improve the conspicuity of small lesions [15].

Variable flip angle sequences also show promise for high-field imaging. These techniques use the desired image contrast and relaxation time-dependent signal evolution to determine the optimal flip angle variation, permitting the use of longer echo train lengths and effective TE without reaching SAR limits. Such techniques include hyperechoes [16], smooth transitions between pseudo steady states (TRAPS) [17] and 3D T2-weighted TSE with high sampling efficiency (SPACE) [18]. In a study by Rosenkrantz *et al.* comparing T2-weighted imaging using a breath-hold fat-suppressed 2D TSE versus a respiratory-triggered 3D T2-weighted SPACE sequence, SPACE offered better image quality with near elimination of motion and pulsation artifacts with improved tissue contrast; however, the SPACE sequence did suffer from relatively increased B1 inhomogeneity [19].

All these techniques can be used in combination with partial Fourier and parallel imaging to further reduce SAR but at the cost of SNR. Parallel transmission as described above is another promising approach to SAR [11, 13].

Signal-to-noise ratio (SNR)

One of the major advantages of high-field imaging is the potential increase in SNR. Increasing field strength from 1.5T to 3T leads to a theoretical twofold increase in signal while noise is less affected by field strength. This gain in SNR can be used to improve speed and/or spatial resolution (Figure 6.5). And yet, this theoretical increase in SNR in body imaging may not be completely realized in the clinical setting because of other constraints. At high field strength, longitudinal relaxation T1, chemical shift, and susceptibility effects increase, while T2 relaxation times decrease (see below). Higher bandwidths are often required to achieve satisfactory T1 tissue contrast and to reduce chemical shift artifact, decreasing the overall SNR. SAR limitations may also reduce imaging efficiency or image quality. More advanced parallel imaging strategies as discussed above can potentially compensate for the limitations of SAR and maximize the potential gains in SNR at higher fields, but ongoing technologic advances in coil and magnet design are likely required.

Sequence optimization at 3T

T1 and T2 relaxation times at 3T

Takahashi *et al.* [20] determined the relaxation time of phantoms with different concentrations of gadolinium contrast material at both 1.5T and 4T, and showed that T1 relaxation times were prolonged (1.10–1.47 times) at 4T compared with those at 1.5T, while T2 values were identical or slightly shortened. In human volunteers, de Bazelaire *et al.* [21] measured relaxation times of abdominal organs at 1.5T and 3T in six volunteers, and showed an overall increase in T1 relaxation times and a slight decrease in T2 relaxation times at 3T when compared with 1.5T, depending on the organ. Specifically, in the liver parenchyma, they reported the following T1 and T2 relaxation times (mean $\pm$ SD, in ms.): 586 ± 39 (T1) – 46 ± 6 (T2) at 1.5T and 809 ± 71 (T1) – 34 ± 4 (T2) at 3T. Owing to the lengthening of T1 relaxation times of liver parenchyma, there is a potential reduction of T1 contrast at 3T. Consequently, for gradient echo imaging, the TR should be longer and flip angle adjusted to optimize image contrast and SNR. T1 relaxation times for gadolinium contrast agents, however, are less affected at higher field strengths. This results in greater image contrast on gadolinium-enhanced images at 3T compared with 1.5T (Figure 6.6).

Because of faster T2 relaxation, FSE or TSE sequences are more affected by blurring artifacts at 3T than at 1.5T [22]. Consequently, a shorter TE and a shorter ETL may be necessary; parallel imaging helps to achieve these goals (Figure 6.7).

Chemical shift imaging, fat–water separation, and fat suppression

At 3T, an increase in precessional frequency of protons is expected resulting in a twofold increase in chemical shift between compounds. Greater chemical

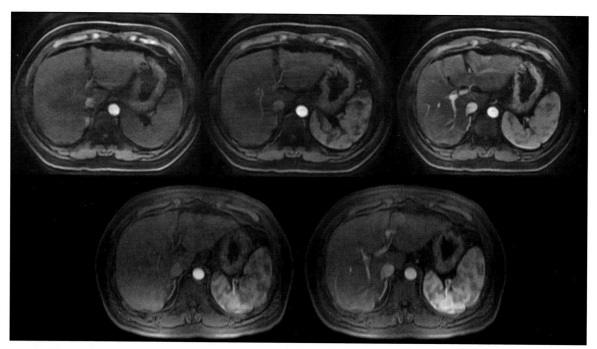

Figure 6.5 Triple post-contrast arterial phase acquisition using 3D fat-suppressed spoiled gradient recalled acquisition in the steady state (SPGR) sequence (LAVA: Liver acquisition with volume acquisition) with a 32-channel coil at 3T in a patient with cirrhosis (top row), compared to dual arterial phase acquisition obtained in the same patient at 1.5T (bottom row, VIBE: volumetric interpolated breath-hold examination). Parameters for 3T acquisition were TR/TE 3.0 ms/1.44 ms, slice thickness 4 mm, number of averages 0.75, matrix 256 × 128, flip angle 12°, parallel imaging factor 2.45, acquisition time 8 seconds each (obtained in a single breath-hold). Good image quality and SNR are possible when combining a 32-channel coil with a 3T system, with high parallel imaging factor, compared to standard 1.5T acquisition.

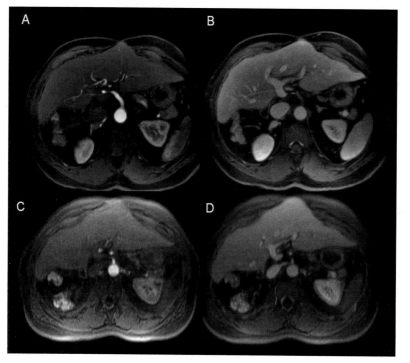

Figure 6.6 Post-contrast 3D GRE images at 1.5T and 3T in the same patient (status post liver transplantation). (A) Arterial phase image at 3T, (B) portal venous phase image at 3T, (C) arterial phase image at 1.5T, (D) portal venous phase image at 1.5T. Parameters for 3T acquisition were TR/TE 3.2 ms/1.5 ms, slice thickness 3 mm, number of averages 0.68, matrix 256 × 192, flip angle 12°, parallel imaging factor 2.12, SAR 2.85 W/kg. For 1.5T, TR/TE 3.0 ms/1.08 ms, slice thickness 3 mm (interpolated), number of averages 1, matrix 256 × 107, flip angle 12°, parallel imaging factor 2, SAR 0.74 W/kg. Higher vessel CNR (contrast-to-noise ratio), calculated as [CNR = (signal intensity = SI) aorta – SI liver/SD noise] was observed at 3T. For the aorta, CNRs were 292/90, for portal vein, CNRs were 80.7/33.7 at 3T and 1.5T, respectively (CNRs were 2.4 to 3.2 times higher at 3T compared with 1.5T).

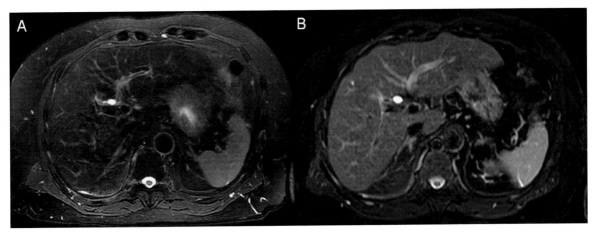

Figure 6.7 Fat-suppressed T2 FSE at 1.5T vs. 3T in a patient with chronic hepatitis B. (A) Respiratory-triggered fat-suppressed T2 FSE at 3T (TR/TE 8500/102, matrix 384 × 256, slice thickness 5 mm, ETL 15, 2 averages, flip angle 90°, SAR 1.48 W/kg), and (B) breath-hold fat-suppressed T2 FSE at 1.5T (TR/TE 2030 ms/76 ms, matrix 256 × 192, slice thickness 6 mm, ETL 28, 1 average, flip angle 132°, SAR 1.78 W/kg). A shorter ETL was used at 3T. In addition, a smaller flip angle was used at 3T to limit SAR deposition.

shift between fat and water also has several implications for routine liver imaging at 3T. First, the greater separation between fat and water lends itself to more successful frequency-selective fat suppression. Second, at 3T chemical shift artifact of the first kind, i.e., mismapping of the frequency-encoded signal of fat into water voxels, is more pronounced at higher receiver bandwidths than at 1.5T. In order to minimize this effect at the interface between fat and water, higher bandwidths for routine sequences are required at 3T and thus, SNR will be reduced. Third, a consequence of the increased precessional frequency of protons at 3T is that the TEs of in- and opposed-phase imaging are more closely spaced with the first opposed-phase echo at 1.14 ms and in-phase at 2.28 ms, as discussed above.

In order to achieve such short TEs in a single breath-hold, extremely high bandwidths are required which are not technically feasible and result in degradation of SNR. To compensate for signal loss, resolution may be decreased but at the potential expense of image quality. Essentially, achieving the ideal TEs in the favorable sequential order becomes much more difficult at 3T. In addition, the qualitative approach to detecting iron or fat content can be less reliable as the changes may be increasingly subtle and susceptibility effects may confound the reader. Fat detection depends on observing the signal loss between two different TEs and intravoxel signal cancellation between fat and water, but this does not take into account effects of T2* which can lead to misinterpretation particularly at 3T because of the increased

sensitivity to T2* effects. A breath-hold sequence is preferred to avoid misregistration and the opposed-phase acquisition should be performed at the shorter TE to eliminate ambiguity of detecting fat versus iron content. If in-phase images are obtained at a shorter TE when compared with opposed-phase images, signal loss demonstrated on the longer TE (opposed-phase in this scenario) could be resulting from intravoxel fat or the paramagnetic influence of iron storage in the liver whether due to hemosiderin or ferritin related to systemic iron overload due to blood transfusions (i.e., thalassemia major, sickle cell disease) or up-regulated intestinal absorption (i.e., hereditary hemochromatosis).

At 3T, there is an ongoing trade off between maximizing SNR and minimizing susceptibility effects. Certainly, the first and third echo or first and fourth echo could be chosen for in/opposed-phased imaging at 3T, e.g., opposed-phase TE = 1.14 ms, in-phase 4.56 ms but at a relatively long TE of 4.56 ms, tissue contrast is reduced and susceptibility from bowel gas and surgical clips becomes more pronounced when compared with 1.5T. In addition, the threshold for steatosis will need to be adjusted for those selected TEs. While no study has been performed using these combinations of TE for detecting fatty liver at 3T, in one study of adrenal adenomas using a TE combination of 1.5 ms (OP) and 4.9 ms (IP), based on area under the curve a signal intensity (SI) index $[(SI_{IP}-SI_{OP})/(SI_{IP})] \times 100\%$ threshold of 1.7% to distinguish adenomas from non adenomas resulted in a sensitivity and specificity of 100% [23]. At 1.5T, using TE of 2.2 ms (OP) and 4.4 ms (IP), a SI index threshold of 16.5% is typically used although there is variability depending on sequence parameters [24].

While the qualitative and semi-quantitative approaches to detect the presence of liver steatosis on MR imaging have been successful, there is increasing demand for more accurate and reproducible methods of quantification of liver fat for diagnosing, grading, and monitoring of therapy. Nonalcoholic fatty liver disease (NAFLD) is an increasingly common cause of chronic liver disease in children and adults in the United States [25, 26]. NAFLD can progress to nonalcoholic steatohepatitis (NASH), placing a patient at risk for cardiovascular and hepatic complications [27, 28]. Cirrhosis may subsequently develop in patients with NASH, placing these patients at increased risk for liver failure and hepatocellular carcinoma (HCC) [29, 30].

Iron in excessive quantities is hepatotoxic as well [31, 32]. In the setting of genetic hemochromatosis, iron within the hepatocytes may increase the risk of developing cirrhosis and HCC [33]. Excessive iron deposition is also associated with chronic viral hepatitis, alcoholic liver disease, and NASH [31] and may in combination with alcohol and fat deposition, further promote development of liver fibrosis and cirrhosis [34, 35]. Although this subject is beyond the scope of this chapter, it is important to discuss MR methods of assessing fat and iron content in the liver as they are becoming more widely available and are becoming routinely used in liver imaging protocols at 1.5 and 3T. Some of the methods discussed permit not only quantification of fat but may also serve as a method of achieving more homogeneous fat suppression at higher field strengths.

There are essentially three general approaches to fat quantification chemical shift imaging based on the principles first described by Dixon [36], frequency-selective fat-suppressed imaging, and MR spectroscopy. Chemical shift imaging may be performed with two echoes or more, each approach with advantages and disadvantages. The chemical shift method relies on measuring net signal in co-localized regions of interest on in-phase ($= S_{water} + S_{fat}$) relative to the opposed-phase imaging ($= S_{water} - S_{fat}$) and calculating a fat signal relative to water signal (FSF) [29]. When this method is performed with

a dual-echo approach, an FSF map of the entire data set can be generated. The inherent problem with this approach is ambiguity in distinguishing between fat-dominant versus water-dominant fatty tissue because only the magnitude of signal intensity is reconstructed, not the phase data. Other limitations that also need to be considered are that chemical shift imaging is sensitive to the dominant CH_2 peak of fat but not sensitive to other chemical moieties of fat and the two-point method does not correct for T1 and T2* relaxation effects [29].

Multiecho gradient echo sequences show great promise for resolving the fat–water ambiguity issue. With this method, magnitude and phase data are acquired over multiple TE generating in- and opposed-phase data sets which can, in turn, be used to calculate selective fat- and water-only images. From these complex data sets, the entire range of fat fraction may be calculated. If more than three echoes are acquired however, a correction for T2* decay is required. If not corrected, T2* effects can lead to under- or overestimation of fat. The iterative decomposition of water and fat with echo asymmetry and least-squares estimation (IDEAL) method is a multiecho technique that can quantify fat; generates fat only, water only, in- and opposed-phase image data sets from a single acquisition [37]; and may be used to produce an alternative, robust method of fat suppression [38]. When using a gradient echo-based approach, T1 effects also need to be considered. Given lipid has a short T1, stronger T1 weighting i.e., high flip angle will suppress water signal and result in relative amplification of fat signal, and thus, low flip angle imaging is preferable. Dual flip angle techniques can also determine fat or water dominance [39]. Finally, another innovative method, referred to as the multi-interference, also uses the multiecho approach with T2* correction but also corrects for multiple fat peaks based on reference spectroscopic data [40].

Frequency-selective imaging methods are less well studied but show promise and can in principle explore the entire range of fat fractions [41, 42]. Essentially, two images are obtained with one with and one without fat suppression but ideally with otherwise identical imaging parameters. A single-shot FSE sequence is typically used (but may be performed with in-phase gradient echo) to reduce T1 effects and a correction of T2 effects is required. The greater spectral separation at 3T is favorable for this method

Table 6.1 Suggested MR imaging protocol used for liver imaging at 3T. All sequences are breath-hold except for fat-suppressed T2 FSE

Sequence	Plane	TR/TE/flip angle	Slice/gap	Matrix
Single-shot FSE T2	Coronal	900–Infinity/70–80/90°	5/1	256 × 320
2D T1 GRE in- and out-of-phase	Axial	179/1.1–2.3/50°	6/1	144 × 203
T2 FSE fat-suppressed	Axial	8500/100/90°	5/1	256 × 384
Time of flight	Axial oblique	16.3/2.3	10/10	224 × 320
Diffusion-weighted imaging[a]	Axial	2400/50–60	7/1.4	144 × 192
3D T1 fat-suppressed GRE (pre-contrast, arterial × 2, portal venous, equilibrium phases)[b]	Axial	3.2/1.5/12°	3/0	192 × 256

[a]Using b = 0, 500, 750 s/mm^2.
[b]For extracellular contrast media.

but it is vulnerable to inhomogeneity of the main magnetic field. An imprecise fat suppression pulse could inadvertently suppress water peaks, thereby causing inaccuracy of measurement.

With the multiecho approaches T2* maps can also be obtained and thus an iron content in the liver may also be estimated with this method [43–47]. However, at 3T iron quantification becomes even more challenging because of susceptibility effects [48]. While multiecho T2* approaches can be successful at detecting liver fat or iron content when there is combined disease, detection and quantification is more difficult; thus, novel approaches to decomposition are actively being pursued [49, 50].

Finally, proton MR spectroscopy alone is considered the most accurate noninvasive tool for MR imaging quantification of liver fat [26, 51] and may prove useful for oncologic applications to distinguish between benign and malignant lesions, assess tumor grade and response to therapy [52], although in vivo studies are still limited. At 3T, greater spectral separation between metabolite peaks combined with higher SNR is potentially advantageous for MR spectroscopy. Potential drawbacks of high field include increased susceptibility effects, B1 inhomogeneity, and shortened T2 relaxation. Better spectral resolution, smaller voxel size, and shorter scan times are expected with increasing field strength and would facilitate more routine clinical implementation. Respiratory-triggered or-gated acquisitions and parallel imaging methods would offer further benefit.

An optimized protocol for liver imaging is listed in Table 6.1.

Applications of 3T MR imaging in focal and diffuse liver disease

There are no studies that have directly compared 1.5T with 3T for detection of focal and diffuse liver disease, but there are several theoretical advantages to consider. Higher baseline SNR at 3T may be used to achieve higher in-plane spatial resolution or thinner section acquisitions. Both can be particularly advantageous for pediatric imaging, for detection of smaller liver lesions for selective treatment planning, and for visualizing the vascular anatomy. The potential for improved fat suppression may also increase lesion conspicuity. Prolonged T1 relaxation times of the tissues could also translate into better background suppression albeit less optimal tissue contrast on unenhanced T1-weighted images at 3T when compared with 1.5T. At 3T, gadolinium T1 relaxivity is only mildly decreased (by 5–10%) while the effect on the T1 relaxation time of vascular tissues is more pronounced such that increased contrast is expected at 3T for equivalent doses of gadolinium chelate agents [6]. Thus, improved background suppression combined with greater sensitivity to gadolinium chelates may translate into lower contrast dose requirement and better lesion conspicuity. Unfortunately, there is limited literature comparing detection and characterization of liver lesions at 1.5T versus 3T using single contrast technique but there has been some investigation of double contrast methods. The lesion characteristics described at 1.5T generally apply to 3T. Examples of focal liver lesions as seen at 3T are given in Figures 6.8–6.10.

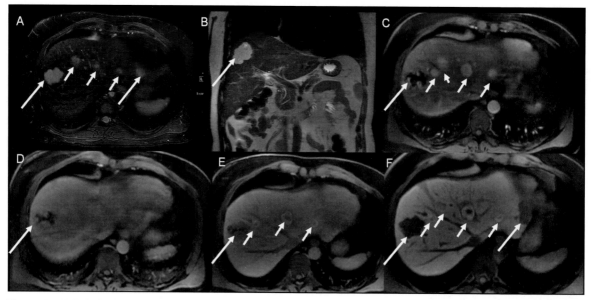

Figure 6.8 Multiple focal nodular hyperplasias (FNHs) and hemangiomas at 3T diagnosed with Gd-EOB-DTPA in a patient with history of colon cancer. (A) Fat-suppressed T2 FSE, (B) coronal single-shot FSE T2, (C–F) 3D SPGR images (LAVA) after injection of Gd-EOB-DTPA (C: arterial, D: portal venous, E: equilibrium, F: delayed hepatocyte phase [20 minutes]). Two hemangiomas are identified (long arrows), in high T2 signal with typical nodular enhancement (seen for the largest one in the right hepatic lobe), both hemangiomas are hypointense of the hepatocyte phase image. Multiple arterial phase-enhancing mildly T2 hyperintense lesions are also present (short arrows), starting to appear hyperintense at the equilibrium phase, with bright signal at the hepatocyte phase, compatible with FNHs. There were no metastatic lesions.

Although increased susceptibility can be a pitfall at 3T, the effect may actually improve lesion conspicuity in cirrhotic livers when using a reticuloendothelial system-specific contrast agent that contains SPIO or ultrasmall superparamagnetic particles of iron oxide (USPIO) nanoparticles. These agents distort the local magnetic field and cause signal loss on T2-weighted imaging such that tumors such as HCC that only demonstrate mild T2 prolongation would become more conspicuous. However, SPIO is currently out of the US market, and USPIO is not FDA approved.

Diffusion-weighted imaging (DWI) shows great promise for liver lesion detection and characterization [53, 54], and for detection of liver fibrosis and cirrhosis [55–58]. While at 3T, the higher SNR could potentially improve DWI and permit acquisition of higher b-values, field inhomogeneity can lead to more distortion artifacts related to susceptibility (Figure 6.11). For example, brain diffusion studies have shown higher SNR but increased image distortion at 3T compared with 1.5T [59, 60], in addition to substantial differences in apparent diffusion coefficient (ADC) values between these field strengths [61]. In a recent study, Dale *et al.* observed a significant increase in liver ADC at 3T using single-shot (SS) EPI DWI, with no significant difference in ADC between 1.5T and 3T for the pancreas and spleen [62]. In our recent experience [63], in eight healthy volunteers assessed at both 1.5T and 3T with SSEPI, we found lower subjective image quality at 3T compared with 1.5T (p = 0.0078–0.0156), and similar ADC values at 1.5T versus 3T for liver parenchyma, except when using b-values of 0, 500, and 600 s/mm^2 and breath-hold technique. We found equivalent ADC reproducibility at both 1.5T and 3T, with equivalent coefficients of variation of ADC between field strengths. Despite the potential advantages of imaging at higher field strength, our results did not show a clear benefit of performing abdominal DWI at 3T. Currently, single-shot spin-echo EPI is commonly used in practice for DWI but spatial resolution is relatively low and sequence is particularly vulnerable to field inhomogeneity because of the relatively long gradient echo train. Improvements in gradient design and parallel imaging are used to reduce geometric distortions and improve resolution. At 3T, alternative sequences for DWI hold promise such as single-shot although limited with respect to spatial resolution.

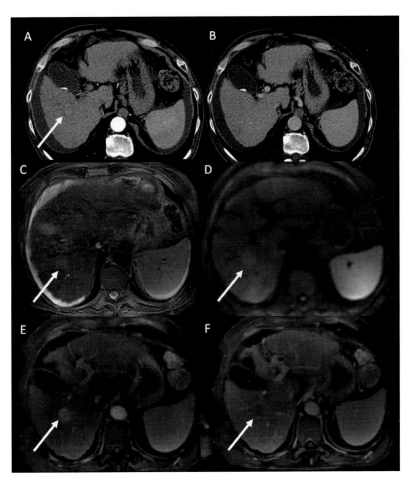

Figure 6.9 HCC better seen at 3T compared to computed tomography (CT). (A, B) Contrast-enhanced multidetector CT (A: arterial, B: portal venous phases). (C) Fat-suppressed FSE T2, (D) single-shot EPI diffusion (b = 500), (E, F) 3D SPGR images (LAVA) after injection of Gd-DTPA (E: arterial, F: portal venous phases). There is a right hepatic lobe HCC (arrow), which is vaguely seen on the arterial phase CT image, not seen on the portal venous phase CT image. The HCC is much more conspicuous on MR imaging, appearing slightly T2 hyperintense, slightly hyperintense on diffusion, with arterial enhancement and portal venous washout.

Non-Cartesian acquisition techniques such as PROPELLER (periodically rotated overlapping parallel lines with enhanced reconstruction) can potentially reduce motion artifacts and increase SNR [64–66]. Steady-state free precession (SSFP) techniques have shown promise for musculoskeletal applications but data are limited for abdominal imaging applications. Although there is potential for high-resolution imaging, this technique is essentially a nonquantitative method [67, 68].

Finally, there is ongoing research in liver MR perfusion for diffuse and focal liver disease particularly in fibrosis and cirrhosis [69, 70]. At 3T, dynamic-enhanced perfusion imaging may be improved because of the potentially greater conspicuity of gadolinium chelates compared to background tissue. However, there are potential drawbacks at 3T because T2* effects are more pronounced, which could lead to decreased signal from gadolinium contrast. Lower dose may be advantageous to reduce T2* effects. Further investigation comparing 1.5T and 3T is required to better understand whether higher field can improve sensitivity or specificity for detecting focal or diffuse liver disease.

Future directions

New solutions for correction of B1 field inhomogeneity such as parallel transmit technology [71] are promising. Optimization of abdominal DWI at 3T is needed. New multichannel coil systems with increased parallel imaging capabilities will also increase the use of 3T and higher field systems.

Conclusion

Three Tesla and higher field systems will likely continue to expand in the future, and 3T systems will likely be the norm in a few years from now. However, knowledge of advantages and pitfalls are necessary to adapt and optimize liver protocols at 3T.

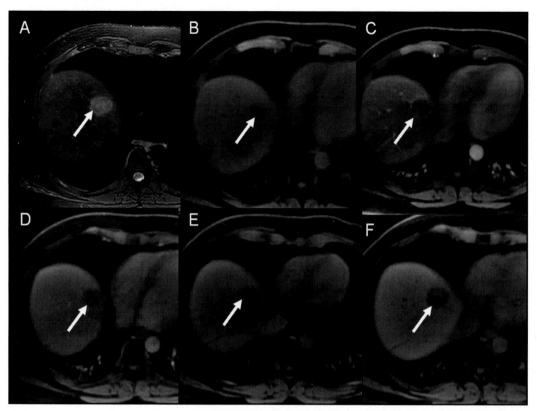

Figure 6.10 Liver metastasis from colon cancer diagnosed at 3T. (A) Fat-suppressed T2 FSE, (B–F) pre- and post-contrast 3D SPGR images (LAVA) before (B) and after injection of Gd-EOB-DTPA (C: arterial, D: portal venous, E: equilibrium, F: delayed hepatocyte phase [20 minutes]). There is a hepatic dome metastatic lesion (arrow), appearing T2 hyperintense, with arterial rim enhancement and internal enhancement at the portal venous phase, and hypointense on the hepatocyte phase.

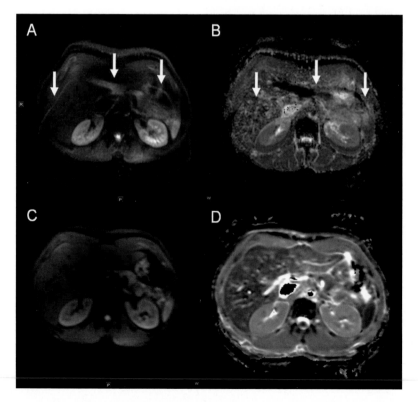

Figure 6.11 Single-shot EPI (SSEPI) diffusion at 3T. (A) Breath-hold SSEPI using TR/TE 2725/83, matrix 192 × 192, slice thickness 7 mm, (B) corresponding apparent diffusion coefficient (ADC) map (using b0–500), (C) breath-hold SSEPI using TR/TE 2400 ms/50.1 ms, matrix 128 × 80, slice thickness 7 mm, (D) corresponding ADC map (using b = 0–500 s/mm^2). Images with high acquisition matrix are severely limited by ghosting artifact (arrows). Better image quality without ghosting is obtained by decreasing the matrix size and the TE, at the expense of lower spatial resolution.

References

1. Lewin JS, Duerk JL, Jain VR, *et al.* Needle localization in MR-guided biopsy and aspiration: effects of field strength, sequence design, and magnetic field orientation. *AJR Am J Roentgenol* 1996; **166**(6): 1337–45.

2. Guo H, Au WY, Cheung JS, *et al.* Myocardial T2 quantitation in patients with iron overload at 3 Tesla. *J Magn Reson Imaging* 2009; **30**(2): 394–400.

3. von Falkenhausen M, Meyer C, Lutterbey G, *et al.* Intra-individual comparison of image contrast in SPIO-enhanced liver MR imaging at 1.5T and 3.0T. *Eur Radiol* 2007; **17**(5): 1256–61.

4. Katz-Brull R, Rofsky NM, Lenkinski RE. Breathhold abdominal and thoracic proton MR spectroscopy at 3.0T. *Magn Reson Med* 2003; **50**(3): 461–7.

5. Futterer JJ, Scheenen TW, Huisman HJ, *et al.* Initial experience of 3 tesla endorectal coil magnetic resonance imaging and 1H-spectroscopic imaging of the prostate. *Invest Radiol* 2004; **39**(11): 671–80.

6. Soher BJ, Dale BM, Merkle EM. A review of MR physics: 3 T versus 1.5T. *Magn Reson Imaging Clin N Am* 2007; **15**(3): 277–90, v.

7. Franklin KM, Dale BM, Merkle EM. Improvement in B1-inhomogeneity artifacts in the abdomen at 3 T MR imaging using a radiofrequency cushion. *J Magn Reson Imaging* 2008; **27**(6): 1443–7.

8. Zapparoli M, Semelka RC, Altun E, *et al.* 3.0-T MR imaging evaluation of patients with chronic liver diseases: initial observations. *Magn Reson Imaging* 2008; **26**(5): 650–60.

9. Collins CM, Wang Z, Mao W, *et al.* Array-optimized composite pulse for excellent whole-brain homogeneity in high-field MRI. *Magn Reson Med* 2007; **57**(3): 470–4.

10. Katscher U, Bornert P, Leussler C, van den Brink JS. Transmit SENSE. *Magn Reson Med* 2003; **49**(1): 144–50.

11. Zhu Y. Parallel excitation with an array of transmit coils. *Magn Reson Med* 2004; **51**(4): 775–84.

12. Vaughan T, DelaBarre L, Snyder C, *et al.* 9.4T human MRI: preliminary results. *Magn Reson Med* 2006; **56**(6): 1274–82.

13. Zhang Z, Yip CY, Grissom W, *et al.* Reduction of transmitter B1 inhomogeneity with transmit SENSE slice-select pulses. *Magn Reson Med* 2007; **57**(5): 842–7.

14. Hargreaves BA, Cunningham CH, Nishimura DG, Conolly SM. Variable-rate selective excitation for rapid MRI sequences. *Magn Reson Med* 2004; **52**(3): 590–7.

15. van den Bos IC, Hussain SM, Krestin GP, Wielopolski PA. Liver imaging at 3.0T: diffusion-induced black-blood echo-planar imaging with large anatomical volumetric coverage as an alternative for specific absorption rate-intensive echo-train spin-echo sequences: feasibility study. *Radiology* 2008; **248**(1): 264–71.

16. Hennig J, Scheffler K. Hyperechoes. *Magn Reson Med* 2001; **46**(1): 6–12.

17. Hennig J, Weigel M, Scheffler K. Multiecho sequences with variable refocusing flip angles: optimization of signal behavior using smooth transitions between pseudo steady states (TRAPS). *Magn Reson Med* 2003; **49**(3): 527–35.

18. Lichy MP, Wietek BM, Mugler JP 3rd, *et al.* Magnetic resonance imaging of the body trunk using a single-slab, 3-dimensional, T2-weighted turbo-spin-echo sequence with high sampling efficiency (SPACE) for high spatial resolution imaging: initial clinical experiences. *Invest Radiol* 2005; **40**(12): 754–60.

19. Rosenkrantz AB, Patel JM, Babb JS, Storey P, Hecht EM. Liver MRI at 3 T using a respiratory-triggered time-efficient 3D T2-weighted technique: impact on artifacts and image quality. *AJR Am J Roentgenol* 2010; **194**(3): 634–41.

20. Takahashi M, Uematsu H, Hatabu H. MR imaging at high magnetic fields. *Eur J Radiol* 2003; **46**(1): 45–52.

21. de Bazelaire CM, Duhamel GD, Rofsky NM, Alsop DC. MR imaging relaxation times of abdominal and pelvic tissues measured in vivo at 3.0T: preliminary results. *Radiology* 2004; **230**(3): 652–9.

22. Constable RT, Anderson AW, Zhong J, Gore JC. Factors influencing contrast in fast spin-echo MR imaging. *Magn Reson Imaging* 1992; **10**(4): 497–511.

23. Schindera ST, Soher BJ, Delong DM, Dale BM, Merkle EM. Effect of echo time pair selection on quantitative analysis for adrenal tumor characterization with in-phase and opposed-phase MR imaging: initial experience. *Radiology* 2008; **248**(1): 140–7.

24. Fujiyoshi F, Nakajo M, Fukukura Y, Tsuchimochi S. Characterization of adrenal tumors by chemical shift fast low-angle shot MR imaging: comparison of four methods of quantitative evaluation. *AJR Am J Roentgenol* 2003; **180**(6): 1649–57.

25. Angulo P. Nonalcoholic fatty liver disease. *N Engl J Med* 2002; **346**(16): 1221–31.

26. Szczepaniak LS, Nurenberg P, Leonard D, *et al.* Magnetic resonance spectroscopy to measure hepatic triglyceride content: prevalence of hepatic steatosis in the general population. *Am J Physiol Endocrinol Metab* 2005; **288**(2): E462–8.

27. Wieckowska A, McCullough AJ, Feldstein AE. Noninvasive diagnosis and monitoring of nonalcoholic steatohepatitis: present and future. *Hepatology* 2007; **46**(2): 582–9.

28. Ekstedt M, Franzen LE, Mathiesen UL, *et al*. Long-term follow-up of patients with NAFLD and elevated liver enzymes. *Hepatology* 2006; **44**(4): 865–73.

29. Cassidy FH, Yokoo T, Aganovic L, *et al*. Fatty liver disease: MR imaging techniques for the detection and quantification of liver steatosis. *Radiographics* 2009; **29**(1): 231–60.

30. Guiu B, Petit JM, Loffroy R, *et al*. Quantification of liver fat content: comparison of triple-echo chemical shift gradient-echo imaging and in vivo proton MR spectroscopy. *Radiology* 2009; **250**(1): 95–102.

31. Alla V, Bonkovsky HL. Iron in nonhemochromatotic liver disorders. *Semin Liver Dis* 2005; **25**(4): 461–72.

32. Ramm GA, Ruddell RG. Hepatotoxicity of iron overload: mechanisms of iron-induced hepatic fibrogenesis. *Semin Liver Dis* 2005; **25**(4): 433–49.

33. Niederau C, Fischer R, Sonnenberg A, *et al*. Survival and causes of death in cirrhotic and in noncirrhotic patients with primary hemochromatosis. *N Engl J Med* 1985; **313**(20): 1256–62.

34. Tsukamoto H, Horne W, Kamimura S, *et al*. Experimental liver cirrhosis induced by alcohol and iron. *J Clin Invest* 1995; **96**(1): 620–30.

35. Facchini FS, Hua NW, Stoohs RA. Effect of iron depletion in carbohydrate-intolerant patients with clinical evidence of nonalcoholic fatty liver disease. *Gastroenterology* 2002; **122**(4): 931–9.

36. Dixon WT. Simple proton spectroscopic imaging. *Radiology* 1984; **153**(1): 189–94.

37. Reeder SB, Hargreaves BA, Yu H, Brittain JH. Homodyne reconstruction and IDEAL water-fat decomposition. *Magn Reson Med* 2005; **54**(3): 586–93.

38. Fuller S, Reeder S, Shimakawa A, *et al*. Iterative decomposition of water and fat with echo asymmetry and least-squares estimation (IDEAL) fast spin-echo imaging of the ankle: initial clinical experience. *AJR Am J Roentgenol* 2006; **187**(6): 1442–7.

39. Hussain HK, Chenevert TL, Londy FJ, *et al*. Hepatic fat fraction: MR imaging for quantitative measurement and display – early experience. *Radiology* 2005; **237**(3): 1048–55.

40. Yokoo T, Bydder M, Hamilton G, *et al*. Nonalcoholic fatty liver disease: diagnostic and fat-grading accuracy of low-flip-angle multiecho gradient-recalled-echo MR imaging at 1.5 T. *Radiology* 2009; **251**(1): 67–76.

41. Qayyum A, Goh JS, Kakar S, *et al*. Accuracy of liver fat quantification at MR imaging: comparison of out-of-phase gradient-echo and fat-saturated fast spin-echo techniques – initial experience. *Radiology* 2005; **237**(2): 507–11.

42. Bernard CP, Liney GP, Manton DJ, Turnbull LW, Langton CM. Comparison of fat quantification

methods: a phantom study at 3.0T. *J Magn Reson Imaging* 2008; **27**(1): 192–7.

43. Gandon Y, Olivie D, Guyader D, *et al*. Non-invasive assessment of hepatic iron stores by MRI. *Lancet* 2004; **363**(9406): 357–62.

44. St Pierre TG, Clark PR, Chua-Anusorn W. Measurement and mapping of liver iron concentrations using magnetic resonance imaging. *Ann N Y Acad Sci* 2005; **1054**: 379–85.

45. St Pierre TG, Clark PR, Chua-anusorn W, *et al*. Noninvasive measurement and imaging of liver iron concentrations using proton magnetic resonance. *Blood* 2005; **105**(2): 855–61.

46. Alustiza JM, Artetxe J, Castiella A, *et al*. MR quantification of hepatic iron concentration. *Radiology* 2004; **230**(2): 479–84.

47. Chandarana H, Lim RP, Jensen JH, *et al*. Hepatic iron deposition in patients with liver disease: preliminary experience with breath-hold multiecho T2*-weighted sequence. *AJR Am J Roentgenol* 2009; **193**(5): 1261–7.

48. Storey P, Thompson AA, Carqueville CL, *et al*. R2* imaging of transfusional iron burden at 3 T and comparison with 1.5T. *J Magn Reson Imaging* 2007; **25**(3): 540–7.

49. Boll DT, Marin D, Redmon GM, Zink SI, Merkle EM. Pilot study assessing differentiation of steatosis hepatis, hepatic iron overload, and combined disease using two-point dixon MRI at 3 T: in vitro and in vivo results of a 2D decomposition technique. *AJR Am J Roentgenol* 2010; **194**(4): 964–71.

50. Hines CD, Yu H, Shimakawa A, *et al*. T1 independent, T2* corrected MRI with accurate spectral modeling for quantification of fat: validation in a fat-water-SPIO phantom. *J Magn Reson Imaging* 2009; **30**(5): 1215–22.

51. Thomsen C, Becker U, Winkler K, *et al*. Quantification of liver fat using magnetic resonance spectroscopy. *Magn Reson Imaging* 1994; **12**(3): 487–95.

52. Kuo YT, Li CW, Chen CY, *et al*. In vivo proton magnetic resonance spectroscopy of large focal hepatic lesions and metabolite change of hepatocellular carcinoma before and after transcatheter arterial chemoembolization using 3.0-T MR scanner. *J Magn Reson Imaging* 2004; **19**(5): 598–604.

53. Taouli B, Koh DM. Diffusion-weighted MR imaging of the liver. *Radiology* 2010; **254**(1): 47–66.

54. Parikh T, Drew SJ, Lee VS, *et al*. Focal liver lesion detection and characterization with diffusion-weighted MR imaging: comparison with standard breath-hold T2-weighted imaging. *Radiology* 2008; **246**(3): 812–22.

55. Taouli B, Tolia AJ, Losada M, *et al*. Diffusion-weighted MRI for quantification of liver fibrosis: preliminary

experience. *AJR Am J Roentgenol* 2007; **189**(4): 799–806.

56. Lewin M, Poujol-Robert A, Boelle PY, *et al.* Diffusion-weighted magnetic resonance imaging for the assessment of fibrosis in chronic hepatitis C. *Hepatology* 2007; **46**(3): 658–65.

57. Taouli B, Chouli M, Martin AJ, *et al.* Chronic hepatitis: role of diffusion-weighted imaging and diffusion tensor imaging for the diagnosis of liver fibrosis and inflammation. *J Magn Reson Imaging* 2008; **28**(1): 89–95.

58. Patel J, Sigmund EE, Rusinek H, *et al.* Diagnosis of cirrhosis with intravoxel incoherent motion diffusion MRI and dynamic contrast-enhanced MRI alone and in combination: preliminary experience. *J Magn Reson Imaging* 2010; **31**(3): 589–600.

59. Hunsche S, Moseley ME, Stoeter P, Hedehus M. Diffusion-tensor MR imaging at 1.5 and 3.0T: initial observations. *Radiology* 2001; **221**(2): 550–6.

60. Kuhl CK, Textor J, Gieseke J, *et al.* Acute and subacute ischemic stroke at high-field-strength (3.0-T) diffusion-weighted MR imaging: intraindividual comparative study. *Radiology* 2005; **234**(2): 509–16.

61. Huisman TA, Loenneker T, Barta G, *et al.* Quantitative diffusion tensor MR imaging of the brain: field strength related variance of apparent diffusion coefficient (ADC) and fractional anisotropy (FA) scalars. *Eur Radiol* 2006; **16**(8): 1651–8.

62. Dale BM, Braithwaite AC, Boll DT, Merkle EM. Field strength and diffusion encoding technique affect the apparent diffusion coefficient measurements in diffusion-weighted imaging of the abdomen. *Invest Radiol* 2010; **45**(2): 104–8.

63. Rosenkrantz AB, Oei M, Babb JS, Niver BE, Taouli B. Diffusion-weighted imaging of the abdomen at 3.0T: image quality and ADC reproducibility compared with 1.5T. *J Magn Reson Imaging* (in press).

64. Deng J, Larson AC. Modified PROPELLER approach for T2-mapping of the abdomen. *Magn Reson Med* 2009; **61**(6): 1269–78.

65. Deng J, Miller FH, Salem R, Omary RA, Larson AC. Multishot diffusion-weighted PROPELLER magnetic resonance imaging of the abdomen. *Invest Radiol* 2006; **41**(10): 769–75.

66. Deng J, Omary RA, Larson AC. Multishot diffusion-weighted SPLICE PROPELLER MRI of the abdomen. *Magn Reson Med* 2008; **59**(5): 947–53.

67. Ding S, Trillaud H, Yongbi M, *et al.* High resolution renal diffusion imaging using a modified steady-state free precession sequence. *Magn Reson Med* 1995; **34**(4): 586–95.

68. Jeong EK, Kim SE, Parker DL. High-resolution diffusion-weighted 3D MRI, using diffusion-weighted driven-equilibrium (DW-DE) and multishot segmented 3D-SSFP without navigator echoes. *Magn Reson Med* 2003; **50**(4): 821–9.

69. Hagiwara M, Rusinek H, Lee VS, *et al.* Advanced liver fibrosis: diagnosis with 3D whole-liver perfusion MR imaging – initial experience. *Radiology* 2008; **246**(3): 926–34.

70. Do RK, Rusinek H, Taouli B. Dynamic contrast-enhanced MR imaging of the liver: current status and future directions. *Magn Reson Imaging Clin N Am* 2009; **17**(2): 339–49.

71. Vernickel P, Roschmann P, Findeklee C, *et al.* Eight-channel transmit/receive body MRI coil at 3 T. *Magn Reson Med* 2007; **58**(2): 381–9.

MR imaging of the pancreas

Sang Soo Shin, Chang Hee Lee, Rafael O. P. de Campos, and Richard C. Semelka

MR imaging technique

New MR imaging techniques that limit artifacts in the abdomen have increased the role of MR imaging in detection and characterization of pancreatic disease. Advantages of imaging at 3T compared with 1.5T include thinner section acquisition (typically 2.5 mm versus 5 mm at 1.5T), higher matrix (typically 340×516 compared with 192×256), and high quality of T1-weighted three-dimensional (3D) gradient echo imaging [1]. Standard sequences at 3T, which include breath-hold T1-weighted 3D gradient echo sequences, fat suppression techniques, and dynamic administration of gadolinium chelate, have resulted in image quality of the pancreas sufficient to detect and characterize focal pancreatic mass lesions smaller than 1 cm in diameter, and to evaluate diffuse pancreatic disease. MR cholangiopancreatography (MRCP) images acquired in a coronal oblique projection to delineate the pancreatic and bile duct is a useful addition. MRCP permits good demonstration of the biliary and pancreatic ducts to assess ductal obstruction, dilation, and abnormal duct pathways. The combination of parenchyma-imaging sequences and MRCP provides comprehensive information to evaluate the full range of pancreatic disease.

MR imaging of the pancreas is optimal at 3T MR system because of a higher signal-to-noise ratio, which facilitates breath-hold imaging, and increased fat–water frequency shift, which facilitates chemically selective excitation-spoiling fat suppression or water excitation [2]. T1-weighted chemically selective fat suppression and T1-weighted breath-hold gradient echo sequences are effective techniques for imaging pancreatic parenchyma. The combination of higher signal-to-noise ratio, greater spectral separation, and increased sensitivity to gadolinium results in the acquisition of images with high quality, and high spatial and temporal resolution. The use of high-spatial-resolution MR imaging at 3T improves the detection of small focal lesions. That is why we prefer to use 3T MR imaging, when evaluating patients for suspected small pancreatic adenocarcinomas and islet cell tumors, as thinner sections may be obtained with the preservation of adequate signal-to-noise ratio.

Our standard MR protocol for the evaluation of the pancreas includes T1-weighted fat-suppressed 3D gradient echo, T1-weighted in-phase and out-of phase gradient echo, T2-weighted single-shot echo-train spin-echo with/without fat suppression, and post-gadolinium imaging in the capillary phase (immediate post-contrast, hepatic arterial dominant phase, 15–20 seconds post-contrast), early hepatic venous phase (45 seconds post-contrast) and interstitial phase (1–10 minutes post-contrast). Table 7.1 provides the typical imaging parameters that we employ. The image quality of post-gadolinium sequences is particularly superior at 3T. The relative enhancement of the pancreas is consistently and significantly higher at 3T than at 1.5T in matched subphases of hepatic arterial enhancement [3]. Therefore, the signal-to-noise ratio and contrast-to-noise ratio benefit of 3T imaging is greatest on contrast-enhanced sequences, particularly on post-gadolinium 3D gradient echo sequence. The advantages in performing post-gadolinium gradient echo imaging as a 3D gradient echo technique include the following reasons: (1) thinner sections can be obtained (3 mm vs. 5 mm for two-dimensional [2D] spoiled gradient echo), (2) the absence of mirror artifact from the aorta, which could be problematic on 2D spoiled gradient echo, and (3) the lesser imaging quality of 2D gradient echo sequences at 3T. Fat suppression is virtually essential to maximize

Body MR Imaging at 3 Tesla, ed. Ihab R. Kamel and Elmar M. Merkle. Published by Cambridge University Press.

Table 7.1 Details of the parameters used for MR imaging on 3T MR scanner

Parameter	T2-weighted half-Fourier RARE	T1-weighted SGE	T1-weighted VIBE	T1-weighted dynamic VIBE
TR (ms)	2000	169	5.2	3.07
TE (ms) (in-phase/out-of-phase)	95	2.5/1.58	2.45/3.67	1.32
Flip angle (°)	150	57	13	13
Matrix (phase × frequency)	204 × 256	204 × 256	224 × 320	224 × 320
FOV (mm^2)	350 × 306	400 × 400	380 × 308	380 × 308
Section thickness (mm)	8	8	3	3
Intersectional gap (mm)	1.6	1.6	0.6	0.6

TR = repetition time, TE = echo time, ms = millisecond, mm = millimeter, FOV = field of view, RARE = rapid acquisition relaxation enhancement, SGE = spoiled gradient echo, VIBE = volumetric interpolated breath-hold examination.

image quality with the 3D gradient echo technique. T2-weighted echo-train spin-echo sequences such as T2-weighted half-Fourier acquisition single-shot turbo spin-echo (HASTE) provide a sharp anatomical display of the common bile duct (CBD) on coronal plane images and of the pancreatic duct on transverse plane images. MRCP images can be acquired oriented in the plane of the pancreatic duct, in an oblique coronal projection, to delineate longer segments of the pancreatic duct in continuity. T2-weighted fat-suppressed images are useful for demonstrating liver metastases and islet cell tumors. T2-weighted images also provide information on the complexity of the fluid in pancreatic pseudocysts, which may reflect the presence of complications such as necrotic debris or infection. MR imaging with the combination of T1, T2, early and late post-gadolinium images, MRCP, and magnetic resonance angiography (MRA) can produce comprehensive information on the pancreas.

MR imaging finding of normal pancreas

The normal pancreas is high in signal intensity on T1-weighted fat-suppressed images because of the presence of aqueous protein in the acini of the pancreas. Normal pancreas is well shown with this technique. The pancreas demonstrates a uniform capillary blush on immediate post-contrast images, which renders it markedly higher in signal intensity than liver, neighboring bowel, and adjacent fat (Figure 7.1). Recognition of the characteristic high signal intensity of normal pancreas on pre-contrast T1-weighted fat-suppressed and immediate post-gadolinium images is useful

in distinguishing pancreas parenchyma from adjacent bowel. For example, pancreatic head is readily distinguished from duodenum or adjacent bowel on immediate post-gadolinium images because the pancreas enhances substantially greater than bowel. By 1 minute after contrast administration, the pancreas shows approximately isointense signal with fat on non-fat-suppressed T1-weighted 3D gradient echo, and moderately higher signal than background fat on fat-suppressed 3D gradient echo sequences. In elderly patients, the signal intensity of the pancreas may diminish and be lower than that of liver. This may reflect changes of fibrosis secondary to the aging process. Fatty replacement of the pancreas occurs frequently as a normal degenerative process and results in a feathery, lobulated appearance on imaging in elderly patients (Figure 7.2).

Developmental anomaly
Pancreas divisum

Pancreas divisum is the most clinically important and common major anatomical variant. Although a misleading term, pancreas divisum is, by definition, a superficially normal-appearing pancreas in which no communication has developed between the duct of the dorsally derived pancreas and the duct of the embryonic ventral pancreas, which normally forms most of the main pancreatic duct. The result of this congenital abnormality is that portions of the pancreas have separate ductal systems: a very short ventral duct of Wirsung drains only the lower portion of

(a)

(b)

(c)

(d)

(e)

(f)

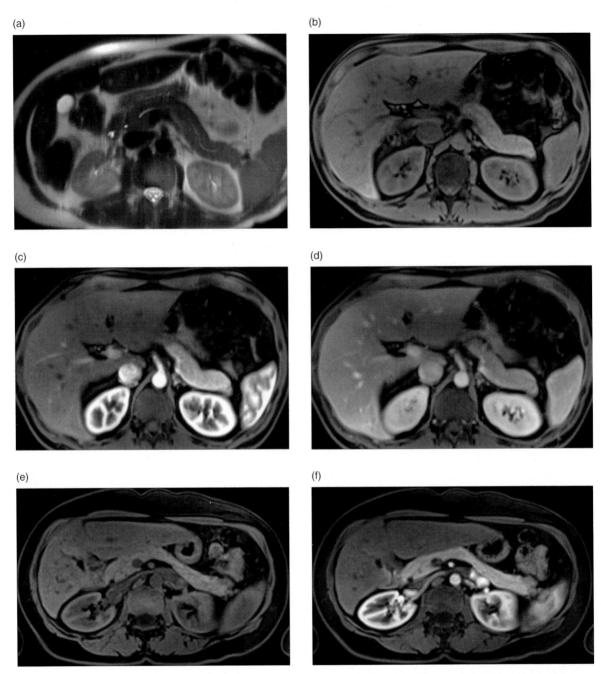

Figure 7.1 Normal pancreas. Axial T2-weighted single-shot echo-train spin-echo (a), T1-weighted fat-suppressed 3D gradient echo (b), immediate post-gadolinium (c) and interstitial phase post-gadolinium (d) T1-weighted fat-suppressed 3D gradient echo images. The pancreas shows relatively high signal intensity on T1-weighted fat-suppressed 3D gradient echo image mainly due to high proteinaceous contents. The pancreas shows a uniform capillary blush on immediate post-gadolinium image and homogeneous architecture on T2-weighted and interstitial phase post-gadolinium images. Normal pancreas in a second patient. Axial T1-weighted fat-suppressed 3D gradient echo (e), immediate post-gadolinium (f) and early hepatic venous phase post-gadolinium (g) T1-weighted fat-suppressed 3D gradient echo images, and MRCP image acquired in a coronal oblique projection (h). Note again the high signal intensity on T1-weighted noncontrast image (e) and the uniform capillary blush on immediate post-gadolinium image (f). MRCP is optimal at 3T. Note that it is possible to obtain excellent delineation of the pancreatic and bile duct (h).

(g)

(h)

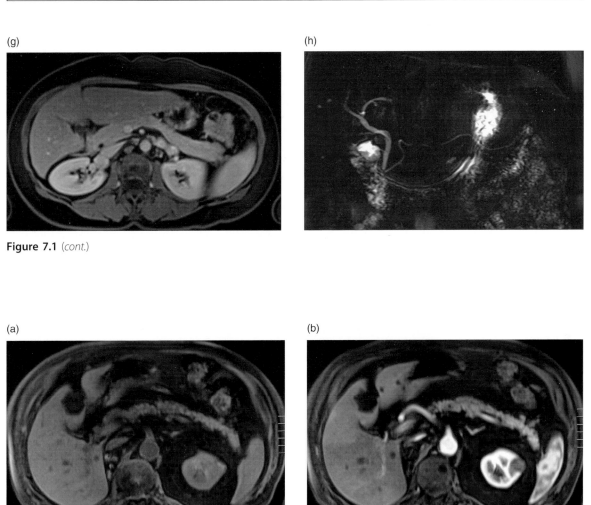

Figure 7.1 (*cont.*)

(a)

(b)

(c)

(d)

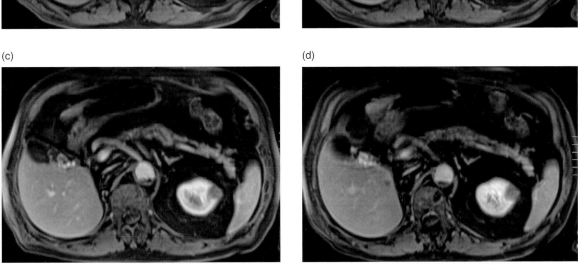

Figure 7.2 Normal pancreas in an elderly patient (82 years) with no history of pancreatic disease. Axial T1-weighted fat-suppressed 3D gradient echo image obtained in the pre-contrast phase (a) and in the hepatic arterial dominant phase (b), early hepatic venous phase (c), and interstitial phase (d) post-gadolinium. Compare with the pancreas demonstrated in Figure 7.1 and note that this pancreas has a smaller thickness, a marbled and lobulated appearance. These findings are normal with aging.

(a)

(b)

(c)

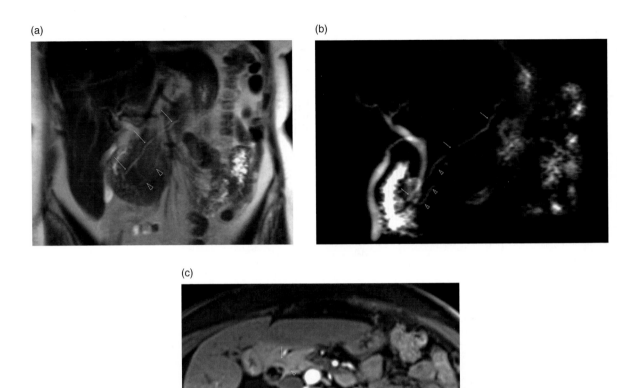

Figure 7.3 Pancreas divisum. Coronal T2-weighted single-shot echo-train spin-echo (a), MRCP acquired in a coronal oblique projection (b), and axial T1-weighted fat-suppressed 3D gradient echo in the hepatic arterial dominant phase post-gadolinium (c). There is a short ventral duct of Wirsung (arrowheads) and a more prominent dorsal duct of Santorini (arrows), with no communication between them and with separate entries into the duodenum.

the head, whereas the dorsal duct of Santorini drains the tail, body, neck, and upper aspect of the head. The incidence of this anomaly varies between 1.3% and 6.7% of the population. On MRCP images, separate entries of the ducts of Santorini and Wirsung into the duodenum are consistently demonstrated because of the good conspicuity of the linear high-signal-intensity tubular structures (Figure 7.3).

Pancreas divisum has been reported to be a pre-disposing factor in recurrent pancreatitis. It is postu-lated that in some people the disproportion between the small caliber of the minor papilla and the large amount of secretion from the dorsal part of the gland leads to a relative outflow obstruction from the dorsal pancreas, resulting in pain or pancreatitis. Compared with patients with pancreatitis and normal duct anatomy, the pancreas in pancreas divisum may appear normal in signal intensity on T1-weighted fat-suppressed images and immediate post-gadolinium gradient echo images because the attacks of recurrent pancreatitis tend to be less severe and changes of chronic pancreatitis may not develop.

Neoplasms

Pancreatic mass lesions can be detected and succ-essfully characterized with a pattern recognition approach using T1, T2, and immediate and late post-gadolinium images.

Adenocarcinoma

Pancreatic ductal adenocarcinoma, referring to car-cinoma arising in the exocrine portion of the gland, accounts for 95% of malignant tumors of the pancreas

(a)

(b)

(c)

(d)

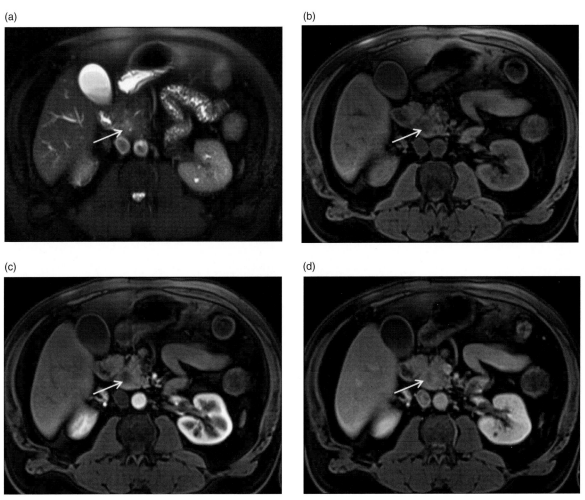

Figure 7.4 Small pancreatic cancer arising in the head. Axial T2-weighted fat-suppressed single-shot echo-train spin-echo (a), T1-weighted fat-suppressed 3D gradient echo (b), immediate post-gadolinium (c), and interstitial phase post-gadolinium (d) T1-weighted fat-suppressed 3D gradient echo images. A small cancer is present in the pancreatic head (arrow), which is clearly defined as a mass on the T1-weighted fat-suppressed image (arrow; b). The tumor appears as a hypoenhancing mass (arrow; c and d) on the post-contrast images and is more distinguished on the immediate post-gadolinium image. On the interstitial phase the tumor has decreased in conspicuity because of progressive enhancement of the lesion and pancreatic parenchymal washout.

and is the fourth most common cause of cancer death in the United States [4]. The tumor has a poor prognosis, with a 5-year survival rate of only 5%. Surgery remains the sole curative treatment of patients with pancreatic carcinoma; therefore, earlier detection of potentially resectable disease may result in improved patient survival.

Tumor detection

Due to the critical importance of detecting cancers when they are small, with suspected small pancreatic cancers our preference is always MR imaging over computed tomography (CT), and 3T over 1.5T MR

imaging. On MR images, pancreatic cancer appears as a low-signal-intensity mass on noncontrast T1-weighted fat-suppressed images and enhances to a lesser extent than the surrounding normal pancreatic tissue on immediate post-contrast images (Figures 7.4, 7.5, and 7.6). These MR imaging features are related to their abundant fibrous stroma and relatively sparse tumor vascularity. The appearance of cancers on interstitial phase images is variable and reflects the volume of extracellular space and venous drainage of cancers compared with the pancreatic tissue. Large pancreatic tumors tend to remain low in signal intensity on interstitial phase images, whereas the signal intensity of

(a)

(b)

(c)

(d)

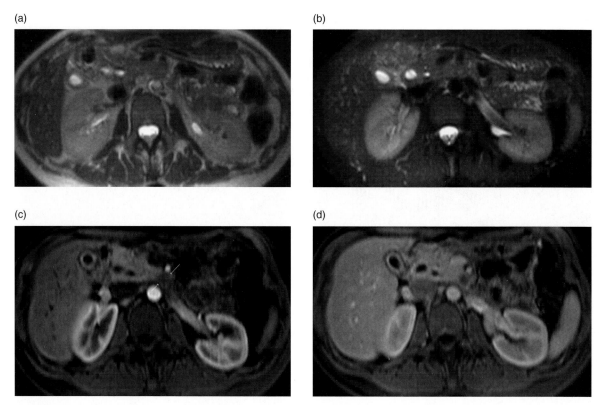

Figure 7.5 Small pancreatic cancer arising in the head. Axial non-fat-suppressed (a) and fat-suppressed (b) T2-weighted single-shot echo-train spin-echo, immediate (c) and interstitial (d) post-gadolinium T1-weighted fat-suppressed 3D gradient echo images. Note a small hypoenhancing mass arising from the tip of the uncinate process. This mass is not identified on T2-weighted images and is clearly seen only on the immediate post-gadolinium 3D gradient echo image (arrows; c).

smaller tumors may range from hypointense to hyperintense on this phase. On T2-weighted images, tumors are usually minimally hypointense to minimally hyperintense relative to the pancreas and are therefore difficult to detect (Figures 7.4 and 7.5).

Although pancreatic adenocarcinoma usually appears as a focal low-signal-intensity mass that is relatively well demarcated from the adjacent normal pancreatic parenchyma on immediate post-contrast images, some tumors can be seen as poorly marginated lesions with decreased enhancement on immediate post-contrast images and slightly increased enhancement on interstitial phase images [5]. This appearance is commonly observed in pancreatic cancer that has been treated with chemotherapy and radiation therapy but may also be seen at initial presentation in up to 27% of patients and has a significant association with well to moderately differentiated histologic pattern [5].

Pancreatic cancer involving the head region can cause stenosis of both the common bile duct and the main pancreatic duct with upstream ductal dilation. Because of obstruction of the main pancreatic duct, the patients often develop tumor-associated pancreatitis. Pancreatic tissue distal to pancreatic cancer is often atrophic in volume and lower in signal intensity than normal pancreatic parenchyma because of chronic inflammation with progressive fibrosis and diminished proteinaceous fluid of the gland (Figure 7.6). In these cases, the tumors are difficult to detect on noncontrast T1-weighted images. However, immediate post-contrast images are able to define the size and extent of cancers that obstruct the pancreatic duct, as tumors almost invariably enhance less than adjacent chronically inflamed pancreas.

Chronic pancreatitis may cause a focal mass-like lesion, usually in the pancreatic head, which appears as a low-signal-intensity mass on noncontrast and immediate post-contrast T1-weighted images. Thus, it may be difficult to distinguish pancreatic cancer from chronic pancreatitis on the basis of the extent of enhancement of the lesion. One study evaluated the

(a)

(b)

(c)

(d)

(e)

(f)

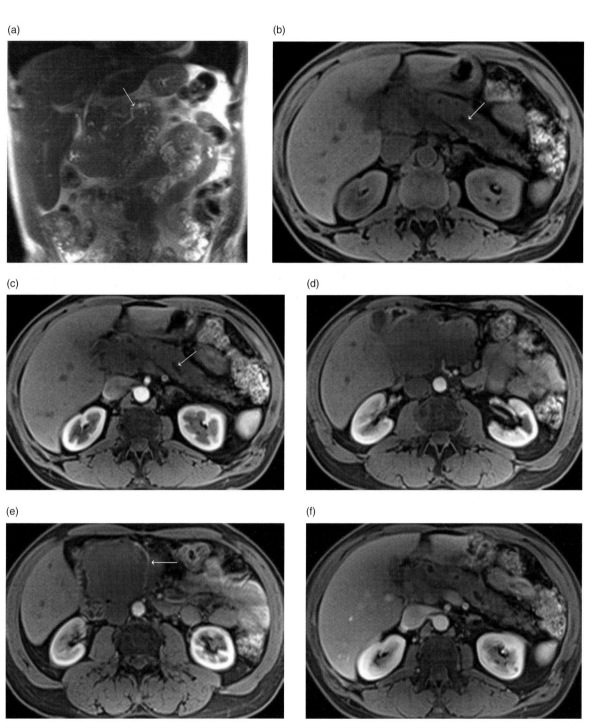

Figure 7.6 Large pancreatic head cancer with pancreatitis occurring distal to the mass. Coronal T2-weighted single-shot echo-train spin-echo (a), axial T1-weighted fat-suppressed 3D gradient echo (b), immediate post-gadolinium (c, d, e) and interstitial phase post-gadolinium (f) T1-weighted fat-suppressed 3D gradient echo images. A very large tumor in the head of the pancreas resulting in obstruction of the pancreatic duct. The dilated pancreatic duct is seen (arrow; a, b, c). On the immediate post-gadolinium images (c, d, e), note the marked low signal intensity of the mass. The evaluation of tumor invasion of the arteries is best done in this phase of enhancement. Note the gastroduodenal artery encasement (arrow, e). The pancreatic tissue distal to the tumor is low in signal intensity on the noncontrast T1-weighted fat-suppressed (b) image and has a diminished enhancement on post-contrast images (c, f), consistent with pancreatitis which is secondary to the tumor in the head of the pancreas.

accuracy of MR imaging, emphasizing a T1-weighted 3D gradient echo sequence, for differentiating pancreatic carcinoma from chronic pancreatitis in patients with focal pancreatic mass [6]. The results showed a sensitivity of 93% and a specificity of 75%, and the most discriminative finding for pancreatic adenocarcinoma was a relatively well-defined margin with relatively lower signal intensity and decreased enhancement compared with the background pancreas on immediate and early hepatic venous phase post-contrast T1-weighted images. In contrast, the discriminative feature of chronic pancreatitis was an ill-defined margin with relatively increased signal intensity and enhancement compared with the background pancreas on early hepatic venous phase images, reflecting a more progressive enhancement of inflammatory tissue than cancer from early to late post-contrast images. An additional helpful imaging feature is effacement of the fine, lobular architectural pattern of the pancreas in pancreatic adenocarcinoma. The presence of lymphadenopathy, encasement of the celiac axis or superior mesenteric artery (SMA), and liver metastases can also be helpful to establish the diagnosis of pancreatic cancer.

Because of the superior soft tissue contrast and more different types of data acquired, MR imaging is more reliable than CT in the detection of pancreatic cancer, particularly small non-contour-deforming pancreatic cancer, which may be difficult to identify even with multi-detector row CT. According to a previous study, immediate post-contrast gradient echo sequence was found to be the most sensitive approach to detect pancreatic cancer, particularly in the head region compared with spiral CT (Figure 7.7) [7]. Both immediate post-contrast gradient echo and noncontrast T1-weighted fat-suppressed sequences performed well at excluding cancer, and both were significantly superior to spiral CT imaging.

Local extension

Because tumors in the head of the pancreas readily encase the common bile duct, they tend to develop clinical symptoms, such as painless jaundice, earlier, and present smaller than tumors in the body or tail, these latter usually grow insidiously and present at a very advanced stage with local invasion. Low-signal-intensity tumors that extend beyond the pancreas and invade adjacent organs are well shown in a background of high-signal intensity fat tissue on non-fat-suppressed T1-weighted images. Gadolinium-enhanced

fat-suppressed gradient echo images acquired in the interstitial phase demonstrate intermediate-signal-intensity tumor with enhancement extending into low-signal-intensity suppressed fat. Thus, a combination of both sequences is of value to detect the local tumor extension beyond the pancreas (Figure 7.8).

Vascular encasement

Pancreatic cancer has a great propensity to encase the adjacent vessels including the main portal vein, the superior mesenteric vein, the celiac trunk and its branches, and the SMA. On MR imaging, vascular encasement is observed as a loss of the fat plane around vessels and as an encasing soft tissue lesion with luminal narrowing of the involved vessel. Immediate post-contrast 3D gradient echo images are useful for depicting arterial patency (Figures 7.6 and 7.8), and early hepatic venous phase post-contrast gradient echo images are useful for evaluating venous patency (Figure 7.8). Vascular encasement is best shown with thin-section 3D gradient echo images, which can be analyzed both as source images in the transverse plane and reformatted images in the coronal plane [8]. Right anterior coronal oblique images are useful for showing the relationship between a tumor and the portal vein as it enters the porta hepatis and between a tumor and the superior mesenteric vein along the medial margin of the pancreatic head. The thinner section that can be acquired at 3T compared with 1.5T, with preserved high signal-to-noise ratio, facilitates the evaluation of vascular patency. When vascular encasement is a critical determination, our preference is to image at 3T.

Lymph node metastases

In pancreatic carcinoma, rich lymphatic network and lack of a capsule account for the early spread of cancer to regional lymph nodes. The nodal groups involved consist of parapancreatic, paraportal, celiac, paracaval, and para-aortic groups. Lymph nodes are well demonstrated on T2-weighted fat-suppressed images and interstitial phase post-contrast fat-suppressed T1-weighted images and are shown as moderately high-signal-intensity foci in a background of low-signal-intensity suppressed fat on both sequences (Figure 7.9). Furthermore, T2-weighted fat-suppressed imaging is particularly useful for the demonstration of lymph nodes that are in close approximation to the liver or in the region of porta hepatis because of the signal intensity difference between moderately high-signal-intensity nodes and moderately low-signal-intensity

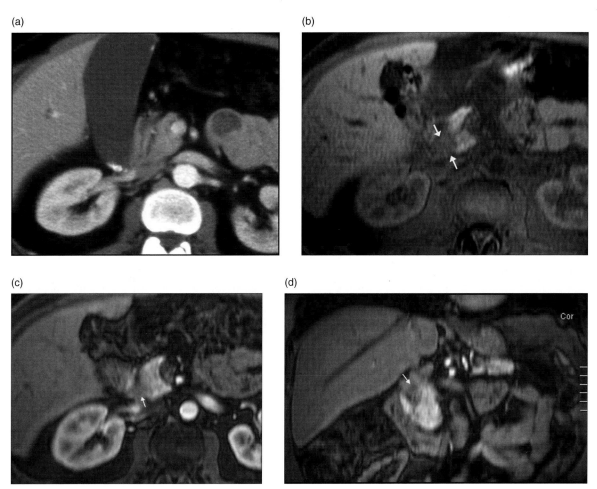

(a) (b)

(c) (d)

Figure 7.7 Small pancreatic cancer depicted on MR imaging and poorly seen on CT. Dynamic contrast-enhanced CT (a), T1-weighted fat-suppressed gradient echo (b), immediate post-gadolinium T1-weighted fat-suppressed 3D gradient echo (c), and coronal reformat of the immediate post-gadolinium T1-weighted fat-suppressed 3D gradient echo (d) images in a patient with small pancreatic cancer. A small cancer is present in the pancreatic head (arrow; c, d), and is more clearly defined as a mass with demarcated borders on T1-weighted fat-suppressed images (arrow; b). The small, non-organ-deforming tumor is not apparent on CT image. The tumor appears as a hypoenhancing mass (arrow; C) on the immediate post-gadolinium image (c) with demarcated margins.

liver (Figure 7.9). Non-fat-suppressed T1-weighted images, in which lymph nodes are seen as low-signal-intensity foci in a background of high-signal-intensity fat, are useful to detect mesenteric or retroperitoneal nodes in the setting of abundant fat in these locations. Coronal plane images can provide good visualization of these nodal groups as well (Figure 7.9).

Pancreatic endocrine tumors

Pancreatic endocrine tumors have been traditionally called islet cell tumors, which were thought to have evolved from the islets of Langerhans. However, more recent evidence suggests that these tumors arise from pluripotential stem cells in the ductal epithelium [9].

They are rare tumors, which occur in approximately 1 in 100 000 individuals, or represent 1–2% of all pancreatic neoplasms. Usually, endocrine tumors of the pancreas are classified into functioning and nonfunctioning tumors. The functioning tumors may present with an endocrine abnormality resulting from the secretion of hormones. The results of special immunohistochemical techniques such as fluorescence-labeled antibody specific for a peptide permit the designation of neoplasm as specific pancreatic endocrine tumors such as insulinoma, gastrinoma, etc. A certain proportion of pancreatic endocrine tumors will secrete no identifiable substance and remain uncategorized after special immunohistochemical

(a)

(b)

(c)

(d)

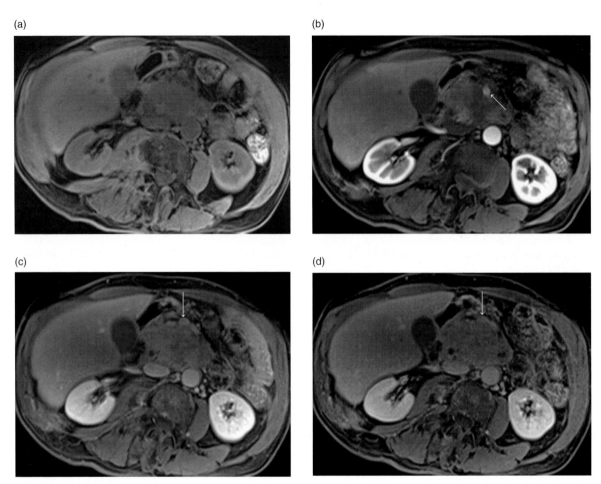

Figure 7.8 Large pancreatic head cancer with duodenal invasion and vascular encasement. Axial T1-weighted fat-suppressed 3D gradient echo image obtained in the pre-contrast phase (a) and in the hepatic arterial dominant phase (HADP) (b), early hepatic venous phase (EHVP) (c), and interstitial phase (IP) (d). The pancreatic mass is low in signal intensity and poorly marginated on the noncontrast T1-weighted image (a). There is diminished and mildly heterogeneous enhancement in the HADP image (b) and progressive tumor enhancement in the EHVP (c) and IP (d) images. Encasement of the superior mesenteric artery is clearly displayed on the HADP image (arrow, b) but difficult to evaluate on the EHVP and IP images (c, d). On the contrary, the superior mesenteric vein (SMV) is clearly displayed on the EHVP and IP images (arrow; c and d) but not on the HADP image. Note that the tumor abuts the SMV, which is anteriorly dislocated and mildly deformed (arrow; c and d). The high quality of the MR images acquired at 3T renders a confident staging of the tumor.

procedures. The most common pancreatic endocrine tumors are insulinomas and gastrinomas, followed in frequency by nonfunctional or untyped tumors. In the authors' experience, most clinically or immuno-histochemically verified pancreatic neuroendocrine tumors are gastrinomas [10]. Hormonally, functional tumors tend to present when they are small because of symptoms related to the hormones secreted by the tumors. Nonfunctional tumors account for at least 15–20% of pancreatic endocrine tumors and tend to present with symptoms owing to large tumor mass or metastatic disease. Malignancy cannot be diagnosed on the basis of the histologic appearance of pancreatic endocrine tumors. Instead, malignancy is determined by the presence of metastases or local invasion beyond the pancreas. Insulinomas are most commonly benign tumors, gastrinomas are malignant in approximately 60% of cases, and almost all other types, including nonfunctioning tumors, are malignant in most cases. The liver is the most common organ for metastatic spread. There is also a modest propensity for splenic metastases.

Tumors are moderately low in signal intensity on T1-weighted fat-suppressed images; demonstrate homogeneous, ring, or diffuse heterogeneous enhancement on immediate post-gadolinium gradient echo; and are

(a)

(b)

(c)

(d)

(e)

(f)

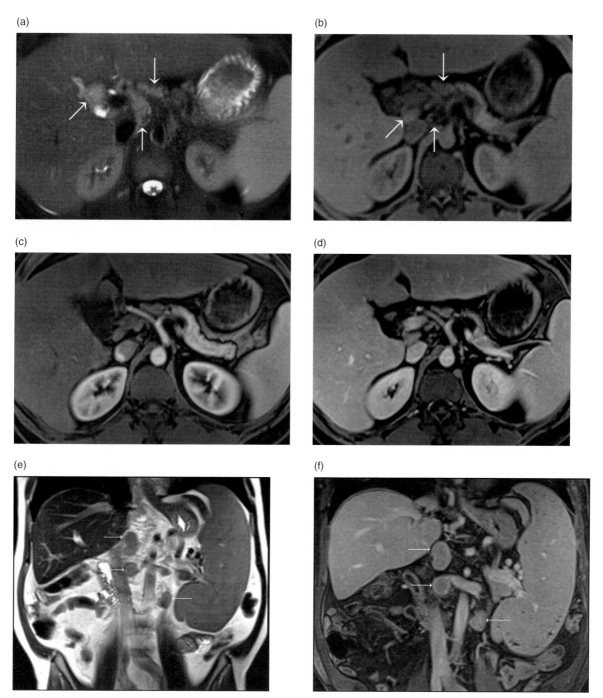

Figure 7.9 Demonstration of lymph nodes in MR imaging. Axial T2-weighted fat-suppressed single-shot echo-train spin-echo
(a), T1-weighted fat-suppressed 3D gradient echo (b), immediate post-gadolinium (c), and interstitial phase post-gadolinium (d) T1-weighted
fat-suppressed 3D gradient echo images. Lymph nodes appear hyperintense on the T2-weighted image and slightly hypointense on T1-
weighted image (arrows). In the region of porta hepatis, the lymph nodes are usually more apparent on the T2-weighted fat-suppressed image
due to the greater contrast between high-signal intensity nodes and low-signal-intensity liver. Coronal T2-weighted single-shot echo-train
spin-echo (e) and interstitial phase post-gadolinium T1-weighted fat-suppressed 3D gradient echo (f) images in a second patient.
Retroperitoneal lymph nodes can be evaluated on coronal images, particularly on the high-quality images acquired at 3T. Note in this case
the large metastatic lymph nodes in the retroperitoneum (arrows; e and f).

(a)

(b)

(c)

(d)

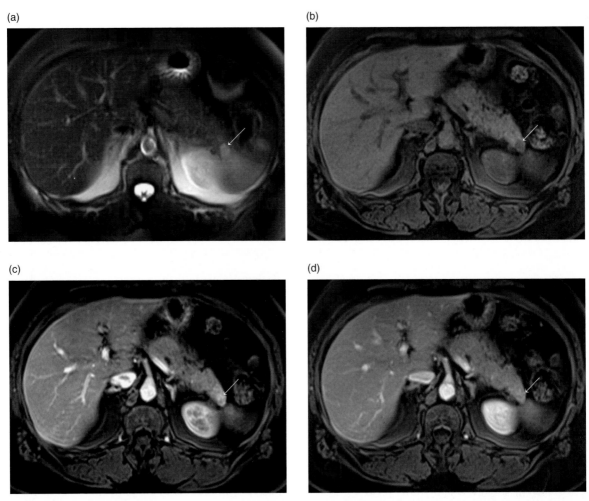

Figure 7.10 Small pancreatic endocrine tumor (insulinoma). Axial T2-weighted fat-suppressed single-shot echo-train spin-echo (a), T1-weighted fat-suppressed 3D gradient echo (b), immediate post-gadolinium (c), and interstitial phase post-gadolinium (d) T1-weighted fat-suppressed 3D gradient echo images. A small nodular lesion is detected in the tip of the pancreatic tail (arrow), which demonstrates homogeneous high signal intensity on the T2-weighted image and low signal on the T1-weighted image. The lesion is hypervascular, displaying diffuse and slightly heterogeneous enhancement on the immediate post-gadolinium image (c). There is homogeneous enhancement on the interstitial phase post-gadolinium image (d), in which the lesion is isointense to background pancreatic parenchyma.

moderately high in signal intensity on T2-weighted fat-suppressed images [10] (Figure 7.10).

Features that distinguish most pancreatic endocrine tumors from ductal adenocarcinomas include high signal intensity on T2-weighted images, increased homogeneous enhancement on immediate post-gadolinium images, hypervascular liver metastases, lack of pancreatic ductal obstruction, and lack of vascular encasement by tumor. The lack of ductal obstruction accounts for the generally normal signal of the pancreas on noncontrast T1-weighted images. In contrast to the frequent occurrence of venous thrombosis in pancreatic ductal adenocarcinoma, thrombosis is rare in the setting of pancreatic endocrine tumor. Peritoneal metastasis and/or regional lymph node enlargement, characteristic features of pancreatic ductal adenocarcinoma, are generally not present in pancreatic endocrine tumors.

Gastrinomas

Gastrinomas occur most frequently in the region of the head of the pancreas including pancreatic head, duodenum, stomach, and lymph nodes in a territory termed the gastrinoma triangle. The anatomical boundaries of the triangle are the porta hepatis as the superior point of the triangle and the second

(a)

(b)

(c)

(d)

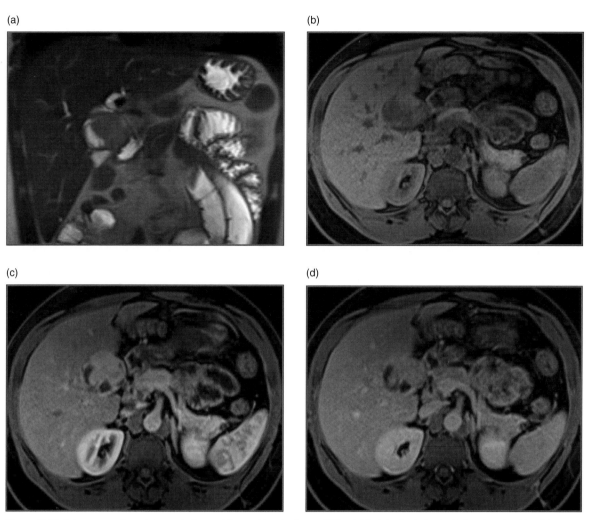

Figure 7.11 Extra-pancreatic gastrinoma in the gastrinoma triangle. Coronal T2-weighted single-shot echo-train spin-echo (a), axial T1-weighted fat-suppressed 3D gradient echo (b), immediate post-gadolinium (c) and interstitial phase post-gadolinium (d) T1-weighted fat-suppressed 3D gradient echo images. There is a lobulated mass at the gastrinoma triangle, pathologically proven as an extra-pancreatic gastrinoma, with slightly high signal intensity on the T2-weighted image (a) and low signal intensity on the T1-weighted image (b). The mass is hypervascular, with intense enhancement on immediate post-gadolinium (c) and delayed fading (d).

and third parts of the duodenum forming the base (Figure 7.11). The Zollinger–Ellison syndrome is defined by the clinical triad of pancreatic islet cell gastrinoma, gastric hypersecretion, and intractable peptic ulcer disease. Ulcers located in the postbulbar region of the duodenum or in the jejunum, particularly if multiple, suggest the diagnosis of a gastrinoma. Although gastrinomas are usually solitary, multiple gastrinomas may occur, especially in the setting of multiple endocrine neoplasia syndrome, type 1. Gastrinomas are not as frequently hypervascular as insulinomas. Gastrinomas are low in signal intensity on T1-weighted fat-suppressed images and high in signal intensity on

T2-weighted fat-suppressed images, demonstrating a peripheral ring-like enhancement on immediate post-gadolinium gradient echo images. These imaging features are observed in the primary lesion and in hepatic metastases. Gastrinomas may occur outside the pancreas, and T2-weighted fat-suppressed images are particularly effective at detecting these high-signal-intensity tumors in a background of suppressed fat.

Insulinomas

Insulinomas are one of the most common pancreatic endocrine tumors and are frequently functionally active. Tumors frequently come to clinical attention

(a)

(b)

(c)

(d)

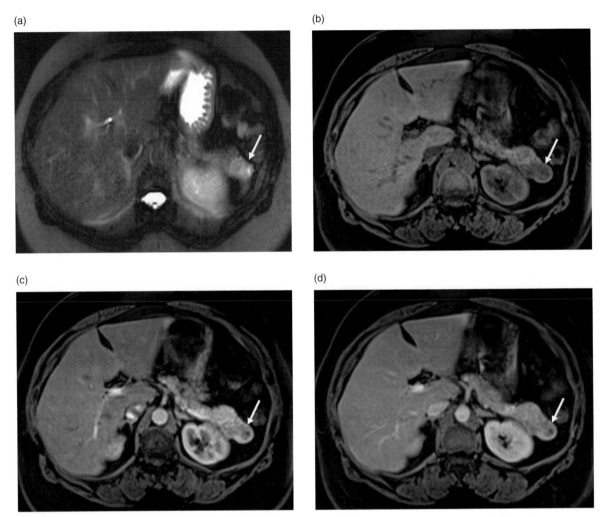

Figure 7.12 Insulinoma in the pancreatic tail. Axial T2-weighted fat-suppressed single-shot echo-train spin-echo (a), T1-weighted fat-suppressed 3D gradient echo (b), immediate post-gadolinium (c) and interstitial phase post-gadolinium (d) T1-weighted fat-suppressed 3D gradient echo images. Note a lobulated mass (arrow) with high signal intensity on the T2-weighted image, low signal intensity on the T1-weighted image, and significant enhancement on post-contrast images mainly on the hepatic arterial dominant phase (c).

when they are small (< 2 cm) because of the severity of the symptoms. Because of the frequently small size and hypervascularity of these tumors at presentation, our preference is to image these patients at 3T. In addition to the heightened ability to detect small lesions, the greater sensitivity to gadolinium enhancement at 3T render this field strength optimal [3]. Patients present with signs and symptoms of hypoglycemia. Insulinomas are usually richly vascular. Angiography has been reported as superior to CT in detecting these tumors because of their small size and increased vascularity. Gadolinium-enhanced MR imaging, especially at 3T, may be superior to angiography for the detection of these tumors, reflecting the

greater number of different types of data acquisition with MR imaging and the high sensitivity for contrast enhancement.

Insulinomas are low in signal intensity on T1-weighted images and high in signal intensity on T2-weighted images. They are well shown on T1-weighted fat-suppressed images. Small insulinomas typically enhance homogeneously on immediate post-gadolinium gradient echo images. Larger tumors, measuring more than 2 cm in diameter, often show ring enhancement (Figure 7.12). Liver metastases from insulinomas typically have peripheral ring-like enhancement, although small metastases tend to enhance homogeneously.

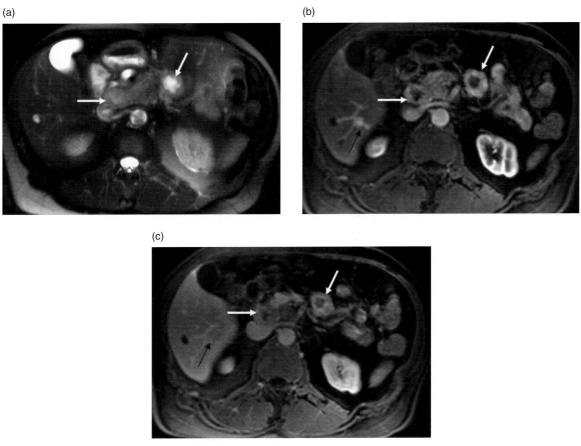

Figure 7.13 Nonfunctioning islet cell tumor. Axial T2-weighted fat-suppressed single-shot echo-train spin-echo image (a), T1-weighted fat-suppressed 3D gradient echo image acquired in the hepatic arterial dominant phase (b) and in the early hepatic venous phase (c) post-gadolinium. A nonfunctioning islet cell tumor (white thick arrow; a–c) is located in both the pancreatic head and in the pancreatic body. Both contain central necrosis. There is also a hypervascular liver metastasis (black arrow; b, c) showing intense enhancement in the hepatic arterial dominant phase and fading in the early hepatic venous phase. Note the liver cyst located in the right lobe of the liver.

Glucagonoma, somatostatinoma, ACTHoma, and VIPoma

These tumors are considerably rarer than insulinomas or gastrinomas. They are usually malignant, with liver metastases present at the time of diagnosis. The primary pancreatic tumors of glucagonoma and somatostatinoma are large and heterogeneous on MR images. They are usually moderately low in signal intensity on T1-weighted fat-suppressed images and moderately high in signal intensity on T2-weighted fat-suppressed images, enhancing heterogeneously on immediate post-gadolinium images. Liver metastases are generally heterogeneous in size and shape, unlike gastrinoma metastases, which are typically uniform. Metastases possess irregular peripheral rims of intense enhancement on immediate post-gadolinium gradient echo images. Peripheral spoke-wheel enhancement may be observed in liver metastases on immediate post-gadolinium images. ACTHomas may present with a large, heterogeneous enhancing primary tumor and small, hypervascular liver metastases. VIPoma may have a characteristic appearance of a small primary tumor despite large and extensive liver metastases.

Pancreatic endocrine tumors: nonfunctioning, untyped, or uncategorized

These tumors do not receive a specific designation when special immunohistochemical stains or serum assays are negative. Tumors are generally large at presentation because they are clinically silent. The imaging appearance of these tumors resembles glucagonomas and somatostatinomas. Liver metastases are generally present at the time of diagnosis (Figure 7.13).

(a)

(b)

(c)

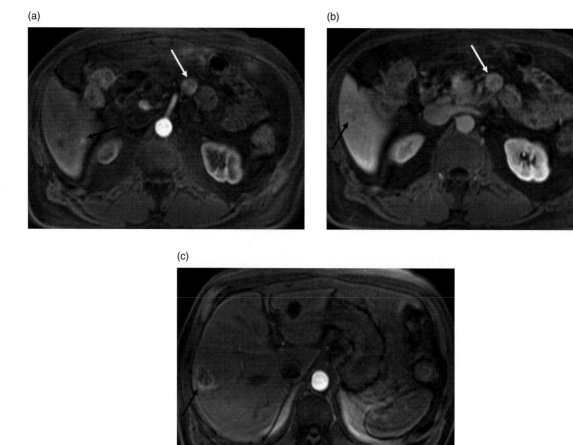

Figure 7.14 Carcinoid tumor of the pancreas with liver metastasis. Axial T1-weighted fat-suppressed 3D gradient echo image acquired in the hepatic arterial dominant phase (a, c) and in the early hepatic venous phase (b) post-gadolinium. There is an exophytic nodule in the body of the pancreas with intense heterogeneous enhancement (white arrow; a, b). There are also hypervascular metastases (black arrow; a–c) in the liver. Note that there is a cyst in the left liver lobe.

Carcinoid tumors

Rarely, carcinoid tumors may originate in the pancreas. Carcinoid tumors are generally large at presentation, with coexistent liver metastases. Focal and diffuse involvements of the pancreas have been observed. Tumors are generally mildly hypointense on T1 and moderately hyperintense on T2 and show diffuse heterogeneous enhancement on immediate post-gadolinium images [10] (Figure 7.14). Enhancement of the primary tumor may be mild, despite extensive enhancement of liver metastases.

Cystic neoplasms

Pancreatic cystic neoplasms generally arise from the exocrine component of the gland. Although secondary cystic change can be seen in most types of pancreatic neoplasms, cystic pancreatic neoplasms are characterized by their dominant cystic configuration.

Serous cystadenoma (microcystic adenoma)

Serous cystadenoma is a benign neoplasm characterized by numerous tiny serous fluid-filled cysts. Serous cystadenomas are usually microcystic and multilocular and consist of multiple small cysts less than 1 cm in diameter (Figure 7.15). Uncommonly, serous cystadenomas may be macrocystic (cysts measurement, 1–8 cm) including multilocular, oligolocular, or unilocular subtypes. This tumor has an increased association with von Hippel–Lindau disease.

Microcystic serous cystadenoma is typically found in women older than 60 years with nonspecific

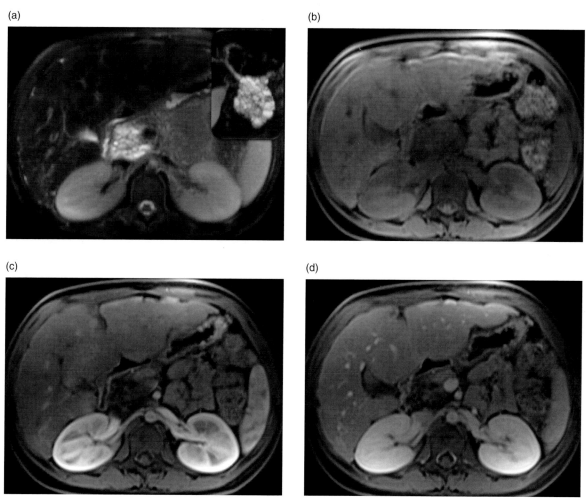

Figure 7.15 Serous cystadenoma. Axial T2-weighted fat-suppressed single-shot echo-train spin-echo image with a cropped maximal-intensity-projection (MIP) coronal cholangiopancreatography image superposed on right top corner (a), axial T1-weighted fat-suppressed 3D gradient echo image obtained in the pre-contrast phase (b), in the hepatic arterial dominant phase (c), and in the early hepatic venous phase (d) post-gadolinium. Note a complex microcystic lesion in the head of the pancreas. There are multiple fine septations with a honeycombed appearance.

complaints of abdominal pain or weight loss or more commonly as an incidental finding. Typical serous cystadenomas are composed of multiple cysts varying in size from 0.2 cm to 2.0 cm, and the size of the tumors ranges in greatest dimension from 1.4 cm to 27 cm. A central stellate scar is commonly present; the central scar may represent compressed contiguous cyst walls of centrally located cysts. Internally, the cyst has a honeycombed appearance compatible with innumerable cysts. On MR images, the tumors are well defined and do not demonstrate invasion of fat or adjacent organs. On T2-weighted images, the small cysts and intervening septations may be well shown

as a cluster of small grape-like high-signal-intensity cysts. This appearance is more clearly shown on breath-hold or breathing-independent sequences such as single-shot echo-train spin-echo because the thin septations blur with longer non-breath-hold sequence. Relatively thin uniform septations and absence of infiltration of adjacent organs and structures are features that distinguish serous cystadenoma from serous cystadenocarcinoma. Tumor septations usually enhance minimally with gadolinium on early and late post-contrast images, although moderate enhancement on early post-contrast images may occur. Delayed enhancement of the central scar may occasionally be observed and is more typical of large tumors. Delayed enhancement of the central scar on post-gadolinium images is apparent in larger tumors, and this enhancement pattern is typical for fibrous tissue in general.

Macrocystic or oligocystic serous cystadenoma is a variant of serous cystadenoma that is very difficult to differentiate from mucinous cystadenoma. Location in the pancreatic head, lobulated contour, and lack of wall enhancement have been reported to be specific for macrocystic serous cystadenoma in comparison with mucinous cystic tumor [11].

Mucinous cystic neoplasm (mucinous cystadenoma/ cystadenocarcinoma)

Mucinous cystic neoplasms are the most common cystic tumors of the pancreas. The large cystic spaces are lined by tall, mucin-producing columnar cells. Mucinous cystic neoplasms may be unilocular or multilocular and are commonly detected only after achieving a large size. Solid papillary excrescences sometimes protrude from the wall into the interior of these tumors. The absence of excrescences does not exclude malignancy. These tumors are divided into benign (mucinous cystadenoma), borderline, and malignant (mucinous cystadenocarcinoma). However, at many institutions, all cases of mucinous cystic neoplasms are interpreted as mucinous cystadenocarcinomas of low-grade malignant potential to reinforce the need for complete surgical resection and close clinical follow-up [12]. Mucinous cystic neoplasms occur more frequently in women, and approximately 50% occur in patients between the ages of 40 and 60 years. These tumors usually are located in the body and tail of the pancreas. Of these tumors, 10% may have scattered calcifications. When the tumors are frankly malignant, there is a great propensity for invasion of local organs and tissues. On gadolinium-enhanced T1-weighted fat-suppressed images, large, irregular cystic spaces separated by septa are demonstrated. Cyst walls and septations are often thicker in mucinous cystadenocarcinomas than those of mucinous cystadenomas. Mucinous cystadenomas are well circumscribed, and they show no evidence of metastases or invasion of adjacent tissues (Figure 7.16). Mucinous cystadenomas described pathologically as having borderline malignant potential may be very large but may not show imaging or gross evidence of metastases or local invasion. Histopathologically, these tumors show moderate epithelial dysplasia. Mucinous

cystadenocarcinoma may be a very locally aggressive malignancy with extensive invasion of adjacent tissues and organs. Absence of demonstration of tumor invasion into surrounding tissue does not, however, exclude malignancy (Figure 7.17). The presence of solid component is also suggestive of malignancy. The higher inherent soft tissue contrast of MR imaging compared with CT results in superior differentiation between microcystic and macrocystic cystadenomas because of sharp definition of cysts that permits evaluation of cyst size and margins. Breathing-independent T2-weighted images are particularly effective at defining the cysts.

Mucin produced by these tumors may result in high signal intensity on T1- and T2-weighted images of the primary tumor and liver metastases. Liver metastases are generally hypervascular and have intense ring enhancement on immediate post-gadolinium images. Metastases are commonly cystic and may contain mucin, which results in mixed low and high signal intensity on T1- and T2-weighted images.

Intraductal papillary mucinous neoplasms (IPMNs)

Intraductal papillary mucinous neoplasm arises in the epithelial cells of pancreatic duct. It has been increasingly diagnosed on various imaging modalities. Histologically, the lesions can represent a wide spectrum of abnormalities, which include simple hyperplasia, adenoma, borderline lesions, and adenocarcinoma. This spectrum of abnormalities may coexist even within the same lesion. Benign lesions such as hyperplasia and adenoma may progress to carcinoma. Owing to its mucin-producing nature, the involved pancreatic duct is filled with mucinous gel-like material and results in varying degrees of ductal dilation. Morphologically, IPMNs can be classified as main duct, branch duct, or combined type, which shows features of both main duct and branch duct types.

Main duct-type IPMN

The main duct type of IPMN is characterized by a dilation of main pancreatic duct of more than 1 cm in diameter, abundant mucin production, and papillary excrescence arising from ductal epithelium. This tumor can be subclassified as diffuse and segmental. Whereas diffuse tumors involve the entire main duct, segmental tumors involve one or more segments of main duct. In general, this type of IPMN is associated with higher prevalence of carcinoma than the branch duct type. Given that these tumors cause large volume

(a)

(b)

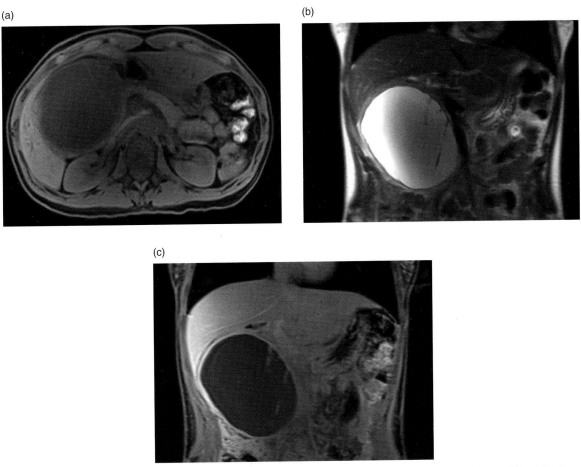

(c)

Figure 7.16 Mucinous cystadenoma. Axial noncontrast T1-weighted fat-suppressed 3D gradient echo image (a). Coronal T2-weighted single-shot echo-train spin-echo (b) and interstitial phase post-gadolinium T1-weighted fat-suppressed 3D gradient echo (c) images. A large well-defined cystic mass arises from the head of the pancreas, displaying low signal intensity on the T1-weighted image (a), high signal intensity on the T2-weighted image (b), and enhancement of septations on the post-gadolinium image (c). There is no evidence of tumor nodules, invasion of adjacent tissue, or liver metastases. Mucinous cystadenoma is potentially a low-grade malignant neoplasm.

of mucin, it is natural that the main pancreatic duct may elaborate copious mucin. Clinically, direct visualization of this phenomenon on endoscopic retrograde cholangiopancreatography can confirm IPMN.

With MR imaging, a prominently dilated main pancreatic duct is noted especially on T2-weighted and MRCP images. Frequently, papillary-growing mural nodules within a dilated main pancreatic duct are demonstrated on post-gadolinium images. Surgical resection is the treatment of choice and a remnant margin free of IPMN should be obtained.

Branch duct-type IPMN

The branch duct type of IPMN involves predominantly side branch ducts and appears as a pleomorphic

cyst. This lesion consists of three or more cysts, including oval, tubular, or clubbed finger-like cysts [13]. This lesion is sometimes described as a cluster of grapes appearance. Typically, the branch duct type of IPMN occurs in the head of the pancreas. This type of IPMN shows an indolent benign course as compared with the main duct type. Direct communication of the lesion with the main pancreatic duct is another important feature that is suggestive of the branch duct type of IPMN. An MR imaging with MRCP images has advantages over multi-detector row CT in the evaluation of IPMN, that is, it has superior soft tissue resolution and allows superior predictability with respect to the ductal communication of the lesion (Figure 7.18) [13]. Thinner section acquisition on

101

(a)

(b)

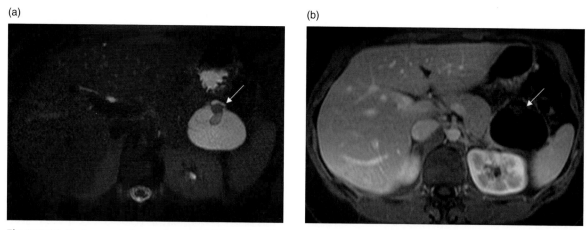

Figure 7.17 Mucinous cystadenocarcinoma. Axial T2-weighted fat-suppressed single-shot echo-train spin-echo (a) and early hepatic venous phase post-gadolinium T1-weighted fat-suppressed 3D gradient echo (b) images demonstrate a large cystic mass originating from the pancreatic tail. It has a complex structure with thin septations and internal cystic structures (arrows). Due to the high protein content these internal cystic structures have low signal on the T2-weighted image and intermediate signal on the post-gadolinium image. While the internal cystic structures do not show appreciable enhancement, the wall of the large cyst shows enhancement.

(a)

(b)

(c)

(d)

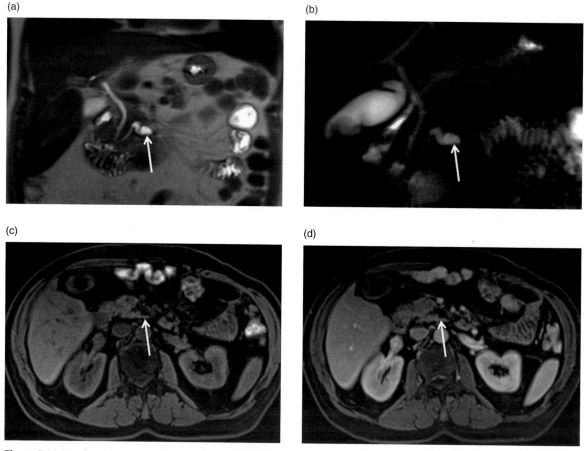

Figure 7.18 Intraductal papillary mucinous neoplasm (IPMN) – branch duct type. Coronal T2-weighted single-shot echo-train spin-echo (a), thick section MRCP (b), fat-suppressed T1-weighted 3D gradient echo (c) and interstitial-phase post-gadolinium fat-suppressed T1-weighted 3D gradient echo (d) images. There is a branch duct type of IPMN in the pancreatic head, which appears as a nonenhancing amorphic cystic mass (arrow), connecting to the pancreatic duct.

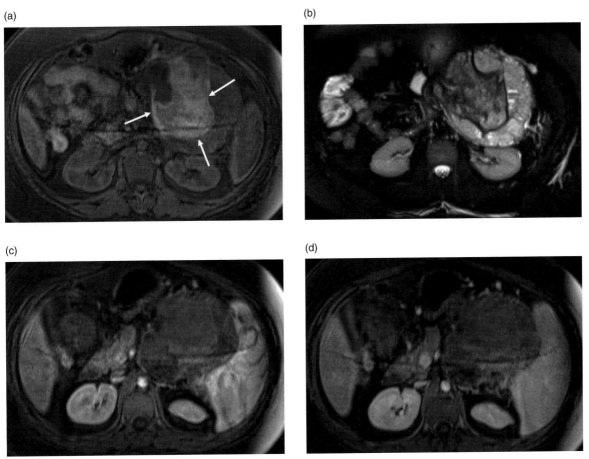

Figure 7.19 Solid pseudopapillary tumor. Axial T1-weighted fat-suppressed 3D gradient echo (a), T2-weighted fat-suppressed single-shot echo-train spin-echo (b), immediate post-gadolinium (c), and interstitial phase post-gadolinium (d) T1-weighted fat-suppressed 3D gradient echo images. A 23-year-old woman with a large heterogeneous mass arising from the pancreatic tail. The tumor contains hemorrhage in the central portion (arrows; a), which appears predominantly hyperintense on the noncontrast T1-weighted image (a) and hypointense on the T2-weighted image (b).

3T systems may show more clearly the communication between the pancreatic duct and the IPMN.

A branch duct type of IPMN that is less than 3 cm in asymptomatic patients is usually benign and grows very slowly. If there are no imaging features concerning for malignancy (presence of solid component, main pancreatic duct dilation, common bile duct dilation, or lymphadenopathy), a branch duct type of IPMN can be safely followed up. In our clinical experience, annual follow-up with repeated MR imaging examination could be the best option in patients with the branch duct type of IPMN compared with other imaging modalities, such as multidetector row CT or endoscopic ultrasound, especially in elderly patients.

Solid pseudopapillary tumor

Generally speaking, this tumor is regarded as benign in nature, with a few examples showing low malignant potential. Solid pseudopapillary tumors mainly occur in women between the second and fourth decades of life [14]. The gross morphologic appearance of this tumor is a large encapsulated mass, consisting of cystic, solid, and hemorrhagic components [14]. The capsule and the peripheral portion of the tumor may contain calcifications. MR images usually show a large well-encapsulated mass, in which there are regions of hemorrhagic degeneration that may appear as fluid-debris levels or high signal intensity on T1-weighted images and low or heterogeneous signal intensity on T2-weighted images (Figure 7.19). According to one report describing MR features, a thick fibrous capsule is seen as a rim of low signal intensity on T2-weighted images. On gadolinium-enhanced dynamic MR imaging, solid components of the tumor show early heterogeneous enhancement with gradual fill-in.

Inflammatory disease

Pancreatitis

Pancreatitis may occur secondary to chronic alcoholism, gallstones, hypercalcemia, hyperlipoproteinemia, blunt abdominal trauma, penetrating peptic ulcer disease, viral infections (most frequently Epstein–Barr), and certain drugs. Pancreatitis can also be hereditary and predisposition may be inherited as an autosomal dominant trait.

Acute pancreatitis

Acute pancreatitis is defined as an acute inflammatory condition typically presenting with abdominal pain and associated with elevations in pancreatic enzymes (particularly amylase and lipase). Acute pancreatitis arises in the majority of cases secondary to alcoholism or cholelithiasis [15]. Alcohol-related acute pancreatitis most frequently results in acute recurrent pancreatitis, whereas gallstone-related pancreatitis typically results in a single attack. The passage of biliary sludge may also cause acute pancreatitis.

Acute pancreatitis results from the exudation of fluid containing activated proteolytic enzymes into the interstitium of the pancreas and leakage of this fluid into surrounding tissue. Trypsin is suspected to be the primary enzyme involved in the coagulative necrosis. Pathologically, acute pancreatitis is characterized by a spectrum of morphologic features, which may be patchy or diffuse. In mild cases, edema predominates, producing so-called edematous or interstitial pancreatitis. There is scattered peripancreatic fat necrosis without parenchymatous or acinar necrosis. In severe cases, extensive pancreatic and peripancreatic fat necrosis, parenchymal necrosis, and hemorrhage occur. In its most devastating form, severe acute pancreatitis may produce an organ that resembles oily mud, where degenerative tissue, fat, and hemorrhage congeal.

Patients with pancreatitis, especially severe disease, may be unable to comply with breath-holding instructions, for example they may be intubated. The superiority of snapshot techniques at 3T renders 3T the preferable field strength to image patients who have reduced breath-holding capacity. The standard single-shot T1-weighted sequence we employ is water excitation magnetization-prepared rapid acquisition gradient echo (WE-MPRAGE). These types of sequences have intrinsically low signal-to-noise, which explains why image quality is superior at 3T [16] (Figure 7.20).

The signal intensity features of the pancreas in uncomplicated mild acute pancreatitis resemble those of normal pancreatic tissue. The pancreas is high in signal intensity on pre-contrast T1-weighted fat-suppressed images and enhances in a normal uniform fashion on immediate post-gadolinium images, reflecting a normal capillary blush (Figure 7.21). The acutely inflamed pancreas shows either focal or diffuse enlargement, which may be subtle. Peripancreatic fluid is well shown on noncontrast or immediate post-gadolinium non-fat-suppressed gradient echo images and appears as low-signal-intensity strands of fluid or fluid collections in a background of high-signal-intensity fat. T2-weighted single-shot echo-train spin-echo imaging employing fat suppression is the most sensitive technique for showing small-volume peripancreatic fluid, which appears as high signal in a background of intermediate- to low-signal pancreas and low-signal fat (Figures 7.20 and 7.21). As a result, MR imaging is sensitive for the detection of subtle changes of acute pancreatitis, particularly minor peripancreatic inflammatory changes even in the setting of a morphologically normal pancreas. CT imaging examinations appear normal in 15–30% of patients with clinical features of acute pancreatitis. The sensitivity of MR imaging exceeds that of CT imaging, suggesting a role for MR imaging in the evaluation of patients with suspected acute pancreatitis and negative CT imaging examination. As the extent of pancreatitis becomes more severe, the pancreas develops a heterogeneous appearance on pre-contrast T1-weighted fat-suppressed images and enhances in a more heterogeneous, diminished fashion on immediate post-gadolinium images.

The percentage of pancreatic necrosis has been considered an important prognostic indicator in patients with acute pancreatitis. Dynamic gadolinium-enhanced gradient echo images may be useful for this determination because MR imaging is very sensitive for the demonstration of the presence or absence of gadolinium enhancement. Complications of acute pancreatitis such as hemorrhage, pseudocyst formation, or abscess are clearly shown on MR imaging (Figure 7.22). Hemorrhagic fluid collections

(a) (b)

(c) (d)

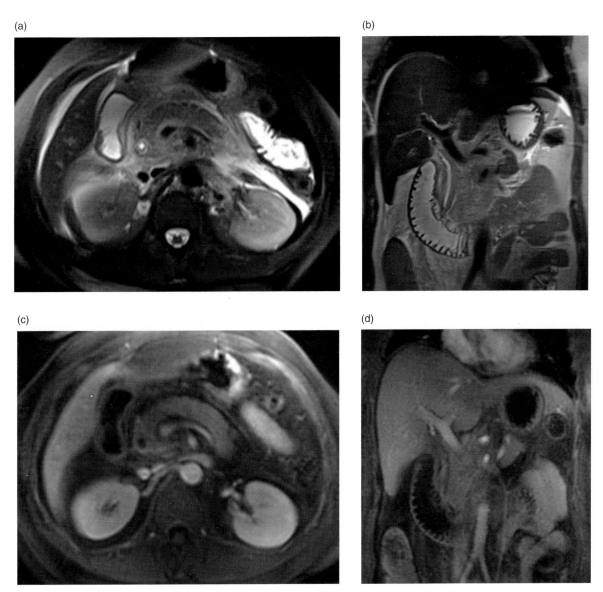

Figure 7.20 Evaluation of pancreatitis in non-cooperative patients. Axial (a) and coronal (b) T2-weighted fat-suppressed single-shot echo-train spin-echo images. Axial (c) and coronal (d) post-gadolinium water excitation magnetization-prepared rapid acquisition gradient echo (WE-MPRAGE) images. This patient had clinically severe acute pancreatitis and was unable to adequately hold his breath. It was possible to obtain very high-quality images using these single-shot techniques. The pancreas has mildly heterogeneous and increased signal intensity on T2-weighted images, with a significant amount of fluid in peripancreatic regions and pararenal spaces (a, b). On the post-contrast WE-MPRAGE images (c, d) it was possible to obtain a satisfactory homogeneous enhancement of the pancreatic parenchyma, thus excluding pancreatic necrosis.

are high in signal intensity on T1-weighted fat-suppressed images, and depiction of hemorrhage is superior on MR images compared to CT images. Martin *et al.* demonstrated correlation between the extent of high signal on noncontrast T1-weighted fat-suppressed SGE and severity of acute pancreatitis, where high signal correlated with hemorrhagic changes [17]. Simple pseudocysts are low in signal intensity or signal void in a background of normal-signal-intensity pancreatic tissue on both non-contrast non-fat-suppressed gradient echo and T1-weighted fat-suppressed gradient echo images. Extrapancreatic pseudocysts are well shown on breath-hold gradient echo images because of high

(a)

(b)

(c)

(d)

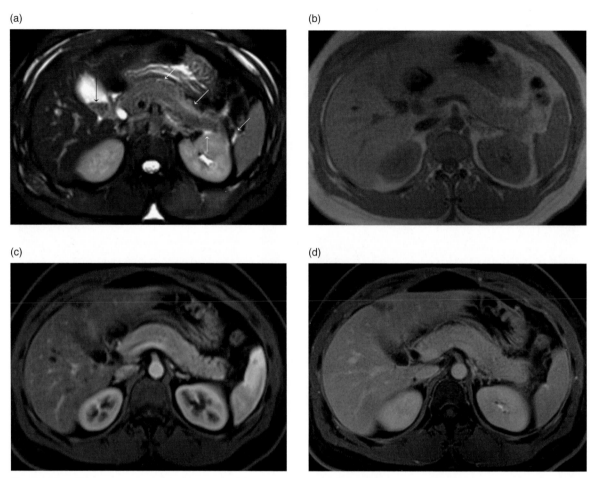

Figure 7.21 Mild acute pancreatitis. Axial T2-weighted fat-suppressed single-shot echo-train spin-echo image (a), T1-weighted non-fat-suppressed gradient echo image (b), post-gadolinium T1-weighted fat-suppressed 3D gradient echo images in the hepatic arterial dominant phase (HADP) (c) and in the interstitial phase (d). There is a small amount of fluid in peripancreatic regions, more clearly seen on the T2-weighted image (white arrows; a). The pancreatic parenchyma has normal signal intensity on the noncontrast T1-weighted image (b) and a normal enhancement on the post-contrast images (c, d). These findings are consistent with mild acute pancreatitis. Note multiple small calculi in the gallbladder on the T2-weighted image (black arrow; a).

contrast with high-signal-intensity fat. Image acquisition in multiple planes permits determination of pseudocyst location in relation to various organs and structures. Pseudocyst walls enhance minimally on early post-gadolinium images and show progressively intense enhancement on 5-minute post-contrast images, consistent with the appearance of fibrous tissue. Simple pseudocysts are relatively homogeneous and high in signal intensity on T2-weighted images. Pseudocysts complicated by necrotic debris, hemorrhage, or infection are heterogeneous in signal intensity on T2-weighted images. Proteinaceous fluid tends to layer in a gradation of concentration with low-signal-intensity concentrated proteinaceous material

in the dependent portion of the cyst. Necrotic material may appear as irregularly shaped regions of low signal intensity in the pseudocyst. This information may provide both therapeutic and prognostic information because pseudocysts that contain necrotic material may not respond to simple percutaneous drainage and thus require open debridement. Breathing-independent T2-weighted sequences such as single-shot echo-train spin-echo may be useful to evaluate these pseudocyst collections, not only because they are the most effective at demonstrating the complexity of fluid but also because many of these patients are very debilitated and unable to cooperate with breath-holding instructions.

(a)

(b)

(c)

(d)

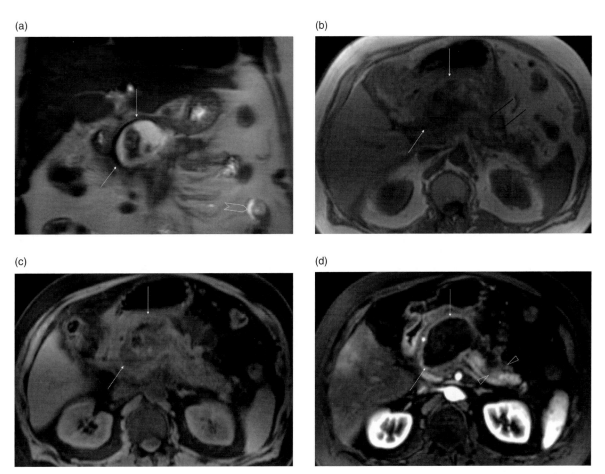

Figure 7.22 Hemorrhagic necrotizing pancreatitis. Coronal T2-weighted single-shot echo-train spin-echo (a), pre-contrast T1-weighted gradient echo (b), pre-contrast T1-weighted fat-suppressed gradient echo (c), and hepatic arterial dominant phase post-gadolinium fat-suppressed T1-weighted 3D gradient echo (d) images. A large pseudocyst (white arrows; a–d) containing blood product is located in the pancreatic head and body region. The blood products show low signal on the T2-weighted image (a) but high signal on the T1-weighted pre-contrast images (b, c). There is mild free fluid (hollow arrow; A) in the abdomen. Peripancreatic tissue is low in signal intensity on pre-contrast images. There are foci of blood products (black arrows; b) and necrosis (arrowheads; d) in the pancreatic parenchyma. Note the associated gastric mucosal inflammation and hepatic inflammation, which are characterized by increased enhancement (d).

Chronic pancreatitis

Chronic pancreatitis is defined pathologically by continuous or relapsing inflammation of the organ leading to irreversible morphologic injury and typically leading to impairment of function. Chronic pancreatitis is acquired either as a disease process distinct from acute pancreatitis or as a complication of repeated attacks of acute pancreatitis. There is a strong association between alcoholism and the development of chronic pancreatitis [18]. Obstruction of the pancreatic duct from various causes, including pancreatic ductal cancer, results in chronic pancreatitis [18]. Acute pancreatitis secondary to gallstone disease rarely results in chronic pancreatitis.

Chronic pancreatitis is associated with decreased endocrine as well as exocrine function [18]. Patients with chronic pancreatitis have an increased risk of developing pancreatic cancer.

Calcification, which is the pathognomonic feature of chronic pancreatitis on CT images, is a late occurrence following development of fibrosis and is observed in only half of these patients. CT imaging is not sensitive at detecting the early changes of fibrosis in chronic pancreatitis. Focal chronic pancreatitis may be difficult to distinguish from adenocarcinoma in the head of the pancreas because both entities may cause focal enlargement, obstruction of the common bile duct and pancreatic duct,

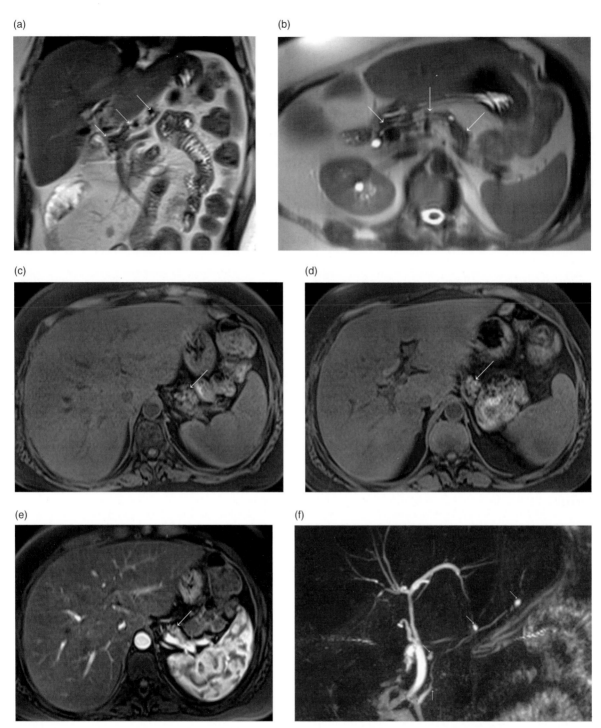

Figure 7.23 Chronic pancreatitis. Coronal (a) and oblique axial (b) T2-weighted single-shot echo-train spin-echo, axial pre-contrast T1-weighted fat-suppressed 3D gradient echo (c, d) images. Post-gadolinium T1-weighted fat-suppressed 3D gradient echo image in the hepatic arterial dominant phase (HADP) (e). Coronal thick-section MRCP (f). This patient is a 47-year-old man with a clinical history of recurrent pancreatitis. Compared to the normal pancreas demonstrated in Figure 7.1, this pancreas has an atrophic appearance (arrows; a–e). The signal intensity of the pancreatic parenchyma on the pre-contrast fat-suppressed T1-weighted images is slightly reduced (c, d). The pancreatic duct is slightly dilated and irregular, with some cystic side branch dilations (small arrows; f). Note also that there is hepatic steatosis.

atrophy of the tail of the pancreas, and obliteration of the fat plane around the SMA.

MR imaging may perform better than CT imaging at detecting changes of chronic pancreatitis in that MR imaging detects not only morphologic findings but also the presence of fibrosis. Fibrosis is shown by diminished signal intensity on T1-weighted fat-suppressed images and diminished heterogeneous enhancement on immediate post-gadolinium gradient echo images (Figure 7.23) [19]. Low signal intensity on T1-weighted fat-suppressed images reflects loss of the aqueous protein in the acini of the pancreas. Diminished enhancement on capillary-phase images reflects disruption of the normal capillary bed and increased chronic inflammation and fibrous tissue. Most cases of chronic pancreatitis show progressive parenchymal enhancement on 5-minute post-contrast images, reflecting the pattern of enhancement of fibrous tissue. Secretin-enhanced MRCP has been used for the evaluation of patients with pancreatic pathologies including chronic pancreatitis. Secretin induces pancreatic duct secretion. Therefore, it has been reported that it improves the visualization of pancreatic ductal system and associated pathologies. Secretin-MRCP has been reported to show early ductal changes (dilatations-strictures) associated with chronic pancreatitis. Secretin-MRCP has also been reported to evaluate and grade pancreatic exocrine function noninvasively. Following secretin stimulation, good duodenal filling should be present in the presence of normal exocrine function.

Autoimmune pancreatitis

Most patients presenting with chronic pancreatitis will have alcohol-related disease. In approximately 30% of patients, the nature and course of chronic pancreatitis are unclear, and these cases may be labeled idiopathic. A subgroup of these cases has been associated with autoimmune disorders such as Sjögren syndrome, primary biliary cirrhosis, and primary sclerosing cholangitis [20]. Histopathologic examination in cases of chronic nonalcoholic pancreatitis, including associated autoimmune disorders, shows periductal chronic inflammation and fibrosis. This process may result in obstruction or destruction of ducts. Recent studies underscore the importance of diagnosing cases of suspected autoimmune-related chronic pancreatitis because these disorders may have a salutary response to steroid therapy. Recent studies have described the MR appearance of autoimmune

chronic pancreatitis as characterized by enlarged pancreas with moderately decreased signal intensity on T1-weighted images, moderately high signal intensity on T2-weighted images, and delayed enhancement of the pancreatic parenchyma after gadolinium administration. Additional findings that may be observed in autoimmune pancreatitis include (1) capsule-like rim surrounding the diseased parenchyma that is hypointense on T2-weighted images and demonstrates delayed enhancement after gadolinium administration, (2) absence of parenchymal atrophy, (3) ductal dilation proximal to the site of stenosis, (4) absence of extra-pancreatic fluid, and (5) clear demarcation of the lesion.

References

1. Edelman RR. MR imaging of the pancreas: 1.5T versus 3T. *Magn Reson Imaging Clin N Am* 2007; **15**: 349–53.

2. Edelman RR, Salanitri G, Brand R, *et al.* Magnetic resonance imaging of the pancreas at 3.0 tesla: qualitative and quantitative comparison with 1.5 tesla. *Invest Radiol* 2006; **41**: 175–80.

3. Goncalves Neto JA, Altun E, Elazzazi M, *et al.* Enhancement of abdominal organs on hepatic arterial phase: quantitative comparison between 1.5- and 3.0-T magnetic resonance imaging. *Magn Reson Imaging* 2010; **28**: 47–55.

4. Jemal A, Siegel R, Ward E, *et al.* Cancer statistics, 2008. *CA Cancer J Clin* 2008; **58**: 71–96.

5. Elias J Jr, Semelka RC, Altun E, *et al.* Pancreatic cancer: correlation of MR findings, clinical features, and tumor grade. *J Magn Reson Imaging* 2007; **26**: 1556–63.

6. Kim JK, Altun E, Elias J Jr, *et al.* Focal pancreatic mass: distinction of pancreatic cancer from chronic pancreatitis using gadolinium-enhanced 3D-gradient echo MRI. *J Magn Reson Imaging* 2007; **26**: 313–22.

7. Semelka RC, Kelekis NL, Molina PL, *et al.* Pancreatic masses with inconclusive findings on spiral CT: is there a role for MRI? *J Magn Reson Imaging* 1996; **6**: 585–8.

8. Birchard KR, Semelka RC, Hyslop WB, *et al.* Suspected pancreatic cancer: evaluation by dynamic gadolinium-enhanced 3D gradient echo MRI. *AJR Am J Roentgenol* 2005; **185**: 700–3.

9. Oberg K, Eriksson B. Endocrine tumors of the pancreas. *Best Pract Res Clin Gastroenterol* 2005; **19**: 753–81.

10. Semelka RC, Custodio CM, Cem Balci N, *et al.* Neuroendocrine tumors of the pancreas: spectrum of

appearances on MRI. *J Magn Reson Imaging* 2000; **11**: 141–8.

11. Khurana B, Mortele KJ, Glickman J, *et al.* Macrocystic serous adenoma of the pancreas: radiologic-pathologic correlation. *AJR Am J Roentgenol* 2003; **181**: 119–23.

12. Buetow PC, Rao P, Thompson LD. From the archives of the AFIP. Mucinous cystic neoplasms of the pancreas: radiologic-pathologic correlation. *Radiographics* 1998; **18**: 433–49.

13. Song SJ, Lee JM, Kim YJ, *et al.* Differentiation of intraductal papillary mucinous neoplasms from other pancreatic cystic masses: comparison of multirow-detector CT and MR imaging using ROC analysis. *J Magn Reson Imaging* 2007; **26**: 86–93.

14. Choi JY, Kim MJ, Kim JH, *et al.* Solid pseudopapillary tumor of the pancreas: typical and atypical manifestations. *AJR Am J Roentgenol* 2006; **187**: W178–86.

15. Steinberg W, Tenner S. Acute pancreatitis. *N Engl J Med* 1994; **330**: 1198–210.

16. Altun E, Semelka RC, Dale BM, Elias J Jr. Water excitation MPRAGE: an alternative sequence for post-contrast imaging of the abdomen in noncooperative patients at 1.5 Tesla and 3.0 Tesla MRI. *J Magn Reson Imaging* 2008; **27**: 1146–54.

17. Martin DR, Karabulut N, Yang M, *et al.* High signal peripancreatic fat on fat-suppressed spoiled gradient echo imaging in acute pancreatitis: preliminary evaluation of the prognostic significance. *J Magn Reson Imaging* 2003; **18**: 49–58.

18. Steer ML, Waxman I, Freedman S. Chronic pancreatitis. *N Engl J Med* 1995; **332**: 1482–90.

19. Semelka RC, Shoenut JP, Kroeker MA, *et al.* Chronic pancreatitis: MR imaging features before and after administration of gadopentetate dimeglumine. *J Magn Reson Imaging* 1993; **3**: 79–82.

20. Irie H, Honda H, Baba S, *et al.* Autoimmune pancreatitis: CT and MR characteristics. *AJR Am J Roentgenol* 1998; **170**: 1323–7.

MR imaging of the adrenal glands

Daniele Marin and Elmar M. Merkle

Introduction

An adrenal "incidentaloma" is an adrenal mass, 1 cm or more in diameter, which is incidentally discovered during a radiologic examination performed for indications other than an evaluation for adrenal disease. With the widespread use of abdominal ultrasonography, multi-detector row computed tomography (MDCT), magnetic resonance (MR) imaging, and positron emission tomography (PET) the incidence of adrenal incidentalomas has substantially increased. According to recent studies, the overall frequency of adrenal masses is approximately 4% at abdominal MDCT [1], which compares favorably with the 6% prevalence rate reported in a large autopsy study [2]. Although the majority of adrenal incidentalomas are clinically benign adenomas, other frequently reported diagnoses include metastases, pheochromocytomas, and adrenocortical carcinomas. The differential diagnosis between benign and malignant adrenal masses has become a common dilemma, which is compounded in patients with known or suspected of having an extra-adrenal malignancy, where approximately 50% of incidentally detected adrenal lesions are metastatic disease [3].

With the widespread use of fast pulse sequences that allow breath-hold imaging of the abdomen during short acquisition times (less than 20 seconds), and substantial reduction in the cost per examination, MR imaging has been advocated by some as the modality of choice in the noninvasive work-up of focal adrenal lesions. Although MR imaging demonstrated high sensitivity for the detection of adrenal masses, lesion characterization remains challenging, thus explaining the less satisfactory specificity of this imaging test. Because morphologic criteria – which include lesion diameter, shape, texture, growth rate,

and contrast enhancement pattern – are often insufficient for adrenal lesion characterization, more functional imaging techniques have been investigated.

In this chapter, we discuss the role of current MR imaging techniques for the management of focal adrenal lesions at both 1.5T and 3T. The indications, major advantages, and shortcomings of different MR techniques are described and illustrated.

MR imaging techniques
Chemical shift MR imaging

Soon after its introduction to clinical MR imaging in the late 1980s, chemical shift MR imaging using a dual gradient echo (GRE) technique with in-phase (IP) and opposed-phase (OP) acquisitions became the method of choice for the characterization of adrenal lesions [4]. Similar to unenhanced CT densitometry, chemical shift MR imaging is a lipid-sensitive technique which exploits the fact that up to 70% of adrenal adenomas contain abundant intracellular fat (mainly cholesterol, fatty acids, and neutral fat), whereas almost all malignant lesions do not.

Using a chemical shift technique, the difference in precessional frequencies (expressed as parts per million of the resonance frequency of the static magnetic field B0) between water and fat protons causes periodic phase interference between fat and water signals, which manifests as an echo time-dependent oscillation of the signal intensity [4]. Depending on the selected echo time, the fat and water signals can either add constructively (IP acquisition) or cancel out (OP acquisition), yielding the classic fat/water cancellation artifact, also known as chemical shift artifact of the second kind [5]. This "artifact" can be seen on routine OP images of the abdomen as a signal void at the boundaries between fatty and nonfatty tissues

Body MR Imaging at 3 Tesla, ed. Ihab R. Kamel and Elmar M. Merkle. Published by Cambridge University Press.

(a)

(b)

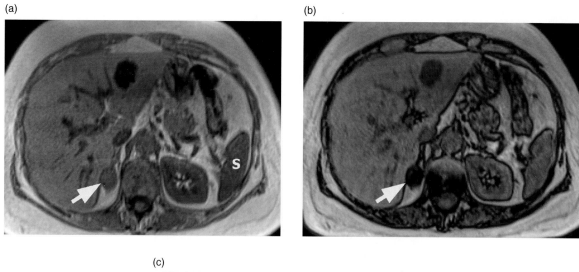

(c)

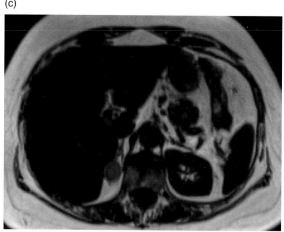

Figure 8.1 A 53-year-old man with incidentally detected adrenal adenoma. (a) Transverse T1-weighted gradient echo IP image at 3T (repetition time [ms]/echo time [ms], 4.5/2.5, 20° flip angle) shows a 2-cm, well-defined, right adrenal lesion (arrow), which demonstrates a signal intensity slightly higher than that of spleen (S) (internal reference organ). (b) T1-weighted gradient echo OP image at 3T (4.5/1.1, 20°) shows marked signal intensity loss of the lesion (arrow) compared with the IP image, a finding suggestive of intralesional fat. Lesion signal intensity is also markedly lower than that of spleen. (c) On the corresponding 2-point Dixon fat-only (FO) image, the lesion shows a signal intensity substantially higher than that of the liver and spleen, which corroborates the presence of intralesional fat.

(etching or India ink pattern) due to volume averaging in voxels containing similar amounts of fat and water signals. This phase-cancellation effect is not limited to the frequency-encoding direction, as in the case of the chemical shift artifact of the first kind, but may be seen in all pixels with similar amounts of water and fat. Because IP and OP images are displayed in a magnitude format, all phase information is lost. This approach, while efficiently reducing the adverse effects from magnet inhomogeneity, also leads to a serious ambiguity as to whether the fat or the water protons contribute the dominant signal within a voxel. Although this limitation can cause

problems in liver imaging and requires the application of time-consuming, phase-sensitive methods, there is evidence those adrenal adenomas contain less than 50% fat [6]. This leads to the general assumption that the fat fraction is always less than the water fraction in adrenal adenomas.

When a chemical shift technique is used to detect fat within an adrenal mass, a diffuse signal intensity loss on the OP image compared with the IP image is indicative of the coexistence of both fat and water signals, which favors a diagnosis of benign adrenal adenoma (Figure 8.1). Previous studies showed a linear inverse correlation between the net signal loss

(a) (b) (c)

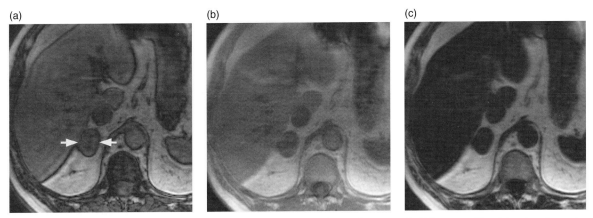

Figure 8.2 A 68-year-old man with surgically confirmed adrenal metastasis from colon cancer. (a, b) Transverse T1-weighted gradient echo (a) OP and (b) IP 3T MR images demonstrate a 2.5-cm, well-defined, right adrenal lesion (arrows), which shows no drop in signal intensity between IP and OP images. (c) On the corresponding FO image, the lesion's signal intensity is low, similar to that of the liver and spleen.

(a) (b)

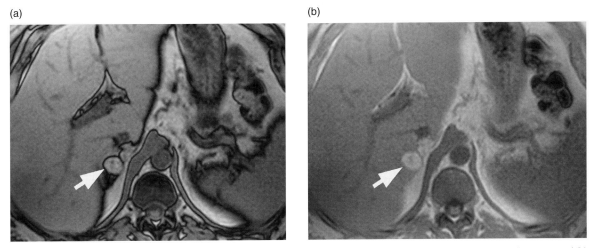

Figure 8.3 A 45-year-old female with incidentally detected adrenal myelolipoma. (a, b) Transverse T1-weighted gradient echo (a) OP and (b) IP 3T MR images demonstrate a 2-cm, well-defined, right adrenal lesion (arrow), which shows a signal intensity similar to that of the subcutaneous fat and higher than that of the liver and spleen. The lesion's signal intensity remains unchanged between IP and OP images.

on OP images and the percentage of fat in an adrenal lesion, with a maximal signal cancellation occurring when fat and water signals have equal intensity. The absence of a signal intensity loss on OP images, on the other hand, is suggestive of a dominant signal from a single proton species, either water or fat. This typically occurs in either malignant, non-fat-containing adrenal tumors, such as metastases or most primary malignant tumors (Figure 8.2), or purely fat-containing, benign adrenal tumors, such as myelolipomas (Figure 8.3). The relative signal intensity on IP images (low in the absence of fat and high in the presence of fat) can differentiate between these two groups of lesions.

In clinical practice, the signal intensity loss of an adrenal lesion between OP and IP images can be assessed using either qualitative or quantitative methods with region-of-interest measurements. Both methods have proved to be effective, particularly if an internal reference tissue (e.g., liver, spleen, or paraspinal muscles) is used to account for the additional signal decay due to T2* effects. Although various equations have been advocated to calculate the lesion's relative signal intensity decrease on OP images – i.e., SI index (SII), the adrenal SI-to-spleen SI ratio (ASR), the adrenal SI-to-liver SI ratio (ALR), and the adrenal SI-to-muscle SI ratio (AMR) [7] – recent evidence suggests that the SI index and ASR using the following equations yield the highest accuracy for adrenal lesion characterization at both 1.5T [7, 8] and 3T [9, 10]:

$$SIIndex = \frac{SI(adrenal)_{in\text{-}phase} - SI(adrenal)_{opposed\text{-}phase}}{SI(adrenal)_{in\text{-}phase}}$$

$$\frac{SIIndex_{adrenal}}{SIIndex_{spleen}} = \frac{SI(adrenal)_{opposed\text{-}phase}}{SI(spleen)_{opposed\text{-}phase}} \times \frac{SI(spleen)_{in\text{-}phase}}{SI(adrenal)_{in\text{-}phase}} - 1.$$

Previous studies have been controversial, however, on the optimal threshold that should be used to achieve the best tradeoff to maximize sensitivity without compromising specificity in the diagnosis of adrenal adenomas. At 1.5T, suggested thresholds ranged from −25 to 0.8 for the ASR and from 1% to 16.5% for the SI index, a variability that is likely related to major differences in MR protocol among studies. For example, while recent studies used MR protocols where both OP and IP images were acquired using the shortest echo time at 1.5T (2.2 ms for OP and 4.4 ms for IP), ensuring that the signal loss on OP images can be attributed primarily to intravoxel fat–water signal cancellation rather than the confounding effect of T2* decay, earlier studies used longer echo times of up to 13 ms. In addition, other sequence parameters such as flip angle and receiver bandwidth may also alter quantitative lesion analysis.

At 3T, the faster phase cycling of spins poses remarkable challenges for the collection of precisely timed OP and IP echo times with the shortest inter-echo interval [9]. Using a 3T MR system, fat and water protons are OP at 1.1, 3.3, 5.5 ms, and so on, and IP at 2.2, 4.4, 6.6 ms, and so on. Applying a two-dimensional (2D) technique, the acquisition of the first OP echo at 1.1 ms and the first IP echo at 2.2 ms within the same breath-hold would require unacceptably high receiver bandwidths at 3T. Although the most intuitive solution of this technical problem is to acquire the first OP echo and first IP echo in different breath-holds, this approach can introduce substantial inaccuracies in the slice selection between OP and IP acquisitions, which would compromise the reliability of quantitative methods for the characterization of adrenal lesions, particularly for smaller adrenal tumors. To avoid data misregistration, most manufacturers developed 2D MR protocols at 3T for sampling both IP/OP echoes

within a single breath-hold. The two most commonly used approaches were (1) the collection of the first IP echo (2.2 ms) followed by the third OP echo (5.5 ms) or (2) the first OP signal (1.1 ms) followed by the second IP signal (4.4 ms) [11]. Although these two approaches were originally thought to be equivalent, this difference in data collection can significantly influence the characterization of adrenal lesions. There is evidence that the use of a shorter echo time for the IP echo than for the OP echo may result in a substantial overlap in the SI index values of adenomas and nonadenomas at both 1.5T [12, 13] and 3T [9]. Previous studies demonstrated that a consistent number of malignant adrenal tumors show a signal loss on OP images, simply due to T2* decay effects on the image with longer echo time. For this reason, radiologists selecting a shorter echo time for the IP echo than for the OP echo are confronted with a diagnostic dilemma when detecting a signal loss in an adrenal lesion on the OP images, because they are unable to distinguish whether signal loss is due to chemical shift effect in a fat-containing adenoma or T2* decay in a malignant lesion with little or no fat.

With the proliferation of robust parallel imaging and 3T whole-body MR systems, three-dimensional (3D) volumetric imaging techniques are rapidly gaining acceptance in clinical practice [14]. Along with improved spatial resolution, these techniques exploit an inherently higher signal-to-noise ratio (SNR) compared with 2D sequences that allows for higher receiver bandwidth without compromising image quality. Recently, dual GRE 3D techniques have been introduced for sampling the shortest possible OP (1.1 ms) and IP (2.2 ms) echo without penalizing SNR at 3T MR imaging. This acquisition scheme minimizes the effects of T2* decay between the two consecutive echo times [11]. Preliminary evidence suggests that, compared with a standard 2D sequence, a dual GRE 3D technique can improve the diagnostic accuracy for the characterization of adrenal lesions, particularly for adrenal lesions with a low lipid-to-water proton ratio (the so-called, lipid-poor adenomas) (Figure 8.4). A further advantage of the 3D technique is its inherently greater SNR, which enables acquisition of thinner sections with no inter-section gap without penalizing image quality. This improves spatial resolution along the z axis, minimizing the effect of partial volume averaging at the edge of a given mass. Partial volume averaging – which

(a)

(b)

(c)

(d)

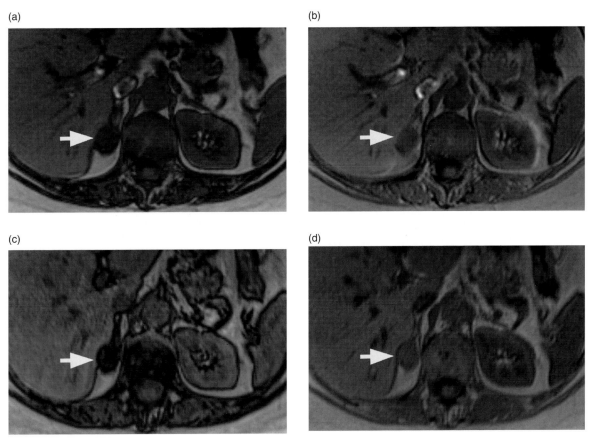

Figure 8.4 Images obtained in a 35-year-old female with an incidentally discovered lipid-poor adrenal adenoma, which was confirmed by surgery. Transverse (a) OP (193/1.6, 22°) and (b) IP (193/4.9, 22° flip angle) MR images with the 2D technique demonstrate a 2-cm, well-defined, left adrenal lesion (arrow), which shows minimal signal intensity variation between the IP and the OP image. Corresponding (c) OP (4.5/1.1, 20°) and (d) IP (4.5/2.5, 20° flip angle) MR images with the 3D technique demonstrate a substantial drop in signal intensity of the lesion (arrow) from the IP to the OP image, which is suggestive of adrenal adenoma.

occurs if the section thickness is more than half the diameter of the lesion being evaluated [15] – is particularly problematic in smaller lesions ($< 1\,\mathrm{cm}$) because it leads to an artificial decrease in the lesion's signal intensity on OP images. This effect may preclude obtaining the accuracy and reproducibility required for successful adrenal lesion characterization at MR. Because of the potential for higher spatial resolution acquisitions, a 3D sequence may result in more accurate signal intensity measurements and better characterization of small adrenal lesions.

A clinically important consideration when using a dual GRE 3D technique to discriminate adrenal adenomas from nonadenomas at 3T is that, for quantitative evaluation methods, the suggested thresholds have to be adjusted compared with the corresponding thresholds with a 2D pulse sequence.

For example, according to a recent study using a 3D technique at 3T [10], the optimal threshold value for the SI index is 6.9%, differing considerably with the corresponding value of 1.7–1.9% suggested with a 2D sequence [9, 10].

Two-point Dixon method

Applying a two-point Dixon method to data generated with a dual GRE acquisition allows for the reconstruction of two additional data sets commonly referred to as "water-only" (WO) and "fat-only" (FO) images without any additional data acquisition time. While the original concept for data processing was described by Dixon in the early 1980s [16], only recent technical developments have made it possible to generate separate WO and FO images from a 3D dual GRE sequence in a clinical setting [17]. At both 1.5T and 3T field strengths, this single breath-hold 3D dual GRE sequence is able to acquire the first OP echo and first IP echo thereby greatly reducing artifacts related to respiratory or other bulk motion and minimizing T2*-related effects. After proper phase correction, summation and subtraction of the raw data sets from IP and OP images permit routine and reliable generation of a WO image and an FO image, respectively, for each slice location.

Compared with a chemical shift technique, where image assessment relies on signal intensity dissimilarities between two different image sets (IP and OP), an FO sequence can simplify the clinical detection of fat by enabling direct visualization of fat signal within tissues. On FO images subcutaneous and visceral fat demonstrate a bright signal, while most abdominal tissues (such as the adrenal glands, liver, pancreas, kidneys, and spleen) show low signal intensity due to selective suppression of water signal. Another advantage of an FO sequence compared with a chemical shift technique is the lack of ambiguity regarding the dominant proton species in a fat–water admixture. This property – related to the capability of an FO sequence to correct for phase errors – may simplify the interpretation of rare adrenal lesions, such as myelolipomas, where the fat component may be equal or greater than 50%.

Recent evidence suggests that, as an adjunct to IP and OP images, FO images may be useful for improving radiologists' confidence in the diagnosis of fat-containing benign adrenal lesions. Benign adrenal tumors, most notably lipid-rich adrenal adenomas, demonstrate typical high signal intensity compared to the background noise on FO images (Figure 8.1). On the other hand, most malignant adrenal tumors show signal intensity similar to that of the liver and spleen on FO images due to the absence of fat (Figure 8.2). Although rarely observed, malignant adrenal tumors may show unexpected high signal intensity on FO images. This finding, which can be explained by uncorrected, iron-related T2* effects often secondary to hemorrhage within an adrenal lesion, may create a pitfall in the evaluation of adrenal masses because it may be erroneously attributed to signal from intralesional fat. Assessment of lesion signal intensity on corresponding IP and OP images is necessary in these equivocal cases.

An FO sequence can be particularly useful in the presence of both fat and iron within a lesion. In this case, while the lesion's signal intensity on IP and OP images may appear normal, the FO images will demonstrate high signal intensity compared with other abdominal organs and the background noise.

Adrenal MR protocol recommendations

While pulse sequences have been optimized for almost 20 years at 1.5T, several issues must be considered when implementing an abdominal MR protocol on a 3T system. Limitations secondary to the greater heterogeneity (often referred to as B1 heterogeneity) of the signal across the field of view; undesired heating of body tissues due to increased energy deposition from higher radiofrequency (RF) excitation pulses; chemical shift and susceptibility artifacts; altered T1 and T2 relaxation times; and electrodynamic effects, such as standing wave phenomenon and eddy currents, need to be accounted for when developing an MR protocol at higher magnetic fields [18]. If not accounted for, these effects can be detrimental and result in suboptimal or nondiagnostic image quality, particularly when examining larger anatomical regions, such as the abdomen or pelvis.

In an attempt to overcome or at least partially offset the technical challenges associated with 3T, several strategies have been advocated: parallel imaging and refocusing flip angle modulation, increase of the receiver bandwidth, the adjustment of repetition times and echo times, and the improvement or development of new shimming techniques, such as the use of additional shimming coils, new shimming algorithms, and higher order shimming of the gradient coils. The application of these methods, however, results in a reduction in SNR that decreases the net gain in signal at 3T, almost invariably less than the expected twofold increase compared with 1.5T. While what constitutes an optimal tradeoff between the gain in SNR and the necessary loss in image quality is still under investigation at higher field strengths, some general recommendations can be made. Table 8.1 summarizes the authors' recommendations for an optimized adrenal MR protocol at 3T. Based on our clinical experience, we recommend that, whenever it is available, a dual GRE 3D technique should replace 2D sequences for chemical shift MR imaging.

Although routine administration of a gadolinium contrast agent is not advocated for adrenal MR imaging, contrast material administration becomes

Table 8.1 3T Adrenal MR imaging sequences and parameters

MR sequence	TR (ms)	TE (OP/IP) (ms)	Flip angle (degrees)	Section thickness (mm)	Intersection gap (mm)	Matrix size	Bandwidth (Hz/pixel)	Field of view (cm)
T2-weighted 2D HASTE	1000	96	109	6	78	256 × 256	490	30–44
T1-weighted 2D dual GRE	193	116/419	22	5	6	192 × 256	930/385	30–44
T1-weighted 3D dual GRE	4.5	1.1/215	20	3	0	192 × 256	1030/1030	30–44

HASTE = half-Fourier acquisition single-shot turbo spin echo, GRE = gradient echo, 2D = two-dimensional, 3D = three-dimensional, TR = repetition time, TE = echo time.

necessary in patients with known or suspected malignant adrenal tumor. In this clinical scenario, a precise assessment of local tumor extension to adjacent vascular and parenchymal organs is critical for optimal treatment planning.

Imaging features of specific adrenal diseases

Adrenocortical adenoma

A nonfunctioning adrenocortical adenoma is the most common cause of an incidental adrenal mass at imaging. There are no specific morphologic features that enable a conclusive diagnosis of adrenal adenomas, as most lesions are small, smooth, and homogeneous when detected. Chemical shift techniques are of utmost importance in the characterization of adrenal adenomas, which demonstrate a substantial signal loss on OP images due to the increased content of intracellular fat (Figure 8.1). Due to a higher sensitivity to smaller amounts of fat, which may result in improved detection of lipid-poor adenomas, a dual GRE 3D technique is preferred over 2D sequences at 3T (Figure 8.4) [10]. A 6-month follow-up with MR or CT is recommended in patients with indeterminate lesions and no history of malignant disease.

Metastasis

The adrenal gland is a common site for metastatic disease, most commonly from carcinoma (lung, breast, and colon), lymphoma, and melanoma. The primary malignancy is usually known at time of diagnosis, and lesion characterization is critical for primary disease staging and treatment planning. Similar

to adrenal adenomas, morphologic features have a limited role in the characterization of adrenal metastases. Metastases should be suspected when adrenal lesions manifest bilaterally, are larger than 3 cm in largest diameter, or show a malignant growth pattern, including irregular borders, necrotic areas, or cystic degeneration. Typical imaging findings of adrenal metastases at MR include hypointense appearance compared with the liver on T1-weighted images, with mild to moderate hyperintensity on T2-weighted images. Unlike most adrenal adenomas, metastases demonstrate no signal loss on OP images due to the absence of intralesional fat (Figure 8.2). Anecdotal reports of adrenal metastases with unexpected signal loss have been described for primary tumors that contain fat, such as liposarcomas, clear cell renal carcinomas, and hepatocellular carcinomas. A similar appearance may be also seen in rare cases of adrenal metastases to an existing adenoma, also known as a "collision" tumor.

Adrenocortical carcinoma

Adrenocortical carcinoma generally presents with abdominal pain and/or a palpable abdominal mass. Because of their indolent course, most adrenocortical carcinomas manifest at an advanced stage, with the average lesion size being larger than 6 cm at the time of diagnosis. Tumors may be functionally active, resulting in endocrine syndromes, such as Cushing syndrome, Conn syndrome, or adrenogenital syndrome. At imaging, adrenocortical carcinomas manifest characteristic findings, including large lesion size and heterogeneous signal intensity on T2- and T1-weighted images before and after contrast material administration, due to areas of hemorrhage, fat, and

(a)

(b)

(c)

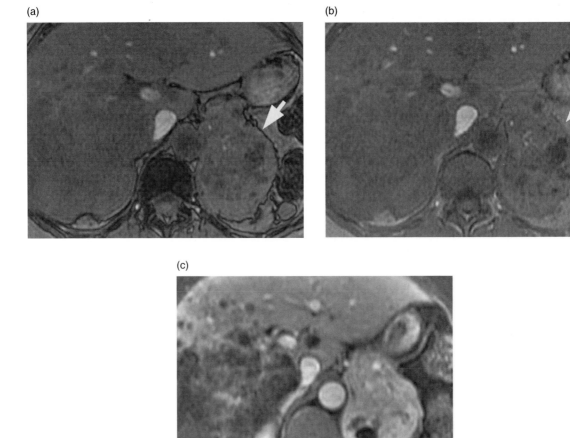

Figure 8.5 A 64-year-old man with abdominal pain and histologically confirmed adrenocortical carcinoma. (a, b) Transverse T1-weighted gradient echo (a) OP and (b) IP 3T MR images demonstrate a large (7-cm), irregular, left adrenal lesion (arrow), which shows heterogeneous signal intensity and lack of signal loss between IP and OP images. (c) Dynamic, gadolinium-enhanced, fat-saturated T1-weighted gradient echo MR image demonstrates heterogeneous enhancement of the lesion due to areas of hemorrhage and necrosis. Also note extensive metastatic involvement of the right liver lobe.

tumor necrosis (Figure 8.5). These findings enable a confident diagnosis at both 1.5T and 3T. Because of the complex anatomical relationships between the primary tumor and the adjacent parenchymal and vascular organs, multiplanar MR imaging is recommended for local tumor staging.

Pheochromocytoma

Pheochromocytomas are rare catecholamine-secreting tumors originating from the adrenal medulla. Pheochromocytomas follow a "10% rule" because, in about 10% of cases, tumors manifest bilaterally or in an extra-adrenal location, follow a

hereditary pattern of transmission, show a malignant behavior, or occur in children. Most pheochromocytomas are larger than 3 cm at the time of diagnosis. With increasing tumor size, intralesional areas of necrosis, hemorrhage, and/or cystic degeneration may appear, mimicking the imaging appearance of adrenocortical carcinomas or large adrenal metastases. Specific MR imaging findings of pheochromocytomas include very high T2 signal intensity (the so-called, "lightbulb sign"), lack of signal loss on OP images, and homogeneous and intense contrast enhancement after intravenous administration of contrast material (Figure 8.6). Rarely, pheochromocytomas manifest as purely cystic lesions

(a)

(b)

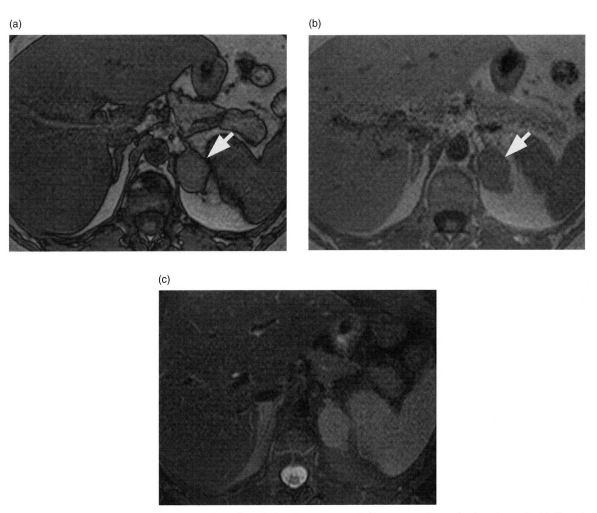

(c)

Figure 8.6 A 48-year-old man with pathologically confirmed pheochromocytoma. (a, b) Transverse T1-weighted gradient echo (a) OP and (b) IP 3T MR images demonstrate a 2.5-cm, solid, left adrenal lesion (arrows), which shows no drop in signal intensity between IP and OP images. (c) On the corresponding half-Fourier acquisition single-shot turbo spin-echo T2-weighted sequence, this lesion demonstrates a bright signal intensity, which is suggestive of pheochromocytoma.

and need to be considered in the differential diagnosis of cystic adrenal lesions. When imaging findings are classic, a confident diagnosis can be made at both 1.5T and 3T.

Myelolipoma

Myelolipomas are rare adrenal tumors that are usually detected incidentally at imaging studies performed for unrelated reasons. Although most lesions are small at the time of diagnosis, with time they can progressively enlarge and manifest with hemorrhage and calcifications. Definitive diagnosis relies on the detection of any degree of macroscopic fat using a fat suppression technique (Figure 8.3).

Fat detection may fail in purely fat-containing myelolipomas using a chemical shift technique due to the absence of a cancellation effect between the fat signal and the missing water signal.

Hemorrhage

Blunt trauma accounts for 80% of adrenal hemorrhages, which are usually unilateral, with a higher prevalence in the right adrenal gland. When a causative factor cannot be identified, an adrenal tumor must be suspected as the potential source for hemorrhage, indicating the need for a short-term follow-up or lesion biopsy. The MR appearance of adrenal hemorrhage includes T1 hyperintensity during the early

(a)

(b)

(c)

(d)

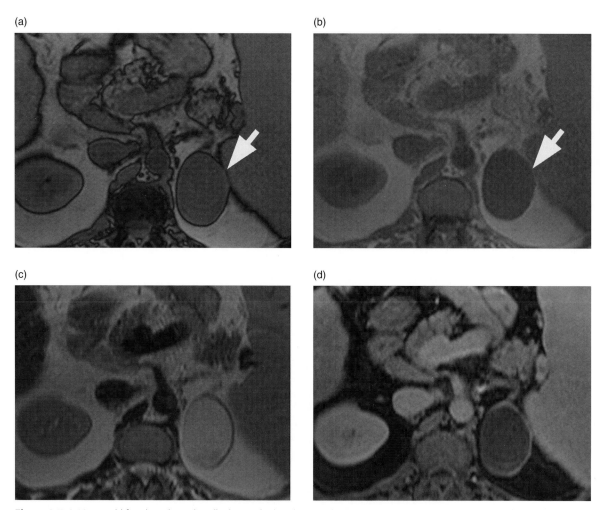

Figure 8.7 A 39-year-old female with incidentally detected adrenal cyst. (a, b) Transverse T1-weighted gradient echo (a) OP and (b) IP 3T MR images demonstrate a 4-cm, well-defined, left adrenal lesion (arrows), which shows low signal intensity and no signal drop between IP and OP images. Corresponding (c) half-Fourier acquisition single-shot turbo spin-echo T2-weighted sequence demonstrates lesion's high signal intensity; (d) gadolinium-enhanced, fat-saturated T1-weighted gradient echo MR image shows absence of lesion enhancement with the exception of a thin peripheral rim of enhancement due to a cystic wall.

phases (methemoglobin) and marked low signal intensity on T2*-weighted images due to iron-related effects. The latter effect becomes increasingly pronounced at higher magnetic field strengths and can be confirmed with a dual GRE sequence as signal loss of the lesion on the image with the longer echo time (the IP image in most circumstances). Hemorrhage may cause increased signal intensity on FO images, mimicking the presence of fat within a lesion.

Cyst

Adrenal cysts are rare lesions that may result from endothelial proliferation, prior hemorrhage, or parasitic disease. Cysts generally demonstrate typical imaging findings, which include homogeneous hyperintensity on T2- and hypointensity on T1-weighted images (Figure 8.7). As a general rule, cysts show no contrast enhancement, with the occasional exception of a thin peripheral rim of enhancement due to a cystic wall.

Ganglioneuroma

Ganglioneuroma is a rare benign adrenal tumor. Lesions may enlarge undetected for a long period of time and manifest as a large mass (occasionally more than 20 cm in largest diameter) that causes

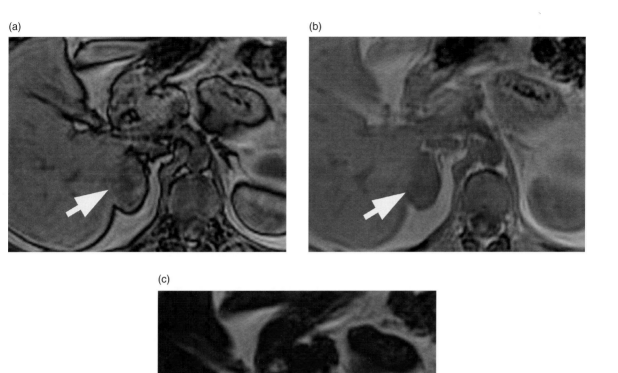

Figure 8.8 A 54-year-old man with pathologically confirmed ganglioneuroma. (a, b) Transverse T1-weighted gradient echo (a) OP and (b) IP 3T MR images demonstrate a 2.5-cm, well-defined, left adrenal lesion (arrows), which shows no drop in signal intensity between IP and OP images. (c) On the corresponding FO image, the lesion's signal intensity is low, similar to that of the liver and spleen. Although suggestive for absence of intralesional fat, these findings are nonspecific.

symptoms of compressive effects on adjacent organs. Ganglioneuroma lack specific imaging features at imaging. Because of the absence of fat, these lesions cannot be differentiated from malignant adrenal tumors and conclusive diagnosis is established at histologic analysis following surgical resection (Figure 8.8).

Conclusion

MR imaging at 1.5T and 3T demonstrates high diagnostic accuracy for the characterization of adrenal lesions using a chemical shift technique. To avoid misclassification of adrenal tumors, the echo time for the OP acquisition should precede that for the

IP acquisition. With the recent introduction of a 3D dual GRE technique, it is now possible to collect the first OP echo followed by the first IP echo during the same breath-hold at 3T. This approach minimizes the effects of T2* decay compared with a standard 2D dual GRE technique, without a penalty in the SNR. Due to dissimilarities in the pulse sequence design, different suggested thresholds need to be selected for various quantitative methods depending on the acquisition technique and the magnetic field strength. As an adjunct to IP and OP images, FO reconstructed images may improve radiologists' confidence in the diagnosis of fat-containing benign adrenal lesions.

References

1. Dunnick NR, Korobkin M. Imaging of adrenal incidentalomas. *AJR Am J Roentgenol* 2002; **179**: 559–68.

2. Kloos RT, Gross MD, Francis IR, Korobkin M, Shapiro B. Incidentally discovered adrenal masses. *Endocr Rev* 1995; **16**: 460–84.

3. Young WF Jr. Clinical practice. The incidentally discovered adrenal mass. *N Engl J Med* 2007; **356**: 601–10.

4. Mayo-Smith WW, Boland GW, Noto RB, Lee MJ. State-of-the-art adrenal imaging. *Radiographics* 2001; **21**: 995–1012.

5. Hood MN, Ho VB, Smirniotopoulos JG, Szumowski J. Chemical shift: the artifact and clinical tool revisited. *Radiographics* 1999; **19**: 357–71.

6. Leroy-Willig A, Bittoun J, Luton JP, *et al.* In vivo MR spectroscopic imaging of the adrenal glands: distinction between adenomas and carcinomas larger than 15 mmol/L based on lipid content. *AJR Am J Roentgenol* 1989; **153**: 771–73.

7. Fujiyoshi F, Nakajo M, Fukukura Y, Tsuchimochi S. Characterization of adrenal tumors by chemical shift fast low-angle shot MR imaging: comparison of four methods of quantitative evaluation. *AJR Am J Roentgenol* 2003; **180**: 1649–57.

8. Mayo-Smith WW, Lee MJ, McNicholas MM, *et al.* Characterization of adrenal masses (< 5 cm) by use of chemical shift MR imaging: observer performance versus quantitative measures. *AJR Am J Roentgenol* 1995; **165**: 91–5.

9. Schindera ST, Soher BJ, Delong DM, Dale BM, Merkle EM. Effect of echo time pair selection on quantitative analysis for adrenal tumor characterization with in-phase and opposed-phase MR imaging: initial experience. *Radiology* 2008; **248**:140–7.

10. Marin D, Soher BJ, Dale BM, *et al.* Characterization of adrenal lesions: comparison of 2D and 3D dual gradient-echo MR imaging at 3T – preliminary results. *Radiology* 2010; **254**: 179–87.

11. Merkle EM, Nelson RC. Dual gradient-echo in-phase and opposed-phase hepatic MR imaging: a useful tool for evaluating more than fatty infiltration or fatty sparing. *Radiographics* 2006; **26**: 1409–18.

12. Reinig JW, Stutley JE, Leonhardt CM, *et al.* Differentiation of adrenal masses with MR imaging: comparison of techniques. *Radiology* 1994; **192**: 41–6.

13. Slapa RZ, Jakubowski W, Dabrowska E, *et al.* Magnetic resonance imaging differentiation of adrenal masses at 1.5T: T2-weighted images, chemical shift imaging, and Gd-DTPA dynamic studies. *MAGMA* 1996; **4**: 163–79.

14. Lee VS, Hecht EM, Taouli B, *et al.* Body and cardiovascular MR imaging at 3T. *Radiology* 2007; **244**: 692–705.

15. Kim JK, Kim SH, Jang YJ, *et al.* Renal angiomyolipoma with minimal fat: differentiation from other neoplasms at double-echo chemical shift FLASH MR imaging. *Radiology* 2006; **239**: 174–80.

16. Dixon WT. Simple proton spectroscopic imaging. *Radiology* 1984; **153**: 189–94.

17. Ma J. Breath-hold water and fat imaging using a dual-echo two-point Dixon technique with an efficient and robust phase-correction algorithm. *Magn Reson Med* 2004; **52**: 415–19.

18. Merkle EM, Dale BM. Abdominal MR imaging at 3T: the basics revisited. *AJR Am J Roentgenol* 2006; **186**: 1524–32.

Magnetic resonance cholangiopancreatography

Byun Ihn Choi and Jeong Min Lee

Introduction

Magnetic resonance cholangiopancreatography (MRCP), in use since the 1990s [1], is an accepted noninvasive imaging technique for the diagnosis of pancreaticobiliary diseases. MRCP images are created with the acquisition of heavily T2-weighted images, and can demonstrate the fluid-filled lumen of the biliary tree and the pancreatic duct with high signal intensity. It is comparable to endoscopic retrograde cholangiopancreatography (ERCP) in the diagnosis of biliary-pancreas pathologic conditions [2–5]. The advantages of MRCP over other imaging techniques include (1) the examination is noninvasive and requires no anesthesia; (2) the examination is not operator dependent, and high-quality images can be obtained consistently; (3) no administration of intraductal or intravenous contrast agent is necessary; (4) no ionizing radiation is used; (5) visualization of ducts proximal to an obstruction is superior to that achieved by ERCP; (6) MRCP can be successfully performed in the presence of biliary–enteric anastomoses; and (7) combination with conventional MR sequences is possible and helpful for the evaluation of duct wall and extraductal disease [6]. For many years, ERCP has been considered the standard of reference for imaging the biliary tract and pancreatic duct owing to its higher spatial resolution and potential for image-guided therapy [7]. However, it has a reported complications rate of up to 5% including duodenal perforation, pancreatitis, bleeding and sepsis [8]. For all of these reasons, MRCP has replaced diagnostic ERCP in the last few years, unless an intervention or tissue sampling is required [9].

In the past decades, MRCP at 1.5T has proven highly accurate for the evaluation of the extrahepatic biliary tree [2–5]. For the evaluation of the intrahepatic biliary system, however, particularly in the absence of obstructive biliary disease, MRCP has some limitations caused by the limited spatial resolution and poor signal-to-noise ratio (SNR) of 1.5T [4]. In recent years, high-field whole-body MR imaging at 3T has gained substantial clinical interest as dedicated torso array receive-only coils for 3T MR systems became available. The main reason for the increased clinical use of 3T units is the desire for an increased SNR at the higher magnetic field strength compared with standard 1.5T [9]. Theoretically, this gain in SNR can be kept or traded for either speed or spatial resolution, or both. Unfortunately, however, several potential disadvantages, such as an increase in imaging artifacts, changes in relaxation kinetics, and specific absorption rate (SAR) constraints, have to be considered [10, 11]. Indeed, certain imaging artifacts are more prominent at 3T compared with 1.5T, mainly because their physical parameters are dependent on the main magnetic field strength (B0). These include chemical shift artifact, susceptibility artifacts, and dielectric resonance artifacts [12]. Those limitations bring technical challenges in transferring 1.5T protocols to 3T, principally to abdominal imaging including MRCP, as results of proper sequence design, incorporating breath-hold issues and large fields of view [12]. In order to decrease those artifacts at 3T, special consideration is required: for example, increasing the receiver bandwidth for decreasing chemical shift artifact, and the use of multiple transmitter coil or radio-frequency (RF) cushion to overcome B1 inhomogeneity artifacts. Nonetheless, recent advancements in 3T MR hardware and software, such as dedicated torso array coils, parallel imaging, and new "low SAR pulses" or variable flip angle refocusing techniques, allow all of the standard MR examinations to be performed on a 3T whole-body MR system. Currently, 3T state-of-the-art MRCP protocols use the same sequence types

Body MR Imaging at 3 Tesla, ed. Ihab R. Kamel and Elmar M. Merkle. Published by Cambridge University Press.

as used at 1.5T, but they are modified to perform well at higher field strength.

Comparison of 3T with 1.5T

Several previous studies which compared MRCP on 3T with 1.5T scanners demonstrated a significantly higher contrast-to-noise ratio (CNR) between the biliary ductal system and the periductal tissue or the liver [13–17]. Although CNR increases at 3T are expected because twice the number of free water protons per voxel contributes to the MR signal at 3T compared with the lower field strength, the CNR at 3T increases, on average, up to 38.1%~ 62% at 3T on MRCP images [14, 15]. This could be attributed to several factors including an alteration of the T1 and T2 relaxation times, the immature hardware and software, B1 inhomogeneity artifacts, and increased susceptibility artifacts [9, 18]. Furthermore, in several previous studies, qualitative image analysis of the visualization of the extrahepatic biliary ductal structures did not reveal any significant preference for 1.5T or 3T [14, 16]. On the contrary, other studies demonstrated superior visualization of the pancreaticobiliary tree at 3T compared with 1.5T on half-Fourier acquisition single-shot turbo-spin echo (HASTE) [15] or three-dimensional (3D) respiratory-triggered rapid acquisition relaxation enhancement (RARE) sequence [17] (Figures 9.1–9.3). In addition, 3T MRCP better demonstrated intrahepatic branches than 1.5T MRCP, and therefore, the 3T

may improve the accuracy of MRCP in diagnosing biliary ductal variants in the preoperative radiologic assessment of living liver lobe donor candidates [19]. Although, in theory, the increased susceptibility artifacts at 3T may decrease depiction of the ductal pancreatic system on MRCP, a previous study demonstrated a clear trend toward improved visualization of the pancreatic duct in volunteers at 3T with a HASTE and a 3D turbo spin echo (TSE) sequence [15]. Until now, MRCP at 3T has to be considered equal, not

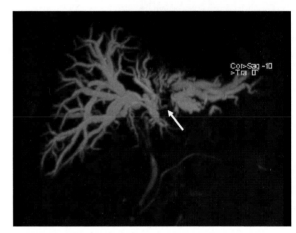

Figure 9.1 Coronal maximum-intensity projection of a respiratory-triggered, 3D turbo spin echo (TSE) MRCP data set acquired at 3T showing a dilated intrahepatic bile duct due to hilar cholangiocarcinoma. Hilar cholangiocarcinoma invades the secondary biliary confluence of the left intrahepatic bile duct (arrow).

(a)

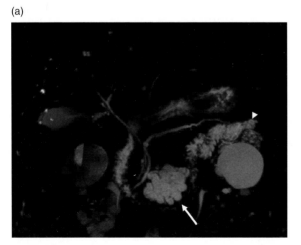

(b)

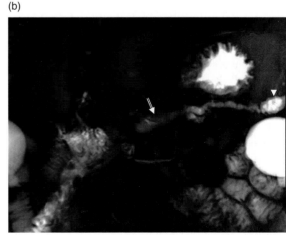

Figure 9.2 (a) 1.5T coronal maximum-intensity-projection MRCP image based on a respiratory-triggered, coronal, 3D T2-weighted TSE sequence demonstrates cystic dilation of the side branches in the uncinate process (arrow), and another lesion in the tail (arrowhead). (b). 3T thick-slab projectional MRCP image obtained 3 years after Whipple's operation shows dilation of the residual pancreatic duct (arrow) and the tail lesion (arrowhead).

(a)

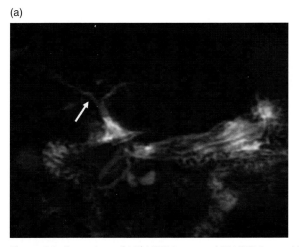

(b)

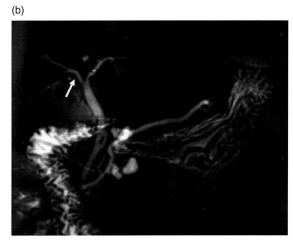

Figure 9.3 Comparison of 1.5T MRCP image and 3T MRCP image. (a) Thick-slab 2D MRCP image acquired at 1.5T. (b) Thick-slab 2D MRCP image acquired at 3T. Note better depiction of the intrahepatic bile ducts (arrow) on 3T MRCP than on 1.5T MRCP, probably due to higher SNR of the bile duct at 3T.

superior to 1.5T; however, with the progressive development of 3T hardware and software, MRCP at 3T holds great promise to improve the diagnosis of pancreaticobiliary disease [9].

Techniques

Current MRCP techniques consist of echo-train spin-echo techniques with two-dimensional (2D) and 3D acquisitions. The HASTE or 2D or 3D RARE sequences are currently the most widely used techniques. In addition, MRCP is performed with thick-slab and thin-slice sequences. A thick-slab single section of 4–8 cm is acquired in various rotations to view the ducts from different angles, obtained in less than 2 seconds for each plane. The thick-slab technique has limitations for the assessment of small intraductal pathologic conditions such as stones or tumors due to their partial volume averaging with intraductal high signal from bile (Figures 9.4 and 9.5). Therefore, in order to evaluate small intraductal pathologies, thin section images with the use of 2D multisection sequence (slice thickness of 3–4 mm) or 3D volumetric imaging (slice thickness of 1–2 mm) are necessary. Using a volumetric, heavily T2-weighted sequence (echotime [TE], approximately 600 ms) in conjunction with respiratory triggering and high matrices, 3D MRCP images are acquired over a period of several minutes, which allows the reconstruction of 3D projection images and thin 2D images (1–2 mm). The advantage of 3D imaging is that it creates isotropic images that can be reformatted in any plane.

Although T2-weighted MRCP has proven to be highly accurate for depiction of stricture or obstruction of the bile duct or the pancreatic duct, it is not able to assess bile excretion dynamics. To overcome this limitation, some investigators advocate the performance of 3D T1-weighted MR cholangiography after the intravenous administration of hepatobiliary MR contrast agents, such as mangafodipir trisodium (Teslanscan), gadobenate dimeglumine (MultiHance®), and gadoxetic acid (Eovist®)[20–22]. Contrast-enhanced MR cholangiography has shown promising results for the assessment of bile duct leaks, intrahepatic anatomy in living liver transplant donor candidates (Figure 9.6), and biliary–enteric anastomoses [20–22] (Figure 9.7).

Clinical applications
Anatomic variant and congenital anomaly

MRCP provides accurate depiction and measurements of the bile and pancreatic ducts in 95% of examinations; associated anatomical variants, such as pancreas divisum and choledochal cysts, can also be visualized [3]. Anatomic variations of the biliary tract occur in up to 37% of individuals [23] (Figure 9.8). MRCP has been shown to accurately detect those biliary variants, for example crossover anomalies such as the dorsocaudal branch of the right hepatic duct entering to the central left hepatic duct, trifurcations, accessory or aberrant ducts that enter the common duct or cystic duct, and cystic duct variant [22, 24]. Awareness of these ductal variants is important in the

(a)

(b)

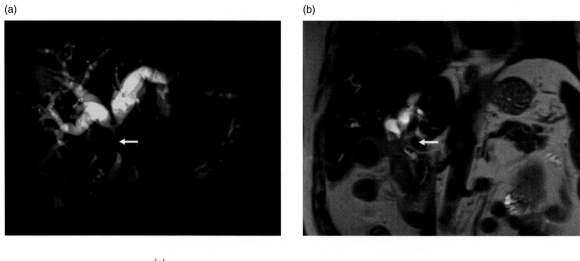

(c)

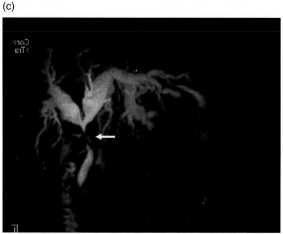

Figure 9.4 MRCP techniques at 3T. (a) Thick-slab 2D projectional MRCP image (60 mm) (b) 2D thin-slice (4 mm) HASTE MRCP image, (c) maximum-intensity-projection 3T MRCP image based on a respiratory-triggered, coronal, 3D T2-weighted TSE sequence. The three MRCP sequences show hilar cholangiocarcinoma clearly (arrows).

planning of laparoscopic cholecystectomy, right lobe living liver transplantation, or complex percutaneous and endoscopic biliary interventions.

Choledochal cysts are segmental aneurysmal dilatations of the common bile duct (CBD) alone or the CBD and common hepatic duct. Choledochal cysts frequently coexist with an anomalous junction of the CBD and the pancreatic cut, and are associated with an increased incidence of gallstone diseases, pancreatitis, and cholangiocarcinoma [6] (Figure 9.9). MRCP is able to provide equivalent diagnostic information for detection of choledochal cysts to that of ERCP without the risk of complications, and has been proposed as the imaging modality of choice in evaluation of choledochal cyst [25, 26]. In addition, MRCP can detect pancreas division, which is usually depicted as two separate drainage systems of the dorsal and ventral pancreas, with a high degree of accuracy, and therefore, it is more frequently used in the evaluation of patients with idiopathic pancreatitis.

Choledocholithiasis

Calculi in the biliary ducts are the most common cause of extrahepatic obstructive jaundice. With the increase of laparoscopic cholecystectomy over recent years, the preoperative diagnosis of choledocholithiasis has become increasingly important because the presence of bile duct stones renders laparoscopic procedures extremely difficult [6]. Common duct stones

(a)

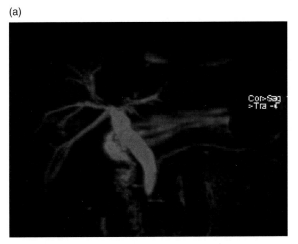

(b)

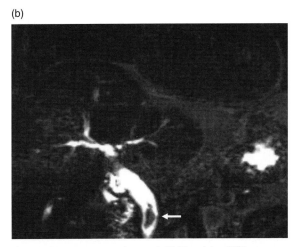

Figure 9.5 Coronal maximum-intensity-projection 3T MRCP image based on a respiratory-triggered, coronal, 3D T2-weighted TSE sequence (a) and coronal source MR image (b). Although the source image shows a filling defect in the distal common bile duct (CBD) (arrow) that represents a stone, the maximum-intensity projection image does not show the stone.

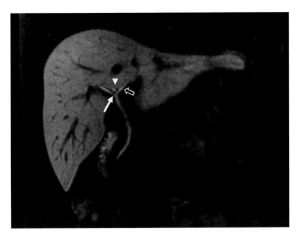

Figure 9.6 3D T1-weighted MR cholangiography image after administration of gadoxetic acid (Eovist) shows a biliary anatomy of trifurcation pattern with a common confluence of right posterior (arrowhead) and right anterior segmental ducts (arrow) and left hepatic duct (open arrow).

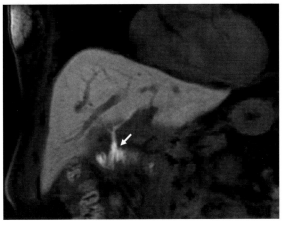

Figure 9.7 3D T1-weighted MR cholangiography image after administration of gadoxetic acid (Eovist) shows contrast passage (arrow) through the anastomosis between the bile duct and the jejunum.

(choledocholithiasis) are displayed by MRCP as a rounded or oval-shaped signal void with a meniscus of fluid above their proximal edge (Figure 9.10). Multiple studies demonstrated that test characteristics of MRCP appear to be similar to ERCP for detecting choledocholithiasis (sensitivity 80–100%, specificity 85–100%) [27, 28]. In the presence of a dilated CBD, MRCP has a 90–95% concordance with ERCP in diagnosing CBD stones over 4 mm in diameter [27, 28]. In addition, MRCP may be particularly effective in detecting intrahepatic calculi, where stones

proximal to strictures may be difficult to visualize by ERCP [29]. There are several pitfalls that mimic stones, which include intraductal air bubbles, blood clots, tumor, sludge, or parasites; flow artifacts; and a pseudostone at the ampulla [6].

Cholangiocarcinoma

MRCP appears to be useful in the evaluation of suspected malignancies of the biliary tract. Multiple studies have demonstrated that MRCP is able to determine the presence, level, and type of malignancy

127

with a high degree of accuracy [30, 31] MRCP is useful in delineating the anatomical extent of perihilar obstruction and interpreting its etiology. Hilar cholangiocarcinomas are the most common manifestation of cholangiocarcinoma and are usually small-volume tumors that result in a high-grade stricture of the confluence of the right and left hepatic ducts. A previous study demonstrated that although both ERCP and MRCP were equally effective in detecting biliary obstruction, MRCP was superior in the investigation of the anatomical extent and the type of

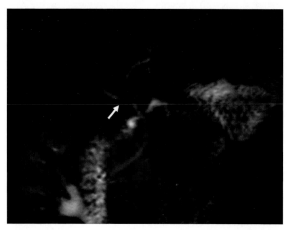

Figure 9.8 Thick-slab 2D projectional MRCP image demonstrates an anatomical variant of the biliary tract in living liver donor candidate. Note the right posterior intrahepatic segmental duct entering the common hepatic duct (arrow).

tumor [32]. Extrahepatic cholangiocarcinomas are seen as strictures or intraductal, polypoid masses resulting in biliary obstruction on MRCP. The imaging features of extrahepatic cholangiocarcinoma at MRCP are dilation of the proximal biliary tree with stricture or abrupt termination at the tumor, typically showing a shoulder sign or irregularity of the ductal wall [5]. MRCP is also very valuable in evaluation of patients with periampullary carcinomas, by demonstrating biliary and pancreatic ductal dilation and the location of strictures (Figure 9.11). Although the role of MRCP in the diagnosis and management of bile duct malignancy is not yet defined, it will probably prove to be a useful noninvasive adjunct to present techniques, since it has the capability to evaluate the bile ducts both above and below a stricture that are often not opacified at ERCP [5]. In addition, MRCP also can demonstrate any intrahepatic mass lesions.

Primary sclerosing cholangitis

The conventional imaging modality to establish the diagnosis of primary sclerosing cholangitis (PSC) is ERCP, which has been regarded as the imaging examination of choice for diagnosing PSC. The imaging findings of PSC are characterized by multifocal, irregular strictures and dilatations of segments of the intrahepatic and extrahepatic biliary tree. The strictures are usually short and annular, alternating with normal or slightly dilated segments, producing a beaded appearance [6].

(a)

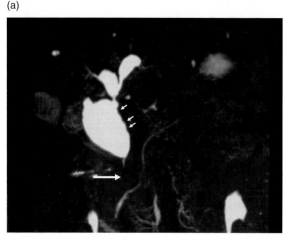

(b)

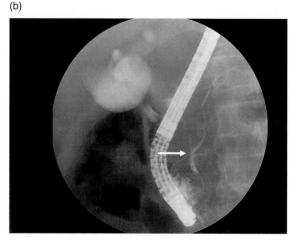

Figure 9.9 (a) Coronal maximum-intensity projection of a respiratory-triggered, 3D TSE MRCP data set showing a Todani-type IVa choledochal cyst in the intrahepatic biliary system and the common bile ductal system. Note an anomalous pancreaticobiliary ductal union (large arrow) and irregular wall of the choledochal cyst of the CBD (small arrows) that suggests coexisting cholangiocarcinoma. (b) ERCP images again show the cystic dilations of the extrahepatic and intrahepatic biliary ductal system and anomalous pancreaticobiliary ductal union (arrow).

(a)

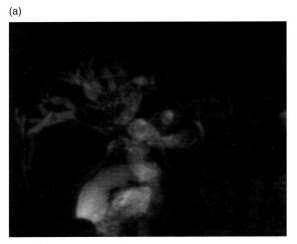

(b)

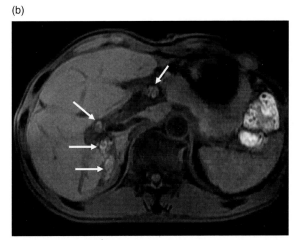

Figure 9.10 Thick-slab 2D MRCP image (a) and axial T1-weighted image (b) show multiple filling defects in the intrahepatic bile ducts that represents stones. Note the stones (arrows) show high signal intensity on T1-weighted image.

Due to technical advances of MR, characteristic changes of PSC are visible on MRCP [33]. However, MRCP provides lower sensitivity for detecting subtle peripheral ductal abnormalities in the liver, due to lower spatial resolution than ERCP. Furthermore, MRCP does not permit therapeutic intervention.

Acute cholecystitis

Ultrasound is often used as an initial modality to evaluate the gallbladder, as it is accurate, relatively inexpensive, and readily available. A previous study by Park *et al.* compared MRCP with ultrasound for the diagnosis of acute cholecystitis [34], and demonstrated that MRCP was superior to ultrasound for detecting stones in the cystic duct (sensitivity 100% versus 14%) but was less sensitive than ultrasound for detecting gallbladder wall thickening (sensitivity 69% versus 96%). With the increase of laparoscopic cholecystectomy over recent years, the preoperative diagnosis of choledocholithiasis in patients with acute cholecystitis has become increasingly important because the presence of bile duct stones renders laparoscopic procedures extremely difficult [6]. At the present time, however, the role of MRCP in the diagnosis of acute cholecystitis is not yet clearly established.

Postoperative alteration of the pancreaticobiliary tract

MRCP has been used successfully in imaging patients following cadaveric and living donor liver transplantation (Figure 9.12), pancreaticoduodenectomy, and creation of

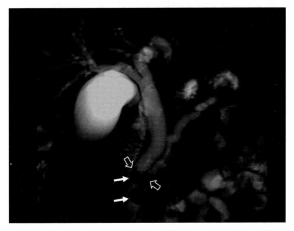

Figure 9.11 Coronal thick-slab 2D MRCP image at 3T shows diffuse dilation of the bile ducts and the main pancreatic duct with filling defects (open arrows) in the distal CBD and the pancreatic duct. Note round and smooth filling defects along the duodenal wall (closed arrows) that represents ampullary cancer.

a biliary–enteric anastomosis. It is very useful in the evaluation of patients with biliary–enteric anastomosis, where ERCP is impossible. Several previous studies have demonstrated the value of MRCP in depicting anastomotic strictures, intraductal stone, and bile plugs in those patients with surgery of the biliary tract [35, 36].

Pancreatitis

MRCP has been evaluated in both acute and chronic pancreatitis. The primary role of MRCP in the setting of acute pancreatitis is the identification of structural abnormalities that predispose to its development, such as CBD stones, pancreas divisum, and tumor obstructing the pancreatic duct [37]. In patients with acute pancreatitis, the combined MR and MRCP is useful for detecting the cause, extent, and complications of this inflammatory process. However, ERCP is preferred in patients with gallstone pancreatitis, obstructive jaundice (with a serum bilirubin concentration above 5 mg/dL) or biliary sepsis since endoscopic papillotomy could be performed during the same procedure. In addition, MRCP is also useful for demonstrating the ductal features of chronic pancreatitis, which include dilation of the main

pancreatic duct and its side branches, mural irregularity, ductoliths, and strictures of the pancreatic duct and CBD. In addition, unenhanced MR imaging, especially T1-weighted, fat-suppressed images, are particularly useful in delineating parenchymal changes such as atrophy and fibrosis by showing decreased signal intensity of the pancreas compared with the liver (Figure 9.13). Secretin-enhanced MRCP may improve visualization of the morphologic features of chronic pancreatitis and is being increasingly studied for evaluation of pancreatic exocrine function and in the early diagnosis of chronic pancreatitis [38].

Pancreatic cancer

MRCP is able to depict both CBD stricture and the malignant strictures (rat-tail appearance) of the main pancreatic duct in patients with pancreatic head cancer, so called "the double duct sign" (Figure 9.14). According to a previous study involving 124 patients who were suspected of having pancreatic cancer and underwent a number of diagnostic studies, including ERCP and MRCP, MRCP appears to be as accurate as ERCP for distinguishing pancreatic cancer from chronic pancreatitis [39]. Although MRCP has not yet replaced ERCP in the patients suspected of having pancreatic cancer in all centers, it may be preferred in patients who have gastric outlet or duodenal stenosis or who have had surgical rearrangement (e.g., Billroth II) or ductal disruption. In addition, it can be valuable for patients in whom attempted ERCP is either totally

Figure 9.12 Coronal maximum-intensity projection of a respiratory-triggered, 3D TSE MRCP data set acquired at 3T showing multifocal strictures (arrows) involving central portion of the intrahepatic ducts in patients with liver transplantation.

(a)

(b)

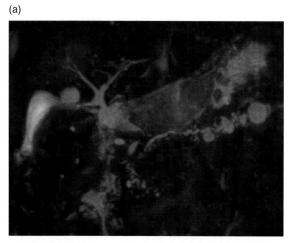
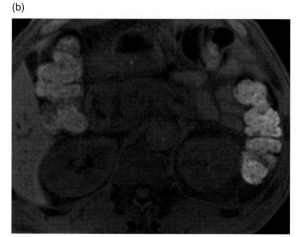

Figure 9.13 (a) Coronal maximum-intensity projection of a respiratory-triggered, 3D fast spin echo MRCP data set acquired at 3T demonstrating a comprehensive image of the pancreaticobiliary tract by demonstrating marked dilation of the main pancreatic duct with multifocal strictures as well as cystic dilation of its side branches. (b) Axial gradient echo opposed-phase image with fat suppression showing significantly decreased signal intensity of the pancreas compared with that of the liver.

(a)

(b)

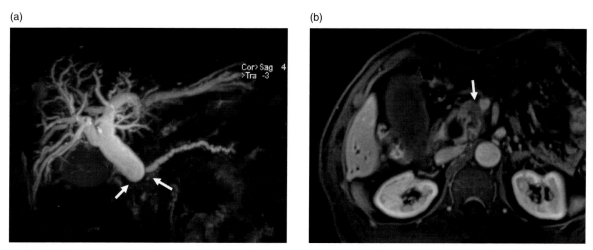

Figure 9.14 (a) Coronal maximum-intensity projection of a respiratory-triggered, 3D TSE MRCP data set acquired at 3T shows a marked dilation of the biliary tree and the pancreatic duct as well as strictures of both the CBD and the main pancreatic duct with so called "double duct sign" (arrows) and (b) gadolinium-enhanced 3D T1-weighted gradient echo image shows a hypointense nodule (arrow) invading the superior mesenteric vein, which are typical imaging features of pancreatic cancers.

(a)

(b)

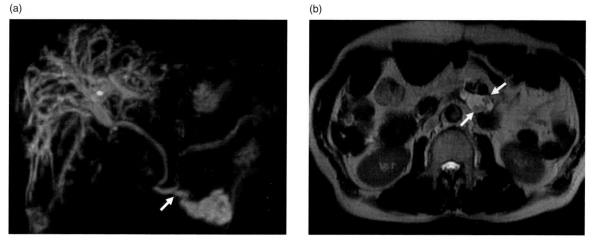

Figure 9.15 (a) Coronal maximum-intensity projection of a respiratory-triggered, 3D fast spin echo MRCP data set acquired at 3T demonstrating a cystic lesion with communication with the pancreatic duct (arrow). Note diffuse dilation of the peripheral portions of the intrahepatic ducts which represents *Clonorchiasis* infestation. (b) Axial T2-weighted HASTE image shows mural nodules (arrows) in the cystic lesion, which was confirmed as noninvasive intraductal pancreatic mucinous carcinoma from pathology evaluation.

unsuccessful or provides incomplete information [40]. Furthermore, MR angiography in conjunction with MRCP is able to provide valuable information for determination of resectability.

Intraductal papillary mucinous neoplasm (IPMN) of the pancreas

IPMN (also referred to as mucinous duct ectasia and intraductal papillary mucinous tumor, IPMT) is a precancerous lesion with a well-described adenoma

carcinoma sequence. Many patients with IPMN do not have invasive cancer and usually have a prolonged course without the development of cancer. IPMNs are classified into main duct type, branch duct type, and combined type, depending on the duct of origin. MRCP can reveal the entire spectrum of IPMNs – main duct dilation, cystic dilation of the side branches, nodules, septa, and intraductal filling defects [37]. Furthermore, it can show communication between the tumor and the pancreatic duct (Figure 9.15). The risk of progression to carcinoma is higher with main duct IPMN than with branch duct IPMN (especially when < 3 cm). In addition, dilation of the main pancreatic duct (≥ 10 mm), cyst size ≥ 30 mm, and the presence of intramural nodules are risk factors for progression and malignancy and are indications for surgical resection [41, 42]. MRCP is more sensitive than ERCP in differentiating mural nodules from mucin globs, which have the same intensity as pancreatic juice [42, 43]. However, MRCP is inferior to ERCP in demonstrating peripheral ductal abnormalities and in the ability to obtain tissue or perform therapeutic interventions.

References

1. Wallner BK, Schumacher KA, Weidenmaier W, *et al*. Dilated biliary tract: evaluation with MR cholangiography with a T2-weighted contrast-enhanced fast sequence. *Radiology* 1991; **181**: 805–8.

2. Romagnuolo J, Bardou M, Rahme E, *et al*. Magnetic resonance cholangiopancreatography: a meta-analysis of test performance in suspected biliary disease. *Ann Intern Med* 2003; **139**: 547–57.

3. Reinhold, C, Bret PM. Current status of MR cholangiopancreatography. *AJR Am J Roentgenol* 1996; **166**: 1285–95.

4. Goldman J, Florman S, Varotti G, *et al*. Noninvasive preoperative evaluation of biliary anatomy in right-lobe living donors with mangafodipir trisodium-enhanced MR cholangiography. *Transplant Proc* 2003; **35**: 1421–2.

5. Park HS, Lee JM, Choi JY, *et al*. Preoperative evaluation of bile duct cancer: MRI combined with MR cholangiopancreatography versus MDCT with direct cholangiography. *AJR Am J Roentgenol* 2008; **190**: 396–405.

6. Bilgin M, Shaikh F, Semelka R, *et al*. Magnetic resonance imaging of gallbladder and biliary system. *Top Magn Reson Imaging* 2009; **20**: 31–42.

7. Masci E, Toti G, Mariani A, *et al*. Complications of diagnostic and therapeutic ERCP: a prospective multicenter study. *Am J Gastroenterol* 2001; **96**: 417–23.

8. Loperfido S, Angelini G, Benedetti G, *et al*. Major early complications from diagnostic and therapeutic ERCP: a prospective multicenter study. *Gastrointest Endosc* 1998; **48**: 1–10.

9. Schindera ST, Merkle EM. MR cholangiopancreatography: 1.5T versus 3T. *Magn Reson Imaging Clin N Am* 2007; **15**: 355–64.

10. Merkle EM, Dale BM. Abdominal MRI at 3.0 T: the basics revisited. *AJR Am J Roentgenol* 2006; **186**: 1524–32.

11. Soher BJ, Dale BM, Merkle EM, A review of MR physics: 3T versus 1.5T. *Magn Reson Imaging Clin N Am* 2007; **200**: 277–90.

12. Ramalho M, Altun E, Heredia V, Zapparoli M, Semelka R. Liver MRI: 1.5T vs. 3T. *Magn Reson Imaging Clin N Am* 2007; **15**: 321–47.

13. Merkle EM, Haugan PA, Thomas J, *et al*. 3.0-versus 1.5-T MR cholangiography: a pilot study. *AJR Am J Roentgenol* 2006; **186**: 516–21.

14. O'Regan DP, Fitzgerald J, Allsop J, *et al*. A comparison of MR cholangiopancreatography at 1.5 and 3.0 Tesla. *Br J Radiol* 2005; **78**: 894–8.

15. Isoda H, Kataoka M, Maetani Y, *et al*. MRCP imaging at 3.0 T vs. 1.5 T: preliminary experience in healthy volunteers. *J Magn Reson Imaging* 2007; **25**: 1000–6.

16. Schindera ST, Miller CM, Ho LM, *et al*. Magnetic resonance (MR) cholangiography: quantitative and qualitative comparison of 3.0 Tesla with 1.5 Tesla. *Invest Radiol* 2007; **42**: 399–405.

17. Onishi H, Kim T, Hori M, *et al*. MR cholangiopancreatography at 3.0 T: intraindividual comparative study with MR cholangiopancreatography at 1.5T for clinical patients. *Invest Radiol* 2009; **44**: 559–65.

18. de Bazelaire CM, Duhamel GD, Rofsky NM, *et al*. MR imaging relaxation times of abdominal and pelvic tissues measured in vivo at 3.0 T: preliminary results. *Radiology* 2004; **230**: 652–9.

19. Kim SY, Byun JH, Lee SS, *et al*. Biliary tract depiction in living potential liver donors: intraindividual comparison of MR cholangiography at 3.0 T and 1.5T. *Radiology* 2010; **254**: 469–79.

20. Kapoor V, Peterson MS, Baron RL, *et al*. Intrahepatic biliary anatomy of living adult liver donors: correlation of mangafodipir trisodium-enhanced MR cholangiography and intraoperative cholangiography. *AJR Am J Roentgenol* 2002; **179**: 1281–6.

21. Hottat N, Winant C, Metens T, *et al*. MR cholangiography with manganese dipyridoxyl diphosphate in the evaluation of biliary-enteric anastomoses: preliminary experience. *AJR Am J Roentgenol* 2005; **184**: 1556–62.

22. An SK, Lee JM, Suh KS. Gadobenate dimeglumine-enhanced liver MRI as the sole preoperative imaging technique: a prospective study of living liver donors. *AJR Am J Roentgenol* 2006; **187**: 1223–33.

23. Huang TL, Cheng YF, Chen CL, *et al*. Variants of the bile ducts: clinical application in the potential donor of living-related hepatic transplantation. *Transplant Proc* 1996; **28**: 1669–70.

24. Fulcher AS, Szucs RA, Bassignani MJ, *et al*. Right lobe living donor liver transplantation: preoperative

evaluation of the donor with MR imaging. *AJR Am J Roentgenol* 1999; **172**: 955–9.

25. Lam WWM, Lam TPW, Saing H, *et al.* MR cholangiography and CT cholangiography of pediatric patients with choledochal cysts. *AJR Am J Roentgenol* 1999; **173**: 401–5.

26. Yu J, Turner MA, Fulcher AS, *et al.* Congenital anomalies and normal variants of the pancreaticobiliary tract and the pancreas in adults. Part 2: pancreatic duct and pancreas. *AJR Am J Roentgenol* 2006; **187**: 1544–53.

27. Chan, YL, Chan, AC, Lam WW, *et al.* Choledocholithiasis: comparison of MR cholangiography and endoscopic retrograde cholangiography. *Radiology* 1996; **200**: 85–9.

28. Lee MG, Lee HJ, Kim MH, *et al.* Extrahepatic biliary diseases: 3D MR cholangiopancreatography compared with endoscopic retrograde cholangiopancreatography. *Radiology* 1997; **202**: 663–9.

29. Kim T, Kim B, Kim J, *et al.* Diagnosis of intrahepatic stones: superiority of MR cholangiopancreatography over endoscopic retrograde cholangiopancreatography. *AJR Am J Roentgenol* 2002; **179**: 429–34.

30. Schwartz LH, Lefkowitz RA, Panicek DM, *et al.* Breath-hold magnetic resonance cholangiopancreatography in the evaluation of malignant pancreaticobiliary obstruction. *J Comput Assist Tomogr* 2003; **27**: 307–14.

31. Kim MJ, Mitchell DG, Ito K, Outwater EK. Biliary dilation: differentiation of benign from malignant causes – value of adding conventional MR imaging to MR cholangiopancreatography. *Radiology* 2000; **214**: 173–81.

32. Yeh TS, Jan YY, Tseng JH, *et al.* Malignant perihilar biliary obstruction: magnetic resonance cholangiopancreatographic findings. *AJR Am J Gastroenterol* 2000; **95**: 432–40.

33. Fulcher AS, Turner MA, Capps GW, *et al.* Half-Fourier RARE MR cholangiopancreatography: experience in 300 subjects. *Radiology* 1998; **207**: 21–32.

34. Park MS, Yu JS, Kim YH, *et al.* Acute cholecystitis: comparison of MR cholangiography and US. *Radiology* 1998; **209**: 781–5.

35. Fulcher AS, Turner MA, Ham JM. Late biliary complications in right lobe living donor transplantation recipients: imaging findings and therapeutic interventions. *J Comput Assist Tomogr* 2002; **26**: 422–7.

36. Tang Y, Yamashita Y, Arakawa A, *et al.* Pancreaticobiliary ductal system: value of half-Fourier rapid acquisition with relaxation enhancement MR cholangiopancreatography for postoperative evaluation. *Radiology* 2000; **215**: 81–8.

37. Fulcher AS, Turner MA. Magnetic resonance cholangiopancreatography. In: Gore RM, Levine MS, eds. *Textbook of Gastrointestinal Radiology*, 3rd edn. Philadelphia, PA, Saunders. 2007; 1383–98.

38. Manfredi R, Costamagna G, Brizi MG, *et al.* Severe chronic pancreatitis versus suspected pancreatic disease: dynamic MR cholangiopancreatography after secretin stimulation. *Radiology* 2000; **214**: 849–55.

39. Adamek HE, Albert J, Breer H, *et al.* Pancreatic cancer detection with magnetic resonance cholangiopancreatography and endoscopic retrograde cholangiopancreatography: a prospective controlled study. *Lancet* 2000; **356**: 190–3.

40. Lopez Hanninen E, Amthauer H, Hosten N, *et al.* Prospective evaluation of pancreatic tumors: accuracy of MR imaging with MR cholangiopancreatography and MR angiography. *Radiology* 2002; **224**: 34–41.

41. D'Angelica M, Brennan MF, Suriawinata AA, Klimstra D, Conlon KC. Intraductal papillary mucinous neoplasms of the pancreas: an analysis of clinicopathologic features and outcome. *Ann Surg* 2004; **239**: 400–8.

42. Irie H, Honda H, Aibe H, *et al.* MR cholangiopancreatographic differentiation of benign and malignant intraductal mucin-producing tumors of the pancreas. *AJR Am J Roentgenol* 2000; **174**: 1403–8.

43. Koito K, Namieno T, Ichimura T *et al.* Mucin-producing pancreatic tumors: comparison of MR cholangiopancreatography with endoscopic retrograde cholangiopancreatography. *Radiology* 1998; **208**: 231–7.

MR imaging of small and large bowel

Manon L. W. Ziech, Marije P. van der Paardt, Aart J. Nederveen, and Jaap Stoker

Introduction

The bowel is an organ which was not easily and accurately assessable until the introduction of cross-sectional imaging and newer endoscopic techniques. The location, length, and bowel peristalsis were major hurdles which were first overcome by the intro-duction of conventional radiology. Barium follow-through examinations and conventional enteroclysis gave valuable information on the presence of stenoses and mucosal lesions while barium enema and double contrast barium enema were used primarily for detec-tion of colorectal cancer and its precursors (adeno-matous polyps). Disadvantages of these techniques were the lack of detailed information on both mural and extramural abnormalities and the resulting medi-ocre accuracy. Furthermore, the ionizing radiation exposure was a major drawback of these examinations especially as these often have to be repeated for treat-ment monitoring or screening of disease recurrence.

Ultrasound and computed tomography (CT) can be used for bowel assessment. They have high spatial resolution, give insight into mural and extramural abnormalities, and are widely available. However, both have their limitations. Ultrasound has a limited field of view in areas where air or bone obscure viewing (e.g., pelvis), while reproducibility is a limitation. The primary drawback of CT is the ionizing radiation, while the contrast resolution is lower than for magnetic resonance (MR) imaging.

MR imaging of the bowel was not possible when MR imaging was first introduced because long acqui-sition times in combination with respiratory move-ment and bowel peristalsis created large artifacts. In the last 10–15 years, fast imaging techniques that can be performed in a breath-hold were developed. Reduction of data-acquisition time, improved image

quality, and optimal resolution are developments in abdominal imaging that have led to the practicability of diagnostic assessment of the bowel with MR imaging. Currently, 1.5T MR imaging scanners are primarily used to evaluate the bowel, but in recent years 3T scanners have been used for MR imaging of the bowel. Because of the anticipated twofold increase in signal-to-noise ratio (SNR) compared with 1.5T, and therefore improvement in temporal or spatial resolution of the images, there is an increasing inter-est in adopting bowel MR protocols for 3T scanners.

Artifacts at 3T

Several different problems are associated with imaging at 3T. In general a direct transition from 1.5T to 3T is not possible. One needs to consider several aspects related to pulse sequence design, such as timings, radiofrequency (RF) pulses, and specific absorption rate (SAR) issues, when imaging at 3T.

Experience gained in, for example, imaging the brain at 3T does not necessarily apply to improve abdominal imaging. Many of the problems that are associated with imaging at 3T differ between regions. The main constraints in 3T imaging are related to changes in tissue T1 and T2 relaxation parameters, SAR limitations, susceptibility artifacts, B1 inhomo-geneity artifacts and steady-state free precession (SSFP) banding artifacts. A problem of the first-generation 3T scanners for abdominal imaging is the reduced field of view in the z-direction, which is often limited to 30 cm. Current 3T MR imaging scanners have fields of view that are comparable to 1.5T scanners.

In general one should be aware of the changes in T1 and T2 values when using 3T. T1 values are pro-longed at 3T, whereas T2 values are slightly shortened [1]. The changes in T1 and T2 relaxation parameters at

Body MR Imaging at 3 Tesla, ed. Ihab R. Kamel and Elmar M. Merkle. Published by Cambridge University Press.
© Cambridge University Press 2011.

3T imply the decrease of T1 contrast in T1-weighted images and the decrease in the SNR of T2-weighted images, if echo time (TE) and repetition time (TR) parameters are used that are identical to the ones used at 1.5T. Direct adoption of imaging parameters used at 1.5T without adjustments will therefore possibly alter the diagnostic quality of the images. Avoiding T1-weighting in spin echo sequences at 3T necessitates the use of higher TR values which has as a drawback an increased scan time.

Energy deposition in tissue due to the RF transmission can be limited by keeping SAR levels below 4 W/kg over the whole body. However, the SAR increases by a factor 4 when going from 1.5T to 3T. Here again, direct transition of sequence parameters (e.g., flip angles) from 1.5T to 3T will not be possible. Sequences working close to SAR limits (e.g., turbo spin echo and SSFP sequences) are consequently limited at 3T. In fast spin echo sequences one might therefore consider using refocusing angles much smaller than 180° and to use parallel imaging factors much larger than 2, thus making use of the increased SNR at 3T.

Susceptibility artifacts are a well-known source of MR imaging artifacts. These artifacts arise in interfaces between different tissues in the body, e.g., bone and soft tissue. A local shortening of T2* can degrade the signal and in more severe cases significant distortion and even signal voids can occur. Those artifacts increase with field strength and consequently at 3T they are more pronounced. Fortunately, in fast imaging sequences with very short TEs susceptibility artifacts only play a minor role, although in echo planar imaging used for diffusion-weighted imaging the effects can be very detrimental. In the latter case, one should use either small fields of view in the phase-encoding direction or high parallel imaging factors to keep the TE as short as possible. In addition, the effectiveness of prepulses, e.g., for fat suppression, can also be decreased by B0 inhomogeneity that is present near tissue interfaces.

B1 artifacts are among the most problematic artifacts hampering clinical routine use of 3T abdominal imaging. Due to the high dielectric constant of tissue (water) the B1 wavelength is decreased from 234 cm in free space to approximately 30 cm in the body. The latter is of the order of magnitude of the field of view of many body imaging protocols and therefore artifacts resulting from the generation of standing waves within the field of view can occur. These artifacts consist of strong signal variations across the image.

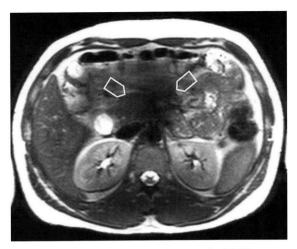

Figure 10.1 Transverse single-shot fast spin echo (SSFSE) image shows large B1 inhomogeneity artifact (drop in signal intensity; arrows).

In areas of high signal intensity constructive interference occurs and areas of signal drop coincide with areas of destructive interference (Figure 10.1). In addition, conductivity effects also tend to increase B1 field inhomogeneity. In regions of highly conductive tissue such as ascites current can be induced by the rapidly changing RF field. The induced current tends to oppose the RF field therefore causing local signal drops in the image. Presently multi-transmit systems are becoming available that largely reduce the effects of B1 homogeneity by use of sophisticated methods for B1 shimming. Several RF transmit coils can be combined whereby the phase and amplitude of the signal emitted by each coil are adjusted in order to obtain a homogeneous B1 field.

Fast three-dimensional (3D) imaging sequences with very short TRs below 10 ms are frequently being used in abdominal imaging because of their imaging speed while still maintaining high SNR and spatial resolution. Pulse sequences falling under the classification of balanced (b)SSFP sequences such as bFFE (balanced fast field echo), TrueFISP (true fast imaging with steady state free precession) and FIESTA (fast imaging employing steady-state acquisition) are very attractive for discrimination between lumen and bowel wall. However, bSSFP sequences suffer from banding artifacts that become more prominent with increasing field strength (Figure 10.2). The bands in the image originate from the dephasing of the transversal magnetization in each TR due to magnetic field inhomogeneities. Furthermore, the combination of

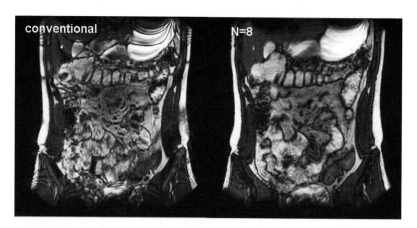

Figure 10.2 bSSFP scan of a patient (left) and a combined image (right) with different phase cycling, i.e., in each acquisition the location of the banding pattern changes. Patient preparation consisted of fasting for 4 hours before the scan followed by drinking 1600 mL mannitol 2.5% in 1 hour before the scan. Scan parameters were: TR/TE = 5.4 ms/ 1.8 ms, Flip angle = 40°; 20 sagittal slices; FOV = 350 × 350 mm^2; voxel size = 2.0 × 2.0 × 2.0 mm^3. Courtesy Sonia I. Gonçalves, AMC, Amsterdam, The Netherlands.

bSSFP with fat suppression can be problematic in terms of SAR, since bSSFP sequences require high flip angles (~45°) to generate the typical contrast between lumen and wall. At present no straightforward solution for the banding artifact is available.

Patient preparation

Oral contrast agents

Bowel pathology can only be accurately assessed when there is adequate luminal distension. Only large masses can be identified without distension. Collapsed bowel segments hamper adequate assessment of bowel wall pathology, as they can imitate or conceal wall-related lesions [2]. Small bowel distension can be achieved either by naso-duodenal intubation (MR enteroclysis) or oral contrast (MR enterography). Both have some drawbacks; enteroclysis is more burdensome and exposes the patient to radiation (during the naso-duodenal intubation under fluoroscopic guidance), whereas enterography is less accurate in showing proximal small bowel lesions. Therefore the authors recommend MR enteroclysis in all new patients and MR enterography for Crohn's disease follow-up.

Distension of the large bowel can be obtained either by rectal insufflation of gas, administration of water-based enemas, or oral contrast agents. Important features of a bowel contrast agent are a high contrast resolution between the bowel wall (and pathology) and the bowel lumen and homogeneous signal intensity of the lumen.

There are three types of contrast agents; positive (bright lumen), negative (dark lumen) and biphasic (bright on one sequence, dark on the other). Bright lumen contrast agents are contrast agents which are gadolinium-based. Gadolinium causes both T1 and T2 shortening. When applying "normal" concentrations, the T1-shortening effect predominates causing high signal intensity on both T1- and T2-weighted images. However, when the gadolinium concentration is much higher, T2 shortening occurs as well, causing signal intensity loss in all sequences. Nevertheless, T2-weighted sequences are more sensitive for this effect, which causes dark-appearing lumen on T2-weighted images (thus making this type of contrast biphasic). With the bright lumen technique, intraluminal lesions (polyps) can be seen as dark-appearing filling defects.

When using negative contrast agents (the dark lumen approach), the lumen of the bowel appears hypointense on both T1- and T2-weighted images. This is caused by local field inhomogeneity induced by the contrast agent causing a signal drop on both T1- and T2-weighted images. When a paramagnetic contrast agent is given intravenously, this causes the bowel wall/lesion to enhance, thus improving the contrast between the bowel wall and lumen.

Biphasic contrast agents differ from bright and dark lumen agents because they appear bright on one sequence, usually T2, and dark on the other, usually T1. Biphasic contrast agents are most commonly applied in small bowel MR imaging. Water is the most easily available biphasic contrast agent, but as water is fast absorbed by the gut, an osmotic agent is often added to improve luminal distension.

For small bowel imaging, the authors prefer to use a biphasic contrast agent (mannitol, 2.5%, 1600 mL) as this results in optimal contrast between bowel wall and lumen at both T1-weighted and T2-weighted sequences. For MR enterography the patient starts to drink the

(A)

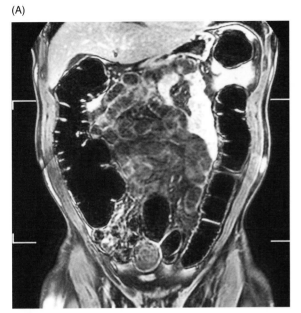

(B)

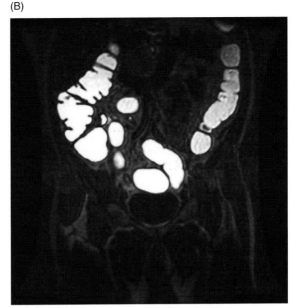

Figure 10.3 (A) Dark lumen MR colonography in a 64-year-old patient. Rectal CO_2 insufflation was used to distend the colon and fecal tagging with an iodinated contrast agent was used to homogeneously label the stool. The coronal 3D T1-weighted gradient echo sequence shows a dark colonic lumen. (B) Bright lumen MR colonography in a 62-year-old male patient. The colon was distended by an oral contrast agent that contained 10 mL gadolinium (0.5 mmol/mL) and rectal administration with a mixture of water and gadolinium-based contrast agent (10 mmol/L). The coronal 3D T1-weighted FFE sequence demonstrates high signal intensity of the colonic lumen.

contrast agent 1 hour before the examination, in aliquots of 1 cup per 5 minutes [3]. When using mannitol, colonoscopy with electrocoagulation should be avoided after the MR imaging, because methane and hydrogen are formed when mannitol dissociates. As an alternative, the sugar alcohol sorbitol (2.5% in 1500 mL water) can be used. For MR enteroclysis, the contrast medium is infused through a naso-duodenal tube at 80–120 mL/min. During the infusion of the contrast, thick-slab SSFSE images are acquired to assess if the contrast has reached the cecum. When this is the case, the MR examination can be performed.

Bowel preparation schemes for 1.5T can also be implemented at 3T. For the same contrast agent concentration, the change in T1 parameter is larger at 3T than at 1.5T, due to the increase of T1 relaxation times at 3T by roughly a factor of 1.5. To obtain images at 3T equivalent to 1.5T less contrast has to be administered. In general one should be aware that increased uptake at 3T should not be straightforwardly interpreted as pathologic [3].

MR colonography is used for diagnostic evaluation of the large bowel and differs from routine abdominal imaging first in the way that it uses colonic distension for optimal visualization of bowel lesions and second it uses either cleansing or fecal tagging for preparation of the bowel [2].

Room air, water, or a barium-containing mixture are generally used as bowel distension agents. Carbon dioxide (CO_2) or room air have been studied as gaseous distending agents in rectal insufflation for MR colonography and result in low signal intensity on T1- and T2-weighted sequences [2] (Figure 10.3). Although most studies report on room-air insufflation, CO_2 has the advantage of less discomfort after the examination, due to faster reabsorption by the gastrointestinal tract than room air. Studies on colonoscopy demonstrated better acceptance by patients of CO_2 than room air [2]. Both automated and manual insufflation is used in gaseous distension, although automated insufflation benefits from monitoring and regulating constant intracolonic pressure as this might vary due to ileocecal reflux and gas incontinence. Up to now, diagnostic performance of MR colonography with gaseous distension varies [2].

Susceptibility artifacts, due to field heterogeneities, are more prone at soft tissue–air interfaces and increase with the increase of the magnetic field strength. As colonic distension by air-based and water-based contrast agents is one of the prerequisites

(A)

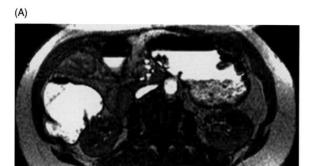

(B)

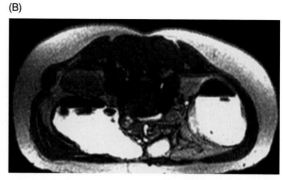

Figure 10.4 Bright lumen MR colonography with supine (A) and prone (B) positioning. The transverse 3D T1-weighted FFE demonstrates that the stool is affected by gravity as the patient changes position; supine and prone.

of MR colonography, the latter is prone to susceptibility artifacts at the interface of gas and bowel wall. The use of fast imaging 3D sequences with very short TEs (3–4 ms) decreases susceptibility artifacts in MR colonography with CO_2 distension. Consequently, susceptibility artifacts at 3T are most pronounced in two-dimensional (2D) gradient echo sequences with TEs in the range of 50–80 ms, therefore the use of 3D sequences is recommended.

Although gaseous distension is akin to colonography with CT (CT-colonography), most studies until now concerned water-based enemas. Bowel distension with water-based enemas consisting of tap water or a mixture of water and gadolinium have been used [2]. Generally a volume of 1 to 3 liters of water-based distension agent is used to maintain constant intracolonic distension. Signal intensity of water is high on T2-weighted images and low on T1-weighted sequences. When labeled with gadolinium, T1-weighted images appear high in signal (bright lumen) (Figure 10.3).

Chemical shift artifacts are increased at high-field imaging due to the increased difference in resonant frequency of water and fat. This artifact has implications for MR colonography which uses water-based enemas for bowel distension. In MR colonography the appearance of dark boundaries due to chemical shift artifacts at fat–water interfaces can hinder visualization of the bowel wall. To overcome these artifacts the bandwidth can be increased, although this reduces SNR. When using effective fat suppression techniques the consequences of this artifact will however be minor.

Fecal tagging

Fecal residue can mimic or obscure bowel pathology and therefore hamper adequate diagnostic assessment

of the large bowel. To overcome this impediment, the colon can be cleansed by purgative solutions as in conventional colonoscopy. In general, sodium phosphate solutions and polyethylene glycol (PEG) electrolyte solutions are used for cleansing.

Fecal tagging as a bowel preparation method was introduced similar to its use in CT-colonography [2]. Fecal tagging refers to consistently labeling stool by oral intake of a contrast agent with a regular meal, in that way providing for sufficient contrast between the colonic wall and the colonic lumen with its fecal content. Furthermore, as bowel purgation was considered burdensome, fecal tagging was also introduced to avoid extensive cleansing of the colon.

Several fecal tagging strategies have been proposed in MR colonography research. Tagging agents containing high concentrations of barium sulfate were studied. Initial results were promising as differentiation of colonic wall and lumen was exceptional, yet subsequent research demonstrated less encouraging results regarding patient acceptance and image quality [2]. Following these results, different solutions containing barium were studied concerning diagnostic accuracy and patient acceptance resulting in improved outcomes [2].

Furthermore, gadolinium-based fecal tagging agents were studied; however, in preliminary research high costs of the tagging agent hindered extensive application [2].

Diagnostic accuracy of bright lumen MR colonography is influenced by false-positive findings caused by residual air and feces. As most lesions are not affected by gravity as opposed to residual air and feces, the examination is performed in both supine and prone position [2] (Figure 10.4). In the dark lumen approach dual positioning is not required to avoid false-positive findings due to air/feces residue as

(A)

(B)

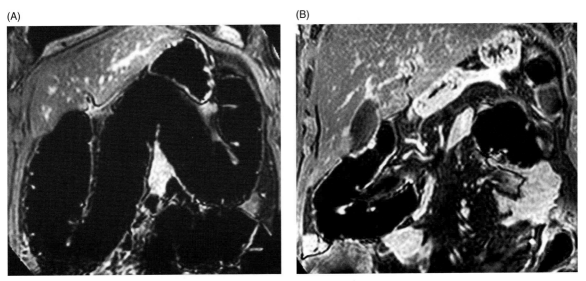

Figure 10.5 Dark lumen MR colonography in a 60-year-old male patient. (A) Coronal 3D T1-weighted gradient echo image in supine position. The transverse colon is well distended. (B) This is contrary to the coronal 3D T1-weighted image in prone position where the colon is not well distended.

(A)

(B)

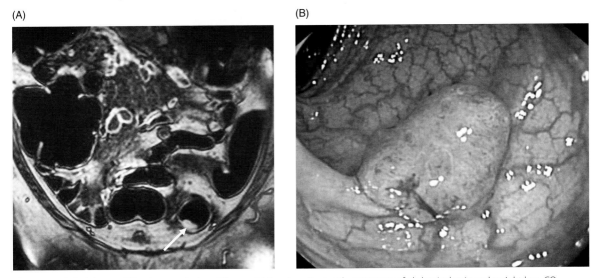

Figure 10.6 Dark lumen MR colonography in a 79-year-old female patient with symptoms of abdominal pain and weight loss. CO_2 insufflation was used for colonic distension and an iodinated oral contrast agent was used for fecal tagging. (A) Coronal 3D T1-weighted gradient echo sequence with fat saturation after intravenously administered paramagnetic contrast agent demonstrates a polyp in the sigmoid (arrow). (B) The presence of a hyperplastic polyp of 12 mm was confirmed at conventional colonoscopy and pathology.

lesions of the bowel wall are enhanced; nevertheless dual positioning is in fact essential for optimal bowel distension (Figure 10.5). To avoid false-positive findings in dark lumen MR colonography, pre-and post-contrast imaging is performed.

For MR colonography, the authors prefer to use the dark lumen approach using automated CO_2 insufflation for bowel distension as this improves adequate colonic distension and patient acceptance (Figures 10.6 and 10.7). As in CT-colonography, fecal tagging with an iodinated contrast agent is applied for adequately labeling the stool, causing high signal intensity of the stool at T1- and T2-weighted sequences. Furthermore, the laxative effect of the iodine provides

(A)

(B)

(C)

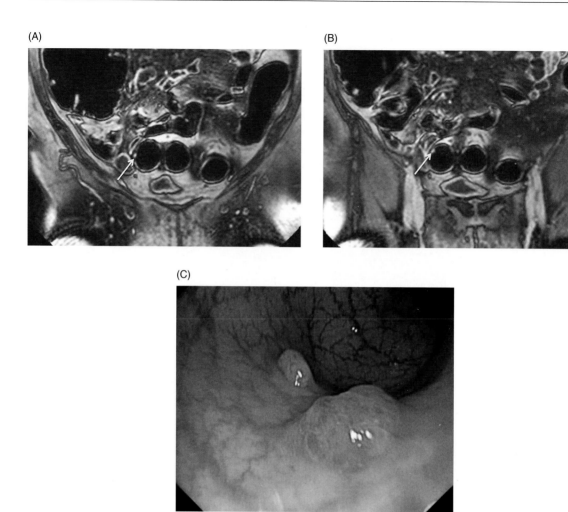

Figure 10.7 Coronal 3D T1-weighted gradient echo, dark lumen MR colonography, in a 79-year-old female patient with symptoms of abdominal pain and weight loss. (A and B) Coronal T1-weighted image with fat saturation demonstrates two sessile polyps in the sigmoid close to each other (arrow). (C) Both polyps were confirmed at conventional colonoscopy, the size was 4 and 5mm, respectively. Histopathology demonstrated one hyperplastic polyp and one adenoma with low-grade dysplasia.

for liquid stool with a good mixture of stool and contrast. To ensure sufficient colonic distension of all bowel segments, prior to data acquisition, the insufflation is performed while changing the patient's position from his/her right lateral side to the left lateral side. The intracolonic pressure is monitored by an automated insufflator. To our knowledge, no MR imaging compatible insufflator exists; therefore long tubing is used for insufflation with the insufflator outside the MR suite.

Sequences at 3T

When transferring bowel imaging MR sequence protocols from 1.5T to 3T, modifications are mandatory because of differences in tissue T1 and T2

relaxation parameters (longer T1 and shorter T2 relaxation times at 3T) and SAR limitations (see specific sequence for details).

All sequences must be performed in 15- to 25-second breath-holds. If the breath-hold is over 15 seconds hyperventilation directly prior to the sequence is recommended. Careful explanation of the procedure and length of the breath-hold is mandatory (see Table 10.1 for recommended scan parameters).

Single-shot fast spin echo (SSFSE)

This sequence is recommended as the initial sequence as it gives an overview of the abdomen. Both coronal and axial sequences must be performed. Since one

Table 10.1 Recommended scan parameters for 3T MR imaging of the bowel

Sequence	SSFSE coronal	SSFSE axial	SSFSE axial with fat saturation	3D T1-weighted gradient echo coronal	3D T1-weighted gradient echo axial
Repetition time (ms)	800	800	1450	2.2	2.2
Echo time (ms)	65	65	70	1.0	1.0
Flip angle (degrees)	90	90	90	10	10
Slice thickness (mm)	4	4	7	2	2
Number of signal averages	1	1	1	1	1
Fat saturation	No	No	yes	yes	yes
Gap (mm)	1	1	1	–	–
Matrix	256 × 200	256 × 200	288 × 233	200 × 200	200 × 200
Field of view (mm^2)	400 × 400	375 × 300	375 × 300	400 × 400	375 × 300

slice is acquired per shot, this sequence is relatively insensitive to motion artifacts although intraluminal flow artifacts can occur. The normal bowel wall has uniform low signal intensity on this sequence; wall edema (e.g., in active inflammation) and mural fat (e.g., in patients with longstanding inflammatory bowel disease) have high signal intensity. To differentiate between edema and intestinal fat, a fat-suppressed sequence is recommended.

Theoretically, 3T MR imaging scanners have twice the SNR compared with a 1.5T scanner. One study has assessed that for SSFSE the ultimate gain in SNR is only 1.7 [4]. This is due to specific problems at 3T, such as SAR limitations. In comparison to 1.5T, the TE of this sequence needs to be shortened. The 180°-refocusing pulses need to be reduced because of SAR limitations, which will lower the SNR. When shortening the TE, the SNR improves but this causes some loss in T2 contrast. In addition, standing wave artifacts can be present in patients with ascites (see Artifacts at 3T).

Three-dimensional T1-weighted gradient echo

The overall enhancement and the enhancement pattern of the bowel wall after intravenous contrast injection is best assessed on this sequence. The authors recommend administering intravenous gadolinium (0.1 mL/kg) and start the scan after 60 seconds. This is specifically important in patients with inflammatory bowel disease where enhancement is one of the features used for determining disease activity. The sequences should be performed in coronal and axial plane if isotropic voxel sizes are not available. Also, the use of fat saturation is recommended to optimize the contrast between enhancing bowel wall and mesenteric fat. Because this sequence is very sensitive to (peristaltic) motion, it is advised to give an antiperistaltic drug, such as N-butyl scopolamine bromide or glucagon. In the USA N-butyl scopolamine bromide is not Food and Drug Administration (FDA) approved for this application and cannot be used.

Three-dimensional spoiled gradient echo sequences (e.g., THRIVE [T1-weighted high-resolution isotropic volume examination], VIBE [volume interpolated breath-hold examination], or FAME [fast acquisition multiecho]) are robust sequences that can be implemented without much adaptation on 3T, with a good SNR and contrast-to-noise ratio [5].

Balanced steady-state free precession (bSSFP)

bSSFP sequences combine their contrast from both T1 and T2 in a ratio (T2/T1). This sequence is often used at 1.5T for assessment of the small bowel wall as it provides a high contrast anatomical overview. Thereby, this breath-hold sequence is not sensitive to motion. At 3T, banding artifacts (appearing as bright and dark stripes in the image) and low SNR substantially degrade the usefulness of this sequence (see Artifacts at 3T). When increasing B0 homogeneity the banding pattern migrates to the borders of the field of view. However, this solution is not very practical at 3T, since the effectiveness of shimming is limited at 3T. Another solution is to vary the location of the banding pattern in consecutive acquisitions [6], as illustrated in Figure 10.2. This can give good results, but the imaging time is increased and the final image is prone to blurring due to differing breath-hold positions. A satisfactory solution to reduce the banding artifact has not been proposed so far.

Diffusion-weighted imaging (DWI)

DWI reflects the changes in water mobility caused by interactions with macromolecules and cell membranes. This can be measured by the apparent diffusion coefficient (ADC value). DWI at 3T can benefit from increased SNR, but also image quality can suffer because of increased magnetic susceptibility. These artifacts can be limited using parallel imaging techniques, thus shortening imaging time and TE.

At 1.5T for detection of active Crohn's disease, DWI showed decreased ADC values in patients with active disease with a sensitivity of 95% and a specificity of 82% [7]. To our knowledge, no study has been performed at 3T.

Developments in DWI demonstrated valuable potential in the field of oncology for detection of cancer and response prediction to therapy. However, to our knowledge, all studies in DWI of the bowel have been performed at 1.5T or lower field strength MR imaging.

Cine imaging

To obtain information about small bowel motion and peristalsis, it can be useful to add a cine MR imaging sequence. Especially, adhesions can be visualized by fixation of bowel loops and lack of normal peristalsis. On 1.5T, this is usually done with the bSSFP sequence. On 3T, SSFSE can be used instead, acquiring two slices per second.

Imaging indications
Inflammatory bowel disease

Crohn's disease and ulcerative colitis are the two main diseases that comprise inflammatory bowel disease (IBD). IBD is characterized by disease remissions and exacerbations. Crohn's disease can be present in the whole gastrointestinal tract, but is most commonly located in the terminal ileum. Colonic

involvement is also often present. Specific for Crohn's disease is the presence of skip lesions where pathologic bowel wall lesions are separated from normal bowel wall. Crohn's disease is a transmural disease, so all bowel wall layers can be involved and extraintestinal manifestations (fistulas, abscesses) can occur.

Ulcerative colitis is a mucosal inflammatory disease and is confined to the colon and rectum with a predilection for the distal colon and rectum, though "backwash ileitis" can mimic terminal ileitis. Because the inflammation occurs only in the mucosal layer of the large bowel, extra-enteric manifestations are very rare.

Diagnosis or follow-up (therapy monitoring) for Crohn's disease is the most important indication for MR imaging of the small bowel. MR imaging is capable of diagnosing Crohn's disease and monitoring therapy response. In a meta-analysis, sensitivity was 93.0% and specificity was 92.8% for detection of Crohn's disease [8]. All studies in this meta-analysis were performed at 1.5T or less. Only one study has been performed that focused on evaluating Crohn's disease activity at 3T [9]. This study demonstrated the feasibility of 3T MR enterography in a small cohort of 20 Crohn's disease patients. Two MR parameters were assessed; correlations were found between the Crohn's disease severity index (CDEIS) and bowel wall thickness and enhancement. As of yet, to our knowledge, no studies have been performed that compared 1.5T with 3T for the accuracy of diagnosing Crohn's disease.

A recent meta-analysis determined the accuracy of MR imaging in grading disease activity. Seven studies were included (one at 3T), of which six examined both the small and the large bowel. MR imaging correctly graded 91% of frank disease and 62% of patients in remission or with mild disease [10]. This low accuracy in grading of mild disease activity (presented often as small mucosal ulcerations) might be due to low spatial resolution in MR imaging or the inability of MR imaging to detect small lesions.

The role of MR colonography in Crohn's disease patients is limited. It has been studied in a few studies and only at 1.5T. Sensitivity for segment-based inflammation was 32% and specificity was 88% [11]. Rimola and colleagues have published an educational exhibit about 50 IBD patients in whom they performed MR colonography, but did not report statistical evidence [12].

The place of MR imaging in ulcerative colitis patients is limited to MR colonography, as ulcerative colitis is limited to the colon. Only the mucosa is affected and especially in mild disease, where only mucosal edema and hyperemia are present, spatial resolution is too low to detect this. When there is severe disease, the colonic wall changes can show ulcerations, wall thickening, and enhancement but less than in Crohn's disease because the inflammation is not transmural [12].

In Crohn's disease patients, current guidelines from the European Crohn's and Colitis Organisation (ECCO) recommend performing ileocolonoscopy for initial diagnosis and to assess the extent of the disease, either by small bowel MR imaging or CT. They add that because of the radiation risk in young patients, MR should be considered where possible. The American College of Radiology recommends performing an abdominal CT, though they indicate that MR imaging may have the same sensitivity and specificity. The choice of examination therefore depends on institutional resources and preferences. For ulcerative colitis, ECCO guidelines do not recommend MR imaging as a routine imaging technique.

Imaging features for IBD

Several imaging features are known to reflect active Crohn's disease activity.

Bowel wall thickening has been used as one of the most important parameters to assess disease activity for a long time [10]. Traditionally, this is best assessed on bSSFP images, but if these are not available, SSFSE can also be used for this purpose (Figure 10.8). There is no consensus in the literature on the exact upper limit of normal bowel wall, however, often a bowel wall > 3 mm is considered as thickened. The thickening can be due either to fibrosis or edema of the bowel wall. In a previous study on a 3T scanner, a significant correlation was found for bowel wall thickness and the CDEIS [9]. False-positive findings mimicking thickened bowel wall can occur when the bowel is not optimally distended; therefore all sequences have to be scrutinized for the images with the most optimal distension. This primarily concerns MR enterography; bowel loop distension is optimized at MR enteroclysis.

Enhancement of the bowel wall. One of the most important findings for disease activity is the enhancement of the bowel wall by intravenous contrast injection. In a meta-analysis, enhancement was one of the most important parameters for Crohn's disease

activity [10]. To our knowledge, only one study assessed enhancement of bowel wall at 3T. In that study, a significant correlation was found between CDEIS and mural enhancement (Figure 10.8) [9].

T1 stratification (layered appearance of bowel wall) can be seen when the bowel wall enhances after intravenous contrast injection. Enhancement can be mucosal (innermost layer of bowel enhancing), homogeneous (all bowel wall enhancing equally) and layered (both mucosal and serosal bowel wall layers enhancing with a central band of relatively reduced enhancement). At 1.5T a multilayered appearance of the bowel wall was associated with inflammatory activity measured at histology [13] (Figure 10.9).

High T2 signal intensity of the bowel wall is most often present when there is inflammation/edema of the bowel wall, such as in active Crohn's disease. Fat suppression is recommended to distinguish edema from fat. At 1.5T, the signal intensity of the bowel wall compared with the signal intensity of cerebrospinal fluid was positively correlated with disease activity measured at histology [13] (Figure 10.9).

Stenosis. A stenosis can be defined as a luminal narrowing of the bowel wall of more than 50%. This can be evaluated on all sequences. If a pre-stenotic dilation is present, this indicates (partial) obstruction. A stenosis can be caused by either fibrosis or inflammation. If the stenosis is due to inflammatory activity, medical therapeutic options should be considered. Therefore it is important to differentiate between fibrosis and inflammation. After intravenous contrast, active Crohn's disease does enhance whereas a fibrotic stenosis does not enhance.

Verification of the degree of obstruction on the different sequences performed during the MR enterography procedure gives important information on the degree of obstruction. The sensitivity of detecting a stenosis with MR enterography at 1.5T is 86% versus 100% for MR enteroclysis [14]. The higher accuracy with MR enteroclysis is due to the better distension, but in daily practice enterography can also be performed because the obstructed flow due to the stenosis gives rise to a pre-stenotic dilation. Also cine imaging can be performed to assess the motility of the bowel wall (see Sequences at 3T).

The presence of the **comb sign** indicates increased blood flow in the vasa recta of a bowel segment. The mesenteric vessels are arranged like the teeth of a comb, hence the name comb sign. This can be seen on bSSFP images or on T1-weighted images.

143

(A)

(B)

(C)

(D)

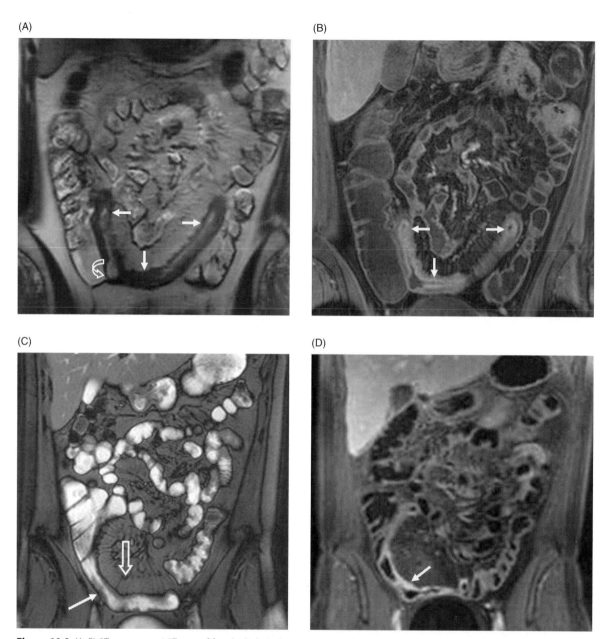

Figure 10.8 (A, B) 3T scan versus 1.5T scan of female Crohn's disease patient. (A) Coronal 3T T2-weighted SSFSE image shows thickened terminal ileum (arrows), with a large ulceration (curved arrow). (B) Coronal 3T T1-weighted gradient echo image with fat suppression after intravenous contrast shows stratified enhancement: enhancing serosa and (sub)mucosa (arrows) of the ileal loop, indicating inflammation. (C, D) Follow-up 1.5T scan of the same patient after 8 months of infliximab therapy. (C) Coronal bSSFP image with fat saturation at 1.5T shows thickened bowel wall (arrow) and the presence of the comb sign (open arrow). (D) Coronal T1-weighted gradient echo image with fat saturation at 1.5T shows homogeneous enhancing bowel wall (arrow).

It is considered to indicate the presence of active disease (Figure 10.8).

Creeping fat or fibro fatty proliferation is the stranding and retracting of mesenteric fat around affected bowel segments. Most often, this phenomenon can be seen in patients with a past episode of active inflammatory bowel disease. The presence of creeping fat can best be assessed on SSFSE images.

Traditionally, the presence of **ulcerations** can best be assessed on bSSFP images, but also on SSFSE. Deep

(A)

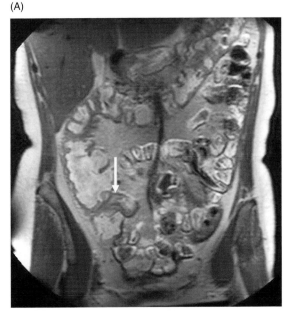

(B)

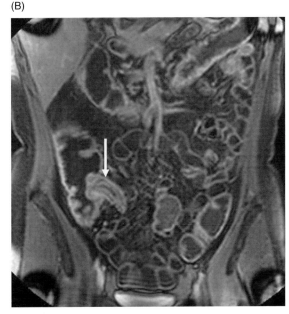

Figure 10.9 A 47-year-old female patient with Crohn's disease. (A) Coronal SSFSE image at 3T shows thickened terminal ileum. The wall is two-layered (arrow), a hypointense mucosa and submucosa and a hyperintense muscularis, which is caused either by edema or intramural fat. (B) Coronal T1-weighted gradient echo image with fat saturation after intravenous contrast shows a layered appearance of the bowel wall (arrow) with enhancement of (sub)mucosa and serosa, which indicates inflammation.

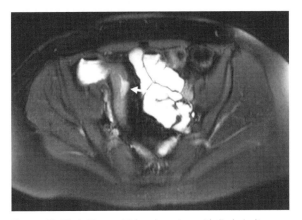

Figure 10.10 A 27-year-old female patient with Crohn's disease. Transverse SSFSE image with fat saturation shows a thickened terminal ileum with an ulceration (arrow).

linear ulcers appear as thin lines of high signal intensity, longitudinally or transversely (fissure ulcers) orientated within the thickened bowel wall (Figure 10.10). On T1-weighted images, ulcerations can be seen as a focal defect in the enhancing bowel wall.

Lymph nodes. Patients with Crohn's disease often have enlarged mesenteric lymph nodes ($> 1\,\text{cm}$). These can best be visualized on bSSFP sequences. At 3T, these can best be seen on a T1-weighted sequence

(Figure 10.11). Lymph nodes may enhance, although the relevance of this finding for determining disease activity is disputed.

Fistula and abscess. Fistulas and abscesses are extraluminal manifestations of Crohn's disease that can best be seen on post-contrast T1-weighted images, because of their enhancement after intravenous contrast due to inflammation (Figure 10.12). A nonactive fibrotic track will not enhance. In abscesses, the center will have a hypointense signal intensity because of the fluid content, whereas the wall of the abscess enhances.

Detection of colorectal polyps and colorectal cancer

Colorectal cancer (CRC) is the second leading cause of cancer-related death in most Western societies. Colorectal adenomas are considered to be the benign precursors in the majority of cases of CRC. Efforts have been made to reduce mortality and incidence by screening and surveillance. CT-colonography has gained clinical acceptance as it is less invasive and burdensome compared with conventional colonoscopy and has proven its role as an alternative to colonoscopy in symptomatic patients. Importantly, it has also been demonstrated to have good accuracy for screening [15].

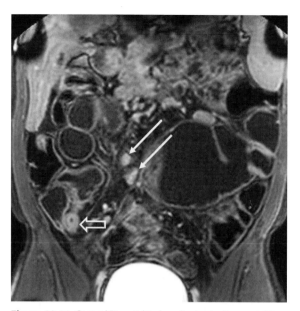

Figure 10.11 Coronal T1-weighted gradient echo image at 3T with fat saturation shows two enlarged lymph nodes (arrows). Also, a thickened pre-terminal ileum loop is visible (open arrow).

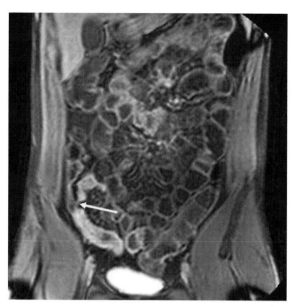

Figure 10.12 Patient with Crohn's disease. Coronal T1-weighted gradient echo image after intravenous contrast with fat saturation shows a fistula between two ileal loops (arrow).

The drawback of CT-colonography is ionizing radiation exposure, which could be prevented by using MR colonography. MR colonography has been studied over the last decade for detection of CRC and the precursor of CRC, colorectal adenomas [16].

Large colorectal lesions are highly suspicious for CRC at MR colonography, especially obstructing masses. For polypoid lesions malignancy cannot be determined at MR colonography. However, the risk of CRC within an adenoma is size-related and therefore polyps are categorized in three categories: large polyps of 10 mm and larger, intermediate polyps of 6–9 mm, and small polyps of 5 mm and smaller. In large polyps a prevalence of advanced histology was demonstrated to be 30.6% and malignancy in approximately 10%. The prevalence of advanced histology in polyps of intermediate size (6–9 mm) was 6.6% with a range of 4.6–11.7% while the chance of malignancy was smaller than 1%. For polyps of ≤ 5 mm advanced neoplasia was demonstrated to be present in 1.7% (range 1.2–2.0%) and the risk of malignancy was demonstrated to be very small (0.06%). In CT-colonography there is consensus that patients are referred for colonoscopy when polyps of 6 mm and larger are demonstrated [2].

Primarily, research has focused on dark lumen MR colonography with the use of bowel cleansing and a water-based enema; the results were encouraging as no false-negative findings were demonstrated. Initial research using the bright lumen method for MR colonography demonstrated high diagnostic accuracy for large lesion detection, though diagnostic performance for smaller lesions varied. Most research was performed at 1.5T or less.

The majority of studies have been performed in patients with symptoms of CRC or patients under surveillance. A systematic review on diagnostic accuracy of detection of (precursors of) CRC with MR colonography showed encouraging results [16]. Thirteen studies, both bright and dark lumen MR colonography studies, were evaluated. Furthermore, two study groups performed MR colonography at 3T MR scanners, however, one study was executed on both 1.5T and 3T MR systems. In this study, unfortunately, differences in diagnostic accuracy, image quality, and patient acceptance were not mentioned. The systematic review on CRC detection with MR colonography showed excellent results as sensitivity was 100%. For the detection of large polyps (10 mm or larger) the per-patient sensitivity was 88% (95% confidence internal [CI]. 63–97%) and specificity 99% (95% CI: 95–100%) and the per-polyp sensitivity was 84% (95% CI: 66–94). No conclusions could be drawn for polyps of intermediate size and smaller than 6 mm, due to heterogeneous data [16].

Although this systematic review demonstrates promising results, it has to be taken into account that data on diagnostic accuracy of MR colonography in detection of CRC and colorectal polyps are heterogeneous and to date, no consensus has been reached on patient preparation method and technique.

The results of MR colonography in symptomatic patients cannot be extrapolated to screening. One prospective study, performed on a 1.5T MR system, has focused on asymptomatic patients with a normal risk profile for CRC [2, 16]. The prevalence for polyps of 10 mm and larger was demonstrated to be 6.3%. Although the overall patient-based sensitivity and specificity was 36.4% and 90.2%, for intermediate-sized lesions and lesions of 10 mm and larger, sensitivity was 60% and 70% respectively and 100% specificity was demonstrated.

Other indications

As of yet, only few studies have been performed that assessed the accuracy of 3T MR imaging of Crohn's disease or colorectal polyp and CRC detection. For other indications for small or large bowel MR imaging discussed here, there are no data on the use of 3T.

As MR imaging permits superior soft tissue resolution, MR imaging is able to detect complications of diverticular disease like abscesses, fistulas, and free abdominal fluid. To date, MR colonography has shown promising results in evaluation of acute diverticulitis; sensitivity was 86% and specificity 92% for detecting diverticular disease with the dark lumen method at 1.5T [17]. The role of 3T MR imaging is not yet established.

MR imaging for acute abdominal pain, specifically appendicitis, was not often used because of long scan times and logistical problems. As faster sequences were developed, more interest has developed for MR imaging for this indication. Most studies have been performed on 1.5T or less and many concern pregnant patients. A systematic review has shown that sensitivity of MR imaging for diagnosing appendicitis is 80% and specificity is 99% [18]. As of yet no data exist on 3T MR imaging for appendicitis.

Peutz–Jeghers syndrome is characterized by the occurrence of hamartomatous small and large polyps and these patients require frequent monitoring because these polyps can degenerate to a malignancy and therefore need to be resected. No studies have

been performed to test the accuracy for polyp detection at 3T MR imaging. For 1.5T, polyps < 5 mm are not detected because of low spatial resolution.

Celiac disease is a gluten-sensitive enteropathy of the small bowel. Because of the lack of specific symptoms, diagnosis can be difficult. Patients whom are referred for small bowel MR for nonspecific gastrointestinal complaints can have celiac disease as their underlying pathology. The most specific sign for celiac disease on MR are fold pattern abnormalities. Ileal jejunization denotes an increase in ileal folds, whereas the folds in the jejunum decrease or completely flatten.

Small bowel malignancies are relatively uncommon. Carcinoid is the most common primary small bowel tumor. At 1.5T carcinoid presents either as a concrete mass that enhanced after intravenous contrast or as a uniform bowel wall thickening which also showed enhancement. Small bowel lymphomas are usually of the non-Hodgkin type. They are mostly located within the bowel wall and enhance after intravenous contrast is given.

1.5T versus 3T

Theoretically, 3T MR imaging scanners have twice the SNR compared with a 1.5T scanner. However, due to specific problems (such as SAR) the ultimate gain in SNR is often less, e.g., 1.7 for SSFSE sequences [4]. The gain in SNR at 3T is used in other fields such as neurovascular imaging to obtain a better imaging quality. In these fields, 3T has become superior to 1.5T imaging.

For bowel imaging, however, imaging at 1.5T is still the standard in most hospitals. In Crohn's disease patients, abdominal MR imaging at 3T is feasible but future research will have to point out if diagnostic accuracy rates are actually higher than at 1.5T.

To our knowledge, the only comparative studies of 3T versus 1.5T for bowel diseases reporting data concern the detection of colorectal polyps and cancer. Wessling et al. demonstrated no significant difference in detection of polyps larger than 6 mm in a phantom (ten sessile polyps: 4×2 mm, 3×3 mm, 1×4 mm, 1×6 mm, 1×8 mm) [19]. This study demonstrated overall sensitivity for polyp detection of 56% at 1.5T and 55% at 3T.

Moreover, a study in 40 patients carried out by Rottgen and coworkers demonstrated no overall significant difference in image quality at 3T compared with 1.5T [20]. Two-dimensional bSSFP images were found to be superior at 1.5T, but there were no significant differences in 3D T1-weighted fat-suppressed gradient echo and SSFSE. Furthermore, a phantom model with polypoid lesions was studied both at 1.5T and 3T. The study demonstrated significantly better visualization of the polyps at 1.5T and visualization of artificial polyps [20]. However, Saar *et al.* demonstrated a sensitivity of 100% for colorectal lesions larger than 6 mm as all carcinomas (4/4) and polyps (16/16) were identified at 3T using two different T1-weighted 3D gradient echo sequences [5]. Diagnostic quality was reported to be excellent in 94% and 92% respectively for the two sequences.

It can be expected that in the future the advantage of 3T MR imaging will be further exploited in techniques such as very fast dynamic contrast-enhanced sequences. In Crohn's disease, it is known that bowel wall enhancement is a marker of disease activity. Dynamic contrast-enhanced MR imaging is a technique that acquires images during the delivery of contrast in the tissue of interest (in this case the bowel), thus highlighting the dynamic response of the tissue to the inflow of blood and the subsequent distribution in the extracellular fluid space. Analysis of the time-dependent changes of signal intensity on dynamic contrast-enhanced MR images might provide valuable information about disease activity in Crohn's disease patients.

Conclusion

The use of abdominal protocols for 3T has increased over the last few years. Although it is feasible to perform MR of the small bowel and MR colonography at 3T, further research has to be performed to determine whether 3T performs better than 1.5T. At this moment, there is no compelling evidence that favors the use of 3T MR imaging over 1.5T MR imaging for imaging bowel diseases. Technologic advances like B1 shimming and increased B0 homogeneity in the *z*-direction of modern 3T scanners, will contribute largely to the clinical acceptance of 3T MR imaging scanners for abdominal imaging.

References

1. de Bazelaire C, Rofsky NM, Duhamel G, *et al.* Combined T2* and T1 measurements for improved perfusion and permeability studies in high field using dynamic contrast enhancement. *Eur Radiol* 2006; **9**: 2083–91.

2. van der Paardt MP, Zijta FM, Stoker J. MR imaging of the colon. *Imaging Med* 2010; **2**: 195–209.

3. Stoker J. *MR Imaging of the Gastrointestinal Tract.* Heidelberg, Springer, 2010.

4. Schindera ST, Merkle EM, Dale BM, *et al.* Abdominal magnetic resonance imaging at 3.0 T what is the ultimate gain in signal-to-noise ratio? *Acad Radiol* 2006; **10**: 1236–43.

5. Saar B, Gschossmann JM, Bonel HM, *et al.* Evaluation of magnetic resonance colonography at 3.0 Tesla regarding diagnostic accuracy and image quality. *Invest Radiol* 2008; **8**: 580–6.

6. Foxall DL. Frequency-modulated steady-state free precession imaging. *Magn Reson Med* 2002; **3**: 502–8.

7. Oto A, Zhu F, Kulkarni K, *et al.* Evaluation of diffusion-weighted MR imaging for detection of bowel inflammation in patients with Crohn's disease. *Acad Radiol* 2009; **5**: 597–603.

8. Horsthuis K, Bipat S, Bennink RJ, *et al.* Inflammatory bowel disease diagnosed with US, MR, scintigraphy, and CT: meta-analysis of prospective studies. *Radiology* 2008; **1**: 64–79.

9. van Gemert-Horsthuis K, Florie J, Hommes DW, *et al.* Feasibility of evaluating Crohn's disease activity at 3.0 Tesla. *J Magn Reson Imaging* 2006; **2**: 340–8.

10. Horsthuis K, Bipat S, Stokkers PC, Stoker J. Magnetic resonance imaging for evaluation of disease activity in Crohn's disease: a systematic review. *Eur Radiol* 2009; **6**: 1450–60.

11. Langhorst J, Kuhle CA, Ajaj W, *et al.* MR colonography without bowel purgation for the assessment of inflammatory bowel diseases: diagnostic accuracy and patient acceptance. *Inflamm Bowel Dis* 2007; **8**: 1001–8.

12. Rimola J, Rodriguez S, Garcia-Bosch O, *et al.* Role of 3.0-T MR colonography in the evaluation of inflammatory bowel disease. *Radiographics* 2009; **3**: 701–19.

13. Punwani S, Rodriguez-Justo M, Bainbridge A, *et al.* Mural inflammation in Crohn disease: location-matched histologic validation of MR imaging features. *Radiology* 2009; **3**: 712–20.

14. Negaard A, Paulsen V, Sandvik L, *et al.* A prospective randomized comparison between two MR imaging studies of the small bowel in Crohn's disease, the oral contrast method and MR enteroclysis. *Eur Radiol* 2007; **9**: 2294–301.

15. Johnson CD, Chen MH, Toledano AY, *et al.* Accuracy of CT colonography for detection of large adenomas and cancers. *N Engl J Med* 2008; **12**: 1207–17.

16. Zijta FM, Bipat S, Stoker J. Magnetic resonance (MR) colonography in the detection of colorectal lesions: a systematic review of prospective studies. *Eur Radiol* 2010; **5**: 1031–46.

17. Ajaj W, Ruehm SG, Lauenstein T, *et al.* Dark-lumen magnetic resonance colonography in patients with suspected sigmoid diverticulitis: a feasibility study. *Eur Radiol* 2005; **11**: 2316–22.

18. Basaran A, Basaran M. Diagnosis of acute appendicitis during pregnancy: a systematic review. *Obstet Gynecol Surv* 2009; **7**: 481–8.

19. Wessling J, Fischbach R, Borchert A, *et al.* Detection of colorectal polyps: comparison of multi-detector row CT and MR colonography in a colon phantom. *Radiology* 2006; **1**: 125–31.

20. Rottgen R, Herzog H, Bogen P, *et al.* MR colonoscopy at 3.0 T: comparison with 1.5T in vivo and a colon model. *Clin Imaging* 2006; **4**: 248–53.

MR imaging of the rectum, 3T vs. 1.5T

Monique Maas, Doenja M. J. Lambregts, and Regina G. H. Beets-Tan

Background

Colorectal cancer is the third most common cancer in men and the second most common cancer in women, with an age-adjusted incidence rate of 46.1 per 100 000 per year in the United Kingdom [1]. The estimated number of deaths in the United States in 2009 was 49 920 [2]. Therefore, colorectal cancer has a high impact on health and society. Until now the precise etiology of rectal cancer has not been clarified. It is currently believed that the etiology is multifactorial, with genetic factors on the one hand and environmental factors, such as diet, smoking, and exercise, on the other hand. Patients usually present with rectal bleeding, weight loss, or abdominal complaints. Based on these symptoms a colonoscopy with biopsy is performed, where a tumor is found. Patients then undergo local staging with MR imaging, which has been proven to be the most accurate modality for staging of rectal cancer [3]. Distant staging is performed with computed tomography (CT) of the abdomen and thorax or a combination of a chest X-ray and an ultrasound of the liver. After staging, the patient is discussed in a multidisciplinary team (MDT) meeting, where the risk profile for recurrence is evaluated. A colorectal MDT consists of surgeons, radiation oncologists, medical oncologists, pathologists, gastroenterologists, and radiologists. Over the years, the role of the radiologist in the MDT has evolved from a reporting role to a full sparring partner in clinical decision-making. Because the aim of imaging of rectal cancer is to determine the risk profile of the patient, which defines the type of treatment the patient will undergo, the radiologist nowadays has a crucial influence on the treatment of the patient.

Local recurrence has been one of the main problems after treatment of rectal cancer. The risk profile for local recurrence is based on risk factors, which can be assessed with MR imaging: (1) tumor stage, (2) nodal stage, (3) involvement of the mesorectal fascia or circumferential resection margin (CRM), and (4) tumor height.

The risk for local recurrence has been reported to be as high as 40%, which was mainly due to a suboptimal surgical technique, with which the mesorectal envelope was bluntly resected, leading to incomplete resections and tumor spill [4]. With the introduction of the total mesorectal excision (TME), which provides an accurate dissection of the whole mesorectal envelope (with the enclosed lymph nodes) along the mesorectal fascia or "the holy plane," the local recurrence rate reduced substantially to 10% in some expert centers [5].

The Swedish rectal cancer trial and Dutch TME trial assessed the influence of neoadjuvant (preoperative) 5×5 gray (Gy) radiation additional to surgery on local recurrence and found that preoperative radiation significantly reduced local recurrence rates from 26%–27% in the nonirradiated group to 9%–11% in the irradiated group [6, 7] Subgroup analyses in the Dutch TME trial revealed that patients with stage I disease (T1–2N0) did not benefit from neoadjuvant 5×5 Gy radiation, because their risk for local recurrence is already very low. Furthermore, patients with stage III disease (TxN+) benefited from preoperative radiation, but still had a relatively high risk for local recurrence in spite of the radiation (11.2%) [7]. For these high-risk patients more intensive neoadjuvant treatment could be considered, such as combined chemo- and radiotherapy (chemoradiation [CRT]). Sauer et al. randomized patients between preoperative and postoperative CRT and found that preoperative

Body MR Imaging at 3 Tesla, ed. Ihab R. Kamel and Elmar M. Merkle. Published by Cambridge University Press.
© Cambridge University Press 2011.

CRT reduced the risk for local recurrence significantly from 13% in the postoperative group to 6% in the preoperative group [8]. In summary, these studies showed that preoperative (chemo)radiation significantly reduces the risk for local recurrence in patients with intermediate- and high-risk tumors.

Based on the results of the aforementioned studies patients can be stratified into three risk groups: (1) the low-risk tumors, which are confined to the bowel wall (T1–2) without nodal metastases (N0), (2) the intermediate-risk tumors, which are T3 tumors without CRM involvement and maximally three nodal metastases (N1) or very distal T2–3Nx tumors, and (3) the high-risk or locally advanced T3–4Nx tumors, which threaten or involve the CRM and/or tumors with more than three nodal metastases (N2). The low-risk patients undergo immediate TME without any neoadjuvant treatment. The patients with an intermediate risk for local recurrence undergo neoadjuvant 5×5 Gy radiation with subsequent TME, and the high-risk group undergoes a long course of CRT followed by TME after an interval of 6–8 weeks. Worldwide there is some variation in the type of neoadjuvant therapy and thus in the risk factors that influence treatment decision-making. In the United States all patients with intermediate and high risk undergo a long course of neoadjuvant CRT and decision-making is mainly based on the T and N stage (T3N+ being stratified for a long course of CRT). In Europe, this neoadjuvant therapy regimen is given to those patients who are at high risk for local recurrence: patients with T3 tumors with a threatened and/or involved mesorectal fascia or with a T4 tumor and/or nodal involvement, for whom surgery only or 5×5 Gy radiation with surgery may not be sufficient. In the latter case, besides the T- and N-stage, involvement of the mesorectal fascia is an important landmark for treatment stratification.

Currently, MR imaging is therefore recommended mostly in European countries while endorectal ultrasound (EUS) is used in the USA. Most widely available and most intensively validated for rectal cancer staging is MR imaging at 1.5T. However, with the introduction of 3T MR units the question whether 3T MR imaging would be more accurate than 1.5T MR imaging is rising. In this chapter rectal MR imaging at 3T, its evidence, the MR anatomy, protocol, and its ability for predicting the risk factors in rectal cancer staging are described.

3T imaging of the pelvis

The increased signal-to-noise ratio (SNR), which can be achieved with 3T MR imaging, can be traded for reduced acquisition time, higher resolution, or both. Until now, much experience has been gained with 3T MR imaging for the brain and skeletal imaging, but in pelvic imaging it has not been widely implemented. Usage of 3T MR imaging in the abdomen and pelvis brings about some high field strength-related challenges, such as more movement and susceptibility artifacts, the latter which also occur next to the gas-filled rectum [9].

Standard MR rectal protocol at 3T

In standard clinical practice phased-array MR imaging is sufficient for rectal cancer staging. Endorectal filling or coils are not recommended, because the rectal distension leads to a smaller distance between the tumor and mesorectal fascia, resulting in an overestimation of CRM involvement [10]. Moreover, the compression of the mesorectum with endorectal filling or coils leads to reduced visibility and more difficult evaluation of lymph nodes. Spasmolytics or bowel preparation are not routinely administered, but in proximal tumors spasmolytics can sometimes be of help in reducing bowel movement artifacts.

A standard MR protocol for rectal cancer imaging at 1.5T consists of two-dimensional (2D) T2-weighted (T2W) fast spin echo (FSE) sequences in three orthogonal directions: axial, coronal, and sagittal. Total examination time is approximately 25 minutes. Based on the sagittal images, the axial sequence is angulated exactly perpendicular to the tumor axis and the coronal sequence is angulated parallel to the tumor axis. These angulations lead to optimal depiction of the relation between the rectal wall, the tumor, and surrounding structures. T2W MR imaging offers a good contrast between the rectal wall and tumor on the one hand and the mesorectal fat and mesorectal fascia on the other hand. Therefore, fat suppression is not recommended. Fat suppression decreases the visibility of the mesorectal fascia and the tumor border, leading to hampered evaluation of the T-stage and of the CRM (Figure 11.1). The recommended slice thickness is generally 3 mm and the field of view should include the anal canal distally, the level of the promontory proximally, and the symphysis and

(a)

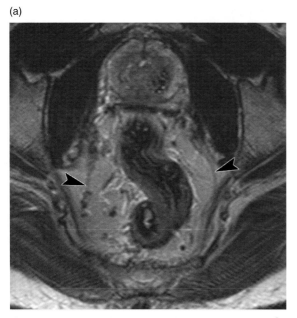

(b)

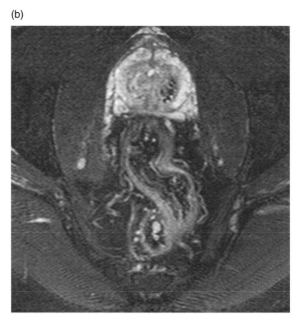

Figure 11.1 (a) An axial T2W image is shown with the mesorectal fascia indicated with the arrowheads. (b) A fat-suppressed image is shown and it is obvious that the mesorectal fascia can no longer be discerned.

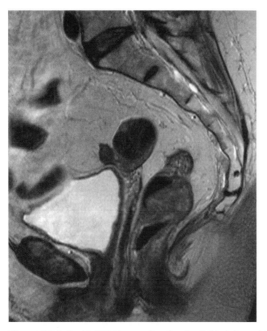

Figure 11.2 Sagittal T2W image showing the field of view which is necessary for rectal cancer staging with MR imaging.

sacrum anteriorly and posteriorly, respectively (Figure 11.2). Some studies have reported the use of T1W with or without gadolinium contrast. At 3T MR imaging Zhang *et al.* have studied a

gadolinium-enhanced T1W three-dimensional (3D) FSE sequence and found that this sequence provided the best depiction of the proximal and distal border between the rectal tumor and the rectal wall compared with the T2W and unenhanced T1W images [11]. Winter *et al.* have reported that a contrast-enhanced (CE) T1W (with gadopentate dimeglumine) sequence provides insufficient depiction of the rectal wall layers and the mesorectal fascia [12].

For rectal cancer imaging at 3T a similar protocol as at 1.5T is recommended. Because 3T MR imaging is known to be more susceptible to artifacts, it is important to keep that in mind whilst developing a sequence at 3T. Long acquisition times increase the risk for movement artifacts, so it is advisable to have sequences with short acquisition times.

Table 11.1 shows the most frequently used scan parameters at 3T MR imaging for rectal cancer in the literature.

Image quality at 3T MR imaging

Several studies have looked into the image quality of 3T MR imaging in rectal cancer.

Zhang *et al.* found that at 3T coronal and axial T2W FSE MR imaging sequences provided the best depiction of tumor margins and had fewer artifacts compared with T1W FSE images ($p < 0.0001$) [11].

Table 11.1 Most commonly applied scan parameters at 3T MR imaging for rectal cancer

Parameter	T2W FSE		
	Sagittal	*Axial*	*Coronal*
TR	2500–5000	2500–5000	2500–5000
TE	100	100	100
Echo train length	6–16	6–16	6–16
Slice thickness (mm)	4–5	3–5	3–5
Matrix	256 × 256 to 512 × 224	256 × 256 to 512 × 224	312 × 312 to 512 × 224
FOV (mm)	200–240	140–240	180–240
NSA	2	2–4	2–4
Duration (min)	3–5	3–4	3–4

TR = repetition time, TE = echo time, FOV = field of view, NSA = number of signal averages.
Winter *et al.* [12], Chun *et al.* [15], Kim *et al.* [27], Kim *et al.* [53].

Winter *et al.* confirmed these findings and showed that image quality at 3T is usually rated as good to very good. Axial T2W FSE images provided the best visualization of the tumor, mesorectal fascia, and rectal wall layers [12].

Anatomy of the rectum at 3T MR imaging

The rectum

The rectum is the part of the bowel between the anorectal and rectosigmoid junction. The rectosigmoid junction is usually defined 15 cm from the anorectal junction, which is approximately situated at the level of the third sacral vertebra. The rectal wall consists of three layers: (1) mucosal layer, (2) submucosal layer, and (3) muscularis propria, of which normally only layer 1 and 3 are visible on T2W MR images (Figure 11.3). In case of edema (for example due to radiation) the submucosal layer can become visible on MR imaging.

The mesorectum and mesorectal fascia

The mesorectum is the compartment which surrounds the rectum and contains lymph nodes and vascular structures. The outer structure of the mesorectum is the mesorectal fascia, which is a thin layer of connective tissue. On T2W MR imaging it can be visualized as a thin hypointense line (Figure 11.4). Anteriorly, the mesorectal fascia is thinner and therefore the relation with prostate and seminal vesicles in men and cervix and vagina in women is very close. The mesorectal compartment narrows towards the distal end of the compartment, which leads to a very close relation between the sphincter complex and the mesorectal fascia in the distal mesorectum (Figure 11.5). Therefore, tumors that are situated more distally in the rectum have a higher risk to have an involved mesorectal fascia and thus an involved CRM. The proximal part of the mesorectum is surrounded by peritoneum. The mesorectal fascia merges with the peritoneum at the level of the seminal vesicles or posterior vaginal wall and cervix, which is called the peritoneal reflection (Figure 11.6). In anteriorly situated tumors the relation between the peritoneal reflection and tumor is very important for surgical treatment planning. Involvement of the peritoneal reflection will lead to more extensive surgery than standard TME.

Blood supply

The rectum's blood supply originates from the superior rectal artery, which branches from the inferior mesenteric artery. The superior rectal artery can be seen as a hypointense structure in the presacral region on T2W images. The superior rectal vein runs lateral and dorsal from the artery. The distal part of the rectum can be supplied additionally by the middle rectal artery, which usually originates from the internal iliac artery.

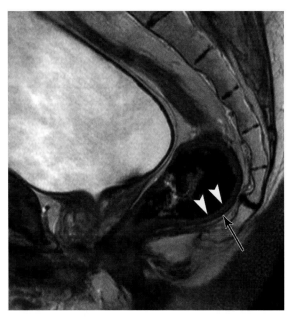

Figure 11.3 The rectal wall with the two visible layers on T2W MR imaging: mucosa (white arrowheads) and muscularis propria (black arrow).

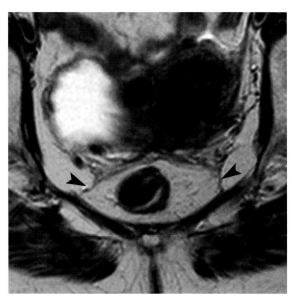

Figure 11.4 Mesorectal fascia at T2W is visible as a thin hypo-intense layer surrounding the mesorectum (arrowheads).

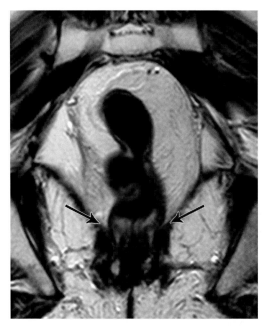

Figure 11.5 Distal tapering of the mesorectum and the mesorectal fascia (arrows). Note the small distance between the fascia and the rectum distally, making prediction of involvement of the mesorectal fascia in distal tumors more difficult than in proximal tumors.

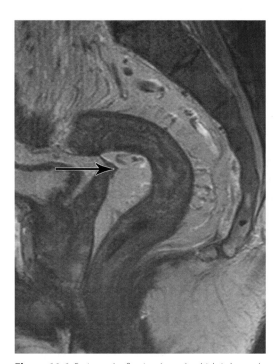

Figure 11.6 Peritoneal reflection (arrow), which is located anteriorly at the level of the seminal vesicles in men or posterior vaginal wall and cervix in women.

Staging of rectal cancer

T-stage

The tumor stage is divided in six categories: T1, the tumor is limited to the submucosa; T2, the tumor is limited to the muscularis propria; T3a, the tumor penetrates the muscularis propria; T3b, the tumor does not penetrate the muscularis propria but has tumor deposits or satellite nodules in the mesorectal soft tissue; T4a, the tumor has a distance of $\leq 2\,\text{mm}$ from the mesorectal fascia; and T4b, the tumor invades another organ (e.g., uterus, sacrum, or prostate) [13]. The overall accuracy of T-staging with phased-array MR imaging at 1.5T is 67–83% [14]. At 3T MR imaging accuracies vary between 63% and 95% [15–17]. This wide range of accuracies can be explained by the fact that the T-stage is often overstaged with MR imaging. First, MR imaging does not have the capacity to discriminate T1 from T2 tumors because not all three layers of the rectal wall are visualized with MR imaging: therefore, T1 and T2 tumors have the same appearance on MR imaging. Second, the distinction between T2 and borderline T3 tumors is very difficult, because benign desmoplasia in a T2 tumor cannot be discerned from malignant desmoplasia in a T3 tumor (Figure 11.7). In a T2 tumor the muscularis propria is intact, which is depicted at MR imaging as an intact hypointense line

(Figure 11.8). When a radiologist sees this intact hypointense line, he or she can be sure that the tumor is limited to the bowel wall and is therefore a T1–T2 tumor. However, when this hypointense line is not sharply delineated due to desmoplasia, it is difficult to stage the tumor correctly as a T2 tumor. Overstaging rates have been reported from 25% to 86% at 3T compared with 25–57% at 1.5T, indicating that 3T does not help in the distinction between T2 and borderline T3 tumors [18, 19].

At the time of writing, there is no consensus in the literature as to whether 3T is beneficial for T-staging in rectal cancer. Controversial results of studies with restricted numbers of patients make it difficult to draw any conclusions. This controversy is reflected in the huge variety of the reported accuracies for T-staging with 3T MR imaging. In addition, no published data have compared 3T with 1.5T within one patient group.

In conclusion, the main issue in T-staging of rectal cancer is to distinguish the tumors which are limited to the bowel wall (T1–T2) from tumors outgrowing the bowel wall (T3–T4). Overstaging errors are often encountered in the differentiation between T2 and early T3 (borderline tumors), because desmoplastic benign reactions from T2 tumors are

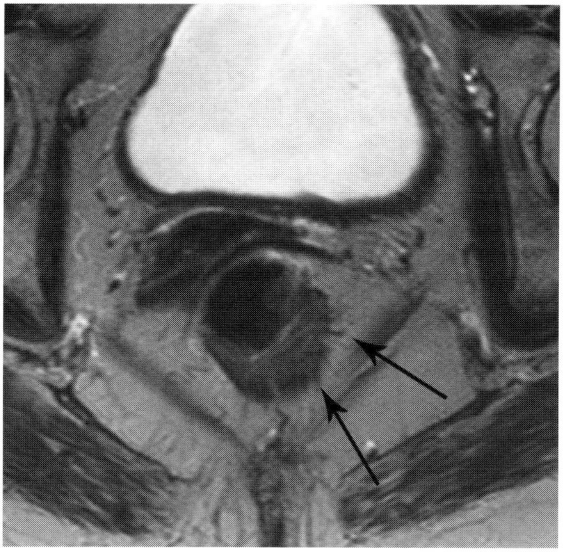

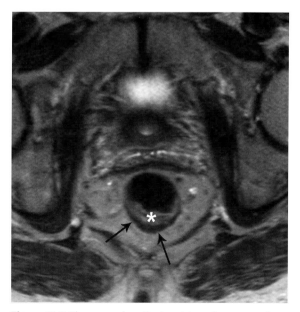

Figure 11.7 Peritumoral stranding (arrows). With MR imaging it is not possible to discriminate stranding with tumor cells from stranding without tumor cells.

Figure 11.8 The arrows show the hypointense line surrounding the tumor (*), which is the muscularis propria. When this line is visible the tumor is limited to the bowel wall and thus a T1 or T2 tumor.

often erroneously interpreted as that of early T3 tumors, wherein the desmoplasia contains tumor cells. There is no consensus in the literature yet as to whether 3T would help to solve this problem and reports show controversial results.

Circumferential resection margin (CRM)

Involvement of the CRM is very important for treatment planning because an involved resection margin leads to increased recurrence rates. When a free CRM is predicted, a standard TME can be performed, but when the CRM is threatened (tumor within 2 mm from the mesorectal fascia) or involved (tumor invasion into or through the mesorectal fascia) the surgeon will have to perform more extensive surgery to ensure that the resection margins will be free from tumor.

MR imaging at 1.5T has proven to be very accurate in the prediction of involvement of the CRM with a specificity of 98% for prediction of a negative CRM, which could be reproduced in a general setting [14, 20]. Evidence also shows that contrast-enhanced MR imaging is not helpful for T-staging or for CRM prediction. Vliegen *et al.* investigated the use of gadolinium-enhanced T1W images for the accuracy of predicting an involved CRM at 1.5T MR imaging. They compared T2W MR imaging with T2W MR imaging combined with CE-T1W images and found that gadolinium CE-T1W images did not improve its accuracy: 87–93% with T2W FSE versus 87% after the addition of the CE-T1W sequence [21]. It is plausible to assume that T2W FSE MR imaging sequences at 3T would be as accurate as at 1.5T in identifying this thin hypointense fascia within the highly intense fat and predicting an involved fascia, because the contrast difference between the fascia and the surrounding fat does not alter at 3T. So far, however, no literature exists focusing on the value of 3T for predicting CRM.

The N-stage

Nodal staging is important because the decision whether or not to administer neoadjuvant therapy is in part based on the nodal status. Nodal stage can be classified into five categories: N0, no involved lymph nodes; N1a, solitary metastasis in a regional lymph node; N1b, metastases in 2–3 regional nodes; N2a, metastases in 4–6 regional nodes; and N2b, metastases in 7 or more regional nodes [13]. Lymph nodes which are located outside the mesorectum, e.g., in the

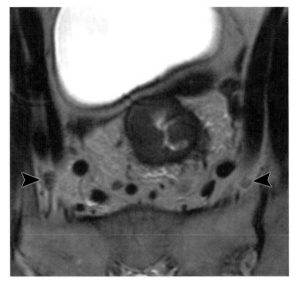

Figure 11.9 The arrowheads show suspicious lymph nodes in the left and right obturator areas.

obturator, para-aortic, or iliacal regions, are called extramesorectal lymph nodes and are also important for treatment planning and prognosis. When there are suspicious extramesorectal nodes (Figure 11.9) at primary staging, they are irradiated and usually also removed with surgery later on. None of the currently available imaging techniques is sufficiently accurate for nodal prediction. Two meta-analyses have shown that accuracies for nodal staging with 1.5T MR imaging range from 55% to 78%, which is comparable to accuracies found with EUS and CT [22, 23]. This low accuracy can be attributed to the criterion which is used for nodal staging: size. Traditionally, a cutoff of 8 mm has been used, leading to many false negatives in nodes smaller than 8 mm, because up to 50% of nodal metastases occur in small nodes (< 5 mm). On the other hand, not all nodes larger than 8 mm are malignant [24]. Therefore, understaging of the small nodes and overstaging of the large nodes occurs, leading to only moderate accuracies. Other criteria have been proposed, such as regularity of nodal border and homogeneity of the nodal signal, which have led to reported sensitivities of 36–85% and specificities of 95–100% [25, 26]. However, these criteria are difficult to evaluate in the smallest 2–3 mm nodes.

For 3T MR imaging the same criteria for nodal staging apply as for 1.5T MR imaging. Accuracies from 64% to 95% have been reported, with most sensitivities in the range of 64–80%. When using 3D

(a)

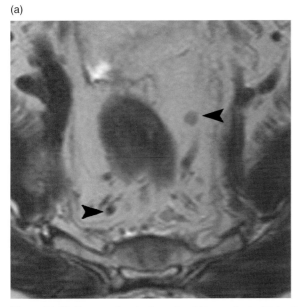

(b)

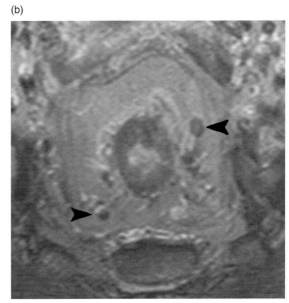

Figure 11.10 Mesorectal nodes (arrowheads) in a patient with locally advanced rectal cancer at 1.5T (a) and 3T (b) MR imaging. Both nodes were predicted malignant and the patient underwent neoadjuvant chemoradiation which sterilized the nodes.

3T images, accuracy for nodal staging was reported to be lower, ranging from 58% to 62% [17]. The number of false-negative findings is relatively high due to understaging of involved nodes based on the aforementioned size criterion. On the other hand, the specificities range from 91% to 98% at 3T MR imaging, indicating that only few patients are overstaged. Kim *et al.* suggest that the criteria for nodal involvement other than size might be more accurately visible at 3T due to enhanced image quality, i.e., improved visibility of the nodal border and signal homogeneity, resulting in fewer false positives [27]. Figure 11.10 shows examples of suspicious mesorectal nodes at 1.5T and 3T MR imaging.

Still, nodal staging with MR imaging remains insufficiently accurate, regardless of the field strength. Some promising results were reported for MR imaging at 1.5T enhanced with ultrasmall superparamagnetic particles of iron oxide (USPIO) for nodal staging [28]. However, no studies have focused on USPIO MR imaging at 3T and moreover USPIO has not been US Food and Drug Administration (FDA) approved for clinical use.

Extramesorectal lymph nodes

In general the same criteria apply for the evaluation of the extramesorectal lymph nodes as for mesorectal lymph nodes. A study by Matsuoka *et al.* in surgical specimens of nodes retrieved from obturator dissections has shown that the short-axis diameter is the best size criterion for prediction of these lateral lymph nodes with the best cutoff value being 4 mm [29]. Unfortunately, validation studies on extramesorectal lymph node prediction with MR imaging at any field strength are lacking.

In summary, nodal staging with MR imaging is important for treatment planning and prognosis. Unfortunately, no currently available technique is sufficiently accurate, because size criteria have been proven unreliable in rectal cancer nodes. Current evidence suggests no benefit for 3T MR imaging above 1.5T MR imaging for predicting nodal stage.

Restaging after chemoradiation

As mentioned in the Background section, the locally advanced rectal tumors are treated with a long course of neoadjuvant CRT, which usually consists of 28 fractions of 1.8 Gy with 5-fluorouracil-based chemotherapy. After completion of the CRT there is an interval of 6–8 weeks before surgery, at the end of which restaging is often performed with MR imaging to evaluate the response to CRT. The same risk factors as mentioned in the Background section are then evaluated. At restaging MR imaging downsizing (i.e., shrinkage of the tumor and nodes) and/

(a)   (b)

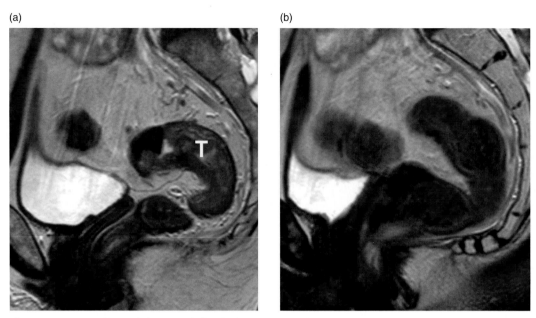

Figure 11.11 A rectal tumor before (a) and after (b) chemoradiation. The tumor (T) is not visible anymore at the restaging MR imaging. This patient was staged as a complete reponse and followed a 'wait-and-see policy'.

or downstaging (a lower T/N-stage compared with primary staging) are assessed. Accurate evaluation of the response to CRT can have important therapeutic consequences. Tumor regression from the resection margins may alter surgical planning. Also, it has been suggested that less extensive surgery (e.g., local excision) could be performed in patients who show a good response to CRT [30]. For patients who have a complete response (no residual tumor cells found at histology [yT0N0], Figure 11.11) it has been suggested to even omit surgery and perform follow-up: the so-called "wait-and-see policy" [31]. Given these recent trends towards less invasive treatment for rectal cancer after CRT, it is important to have imaging techniques which can select these good and complete responders accurately. Predicting the T-stage after CRT (the yT-stage) is difficult. Tumor regression due to CRT leads to fibrotic tissue at the former tumor location, which often results in a diffuse hypointense thickened rectal wall on T2W images (Figure 11.12). MR imaging cannot identify areas with residual tumor in these hypointense areas and therefore radiologists will tend to overstage the hypointense areas as residual tumor to be on the safe side. Because all sites of former tumor often become fibrotic, overstaging rates after CRT are higher than at primary staging [32–34].

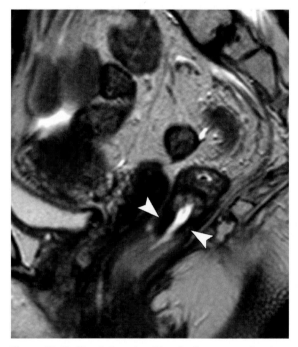

Figure 11.12 Fibrosis (arrowheads) at the former tumor location, which is depicted as a hypointense area on T2W images.

High negative predictive values (NPVs) of 91–100% can be obtained for prediction of tumor regression from the mesorectal fascia at 1.5T MR imaging, but

158

the positive predictive values range from 44% to 68%, again reflecting the difficulty in discriminating fibrosis with malignant cells from fibrosis without malignant cells at the border of the mesorectal fascia [33, 35].

Restaging of nodal involvement is particularly important when minimal invasive treatment for good and complete responders to CRT is considered, because the mesorectum and the lymph nodes are then left *in situ*. If any malignant nodes are left behind, this can lead to recurrences. Nodal restaging with T2W MR imaging is sufficiently accurate with NPVs of 93–100% for MR imaging in predicting nodal metastases [36–38]. The hypothesis for this increased NPV after CRT is that the earlier-mentioned size and morphologic criteria are more reliable after CRT. The small nodes, which are the most difficult to evaluate with T2W MR imaging, disappear after CRT. All nodes shrink after CRT and up to 81% of the malignant nodes sterilize after CRT [39]. Therefore, when nodes are still of large size after CRT, the probability of these relatively larger nodes being malignant will be higher.

To summarize, restaging MR imaging after CRT is important when surgical treatment may be altered in the case of a good response. The great challenge for radiologists in restaging of rectal cancer after CRT is thus to distinguish residual tumor in fibrotic areas. No evidence so far exists for restaging after CRT with 3T MR imaging, so at present 1.5T MR imaging remains the standard technique for restaging after CRT.

Endorectal ultrasound (EUS)

EUS is widely used for rectal cancer staging. Its strength lies mainly in the discrimination between tumors limited to the submucosa (T1) and tumors invading the muscularis propria (T2). Although the initial reports from single-center studies showed high sensitivity, specificity, and accuracy, more recent large single-center and multicenter studies with sonographers with different skills could not confirm these results. Furthermore, regardless of the expertise of the sonographer, EUS, like MR imaging or other imaging modalities, lacks the ability to discriminate between desmoplasia with or without tumor cells and therefore between T2 and T3 tumors [22]. EUS thus shows high sensitivity, but low specificity for prediction of tumor penetration through the rectal wall (T3). Furthermore, because of its limited field of view, EUS is not suitable for the evaluation of larger tumors that

extend to the dorsal pelvic wall. In up to 13% of patients with stenosing tumors the lesion cannot be analyzed accurately with EUS, due to difficulties with insertion of the probe and/or the limited field of view [40]. A major limitation of EUS in rectal cancer is that nodal staging, in specific of the nodes high in the mesorectum and outside the mesorectum in the iliac and obturator loges, is inaccurate. So far, there is only one small study on EUS versus 3T MR imaging [15]. This one study in 24 patients with rectal cancer (T1–T3) found a slightly higher sensitivity of 100% for perirectal invasion for EUS versus 91% for 3T MR imaging. However, specificity for perirectal invasion at 3T MR imaging was higher (93%) compared to EUS (82%). The diagnostic performance for nodal staging was comparable for both modalities, with low sensitivities of 58–63% and high specificities of 82–92%.

In conclusion, EUS is most suitable to distinguish T1 from T2 tumors, where MR imaging has a small role.

Whole-body MR imaging at 3T in colorectal cancer

Distant staging in patients with colorectal cancer requires a multimodality approach, consisting of chest X-ray (or chest CT) and CT, MR imaging, or ultrasound of the liver and abdomen. Recently, whole-body imaging techniques have been promoted as an alternative to such a multimodality approach. Since all information can be obtained within one single examination, a whole-body strategy is potentially more cost-effective and less cumbersome for the patient. So far, fluorodesoxyglucose positron emission tomography (FDG-PET)/CT has most frequently been investigated for whole-body staging in colorectal cancer, although its clinical role is mainly limited to rule out extrahepatic lesions in patients scheduled for resection of their liver metastases and in the follow-up. MR imaging could be an attractive candidate for whole-body screening in rectal cancer, because – unlike CT and FDG-PET – MR imaging does not require the use of ionizing radiation. Moreover, MR imaging is already widely adapted as the standard imaging technique for local tumor staging in rectal cancer. Especially the use of diffusion-weighted MR imaging (DWI) has revealed great potential for detection of malignant tumors throughout the body [41]. DWI adds functional information reflecting tissue cellular structure and can complement the data from standard anatomical MR imaging within one single examination. Clinical

(a)

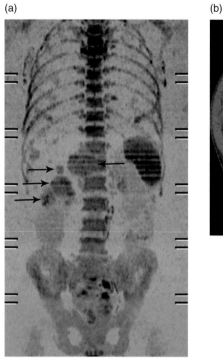

(b)

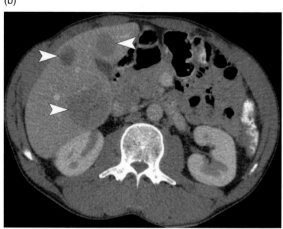

Figure 11.13 Coronal whole-body diffusion-weighted image (a) and corresponding CT image (b) of a male patient with several large malignant lesions in the liver (arrowheads). The lesions are visible as high-signal-intensity nodules on diffusion MR imaging (arrows). The image display of whole-body DWI resembles that of FDG-PET.

studies have already shown that whole-body MR imaging including DWI could be useful for the screening of metastatic bone lesions [42, 43], metastatic lung cancer [44, 45], and malignant lymphoma [46]. Interestingly, the limited number of studies that investigated the use of MR imaging for whole-body screening in rectal cancer were mainly conducted at 3T. These studies mainly focused on detection of recurrent tumor and did not investigate MR imaging for primary tumor staging. Squillaci *et al.* performed whole-body MR imaging at 3T in 20 patients with suspected locally recurrent colorectal cancer or distant metastases [47]. MR imaging was compared to FDG-PET/CT, which – together with clinical follow-up – served as the reference standard. MR imaging showed good results for the detection of liver and bone metastases, but was inferior to FDG-PET for the evaluation of lymph nodes and lung lesions. Schmidt *et al.* compared FDG-PET/CT to whole-body MR imaging at either 1.5T (n = 14) or 3T (n = 10), using clinical and radiologic follow-up as the reference standard [48]. They confirmed the finding of Squillaci *et al.* that MR imaging was inferior to FDG-PET for evaluation of

nodal disease (sensitivity 63% versus 93%). Furthermore, FDG-PET/CT outperformed whole-body MR imaging in the detection of lung metastases and peritoneal tumor metastases. MR imaging, however, revealed more metastases in the liver and bone than could be detected with FDG-PET. Results were comparable for 1.5T and 3T MR imaging, although examination time was considerably shorter at 3T. Since whole-body imaging using MR imaging is fairly time-consuming, a potential benefit of using higher field strengths would be that the higher SNR could be traded for more acceptable acquisition times. Furthermore, use of the built-in quadrature body coil at 3T may already result in acceptable diagnostic quality, so that patient repositioning and the use of multiple surface coils can be avoided.

Figure 11.13 shows an example of whole-body DWI and the corresponding liver CT from a patient with colorectal liver metastases. So far, no studies have specifically focused on DWI for whole-body staging in patients with colorectal cancer. Nevertheless, several studies have shown that DWI might be helpful for the detection of small hepatic lesions [49].

DWI is also known to be a very sensitive technique for the detection of lymph nodes, which could aid in improving the suboptimal results reported with MR imaging [50]. It should, however, be noted that benign and metastatic nodes may have an equal appearance on DWI, making DWI prone to staging errors [51]. So far, only one study by Mürtz *et al.* has compared 1.5T and 3T for whole-body DWI [52]. DWI will generally be more challenging at 3T, since at higher field strengths the technique is more prone to susceptibility artifacts. Mürtz *et al.* reported that at 3T MR imaging the contrast between lesions and background was better, but significantly more image distortions and motion artifacts were observed.

In conclusion, the evidence on whole-body imaging for rectal cancer with MR imaging is limited and future studies will have to determine the clinical value of MR imaging, both at 1.5T and 3T. Functional imaging techniques, such as DWI, will likely prove to be valuable to complement the information derived from anatomical MR imaging.

Conclusion and recommendations

Preliminary results have shown that 3T MR imaging is feasible for staging of rectal cancer patients. However, based on the currently available literature there is no evidence (yet) that 3T MR imaging can improve staging of rectal cancer. Only small studies exist, from which we cannot draw any strong conclusions on its benefit. It is unclear whether the main difficulties in discriminating T2 tumors from small T3 tumors can be solved with 3T MR imaging. Nodal staging with 3T MR imaging remains difficult, because of the unreliable criteria which are currently applied with morphologic imaging. Some factors have not been studied yet at 3T MR imaging, such as CRM involvement and restaging MR imaging after CRT for the locally advanced tumors. In short, at the time of writing it is unclear what the benefits of 3T MR imaging are for staging of rectal cancer patients. Therefore, it is justified to continue staging with 1.5T MR imaging.

References

1. United Kingdom Cancer Research. http://info. cancerresearchuk.org/cancerstats/types/bowel/ incidence/index.htm. Accessed July 27, 2010.

2. National Cancer Institute United States. http://www. cancer.gov. Accessed April 23, 2010.

3. Valentini V, Aristei C, Glimelius B, *et al.* Multidisciplinary Rectal Cancer Management: 2nd European Rectal Cancer Consensus Conference (EURECA-CC2). *Radiother Oncol* 2009; **92**(2): 148–63.

4. Quirke P, Durdey P, Dixon MF, *et al.* Local recurrence of rectal adenocarcinoma due to inadequate surgical resection. Histopathological study of lateral tumor spread and surgical excision. *Lancet* 1986; **2**(8514): 996–9.

5. Heald RJ, Ryall RD. Recurrence and survival after total mesorectal excision for rectal cancer. *Lancet* 1986; **1**(8496): 1479–82.

6. Improved survival with preoperative radiotherapy in resectable rectal cancer. Swedish Rectal Cancer Trial. *N Engl J Med* 1997; **336**(14): 980–7.

7. Kapiteijn E, Marijnen CA, Nagtegaal ID, *et al.* Preoperative radiotherapy combined with total mesorectal excision for resectable rectal cancer. *N Engl J Med* 2001; **345**(9): 638–46.

8. Sauer R, Becker H, Hohenberger W, *et al.* Preoperative versus postoperative chemoradiotherapy for rectal cancer. *N Engl J Med* 2004; **351**(17): 1731–40.

9. Merkle EM, Dale BM. Abdominal MRI at 3T: the basics revisited. *AJR Am J Roentgenol* 2006; **186**(6): 1524–32.

10. Slater A, Halligan S, Taylor SA, *et al.* Distance between the rectal wall and mesorectal fascia measured by MRI: effect of rectal distension and implications for preoperative prediction of a tumor-free circumferential resection margin. *Clin Radiol* 2006; **61**(1): 65–70.

11. Zhang XM, Zhang HL, Yu D, *et al.* 3-T MRI of rectal carcinoma: preoperative diagnosis, staging, and planning of sphincter-sparing surgery. *AJR Am J Roentgenol* 2008; **190**(5): 1271–8.

12. Winter L, Bruhn H, Langrehr J, *et al.* Magnetic resonance imaging in suspected rectal cancer: determining tumor localization, stage, and sphincter-saving resectability at 3-Tesla-sustained high resolution. *Acta Radiol* 2007; **48**(4): 379–87.

13. Sobin L, Gospodarowicz M, Wittekind C. *TNM Classification of Malignant Tumors*, 7th edn. Chichester, Wiley-Blackwell, 2009.

14. Beets-Tan RG, Beets GL, Vliegen RF, *et al.* Accuracy of magnetic resonance imaging in prediction of tumor-free resection margin in rectal cancer surgery. *Lancet* 2001; **357**(9255): 497–504.

15. Chun HK, Choi D, Kim MJ, *et al.* Preoperative staging of rectal cancer: comparison of 3-T high-field MRI and endorectal sonography. *AJR Am J Roentgenol* 2006; **187**(6): 1557–62.

16. Futterer JJ, Yakar D, Strijk SP, *et al.* Preoperative 3T MR imaging of rectal cancer: local staging accuracy using a two-dimensional and three-dimensional

T2-weighted turbo spin echo sequence. *Eur J Radiol* 2008; **65**(1): 66–71.

17. Kim H, Lim JS, Choi JY, *et al.* Rectal cancer: comparison of accuracy of local-regional staging with two- and three-dimensional preoperative 3-T MR imaging. *Radiology* 2010; **254**(2): 485–92.

18. Kim NK, Kim MJ, Park JK, *et al.* Preoperative staging of rectal cancer with MRI: accuracy and clinical usefulness. *Ann Surg Oncol* 2000; **7**(10): 732–7.

19. Maas M, Lambregts D, Wildberger J, *et al.* MR for rectal cancer at 1.5 Tesla is sufficient for T-staging, 3.0 Tesla MR imaging does not necessarily improve radiologist's performance. *Eur Radiol* 2009; **19** (Suppl 2): 650.

20. Brown G, Radcliffe AG, Newcombe RG, *et al.* Preoperative assessment of prognostic factors in rectal cancer using high-resolution magnetic resonance imaging. *Br J Surg* 2003; **90**(3): 355–64.

21. Vliegen RF, Beets GL, von Meyenfeldt MF, *et al.* Rectal cancer: MR imaging in local staging – is gadolinium-based contrast material helpful? *Radiology* 2005; **234** (1): 179–88.

22. Bipat S, Glas AS, Slors FJ, *et al.* Rectal cancer: local staging and assessment of lymph node involvement with endoluminal US, CT, and MR imaging – a meta-analysis. *Radiology* 2004; **232**(3): 773–83.

23. Lahaye MJ, Engelen SM, Nelemans PJ, *et al.* Imaging for predicting the risk factors – the circumferential resection margin and nodal disease – of local recurrence in rectal cancer: a meta-analysis. *Semin Ultrasound CT MR* 2005; **26**(4): 259–68.

24. Dworak O. Number and size of lymph nodes and node metastases in rectal carcinomas. *Surg Endosc* 1989; **3** (2): 96–9.

25. Brown G, Richards CJ, Bourne MW, *et al.* Morphologic predictors of lymph node status in rectal cancer with use of high-spatial-resolution MR imaging with histopathologic comparison. *Radiology* 2003; **227**(2): 371–7.

26. Kim JH, Beets GL, Kim MJ, *et al.* High-resolution MR imaging for nodal staging in rectal cancer: are there any criteria in addition to the size? *Eur J Radiol* 2004; **52**(1): 78–83.

27. Kim CK, Kim SH, Chun HK, *et al.* Preoperative staging of rectal cancer: accuracy of 3-Tesla magnetic resonance imaging. *Eur Radiol* 2006; **16**(5): 972–80.

28. Lahaye MJ, Engelen SM, Kessels AG, *et al.* USPIO-enhanced MR imaging for nodal staging in patients with primary rectal cancer: predictive criteria. *Radiology* 2008; **246**(3): 804–11.

29. Matsuoka H, Masaki T, Sugiyama M, *et al.* Morphological characteristics of lateral pelvic lymph nodes in rectal carcinoma. *Langenbecks Arch Surg* 2007; **392**(5): 543–7.

30. Borschitz T, Wachtlin D, Mohler M, *et al.* Neoadjuvant chemoradiation and local excision for T2–3 rectal cancer. *Ann Surg Oncol* 2008; **15**(3): 712–20.

31. Habr-Gama A, Perez RO, Nadalin W, *et al.* Operative versus nonoperative treatment for stage 0 distal rectal cancer following chemoradiation therapy: long-term results. *Ann Surg* 2004; **240**(4): 711–17; discussion 717–18.

32. Dresen RC, Beets GL, Rutten HJ, *et al.* Locally advanced rectal cancer: MR imaging for restaging after neoadjuvant radiation therapy with concomitant chemotherapy. Part I. Are we able to predict tumor confined to the rectal wall? *Radiology* 2009; **252**(1): 71–80.

33. Vliegen RF, Beets GL, Lammering G, *et al.* Mesorectal fascia invasion after neoadjuvant chemotherapy and radiation therapy for locally advanced rectal cancer: accuracy of MR imaging for prediction. *Radiology* 2008; **246**(2): 454–62.

34. Kuo LJ, Chern MC, Tsou MH, *et al.* Interpretation of magnetic resonance imaging for locally advanced rectal carcinoma after preoperative chemoradiation therapy. *Dis Colon Rectum* 2005; **48**(1): 23–8.

35. Kulkarni T, Gollins S, Maw A, *et al.* Magnetic resonance imaging in rectal cancer downstaged using neoadjuvant chemoradiation: accuracy of prediction of tumor stage and circumferential resection margin status. *Colorectal Dis* 2008; **10**(5): 479–89.

36. Denecke T, Rau B, Hoffmann KT, *et al.* Comparison of CT, MRI and FDG-PET in response prediction of patients with locally advanced rectal cancer after multimodal preoperative therapy: is there a benefit in using functional imaging? *Eur Radiol* 2005; **15**(8): 1658–66.

37. Lahaye MJ, Beets GL, Engelen SM, *et al.* Locally advanced rectal cancer: MR imaging for restaging after neoadjuvant radiation therapy with concomitant chemotherapy. Part II. What are the criteria to predict involved lymph nodes? *Radiology* 2009; **252**(1): 81–91.

38. Suppiah A, Hunter IA, Cowley J, *et al.* Magnetic resonance imaging accuracy in assessing tumor down-staging following chemoradiation in rectal cancer. *Colorectal Dis* 2009; **11**(3): 249–53.

39. Koh DM, Chau I, Tait D, *et al.* Evaluating mesorectal lymph nodes in rectal cancer before and after neoadjuvant chemoradiation using thin-section T2-weighted magnetic resonance imaging. *Int J Radiat Oncol Biol Phys* 2008; **71**(2): 456–61.

40. Ptok H, Marusch F, Meyer F, *et al.* Feasibility and accuracy of TRUS in the pre-treatment staging for

rectal carcinoma in general practice. *Eur J Surg Oncol* 2006; **32**(4): 420–5.

41. Charles-Edwards EM, deSouza NM. Diffusion-weighted magnetic resonance imaging and its application to cancer. *Cancer Imaging* 2006; **6**: 135–43.

42. Gutzeit A, Doert A, Froehlich JM, *et al.* Comparison of diffusion-weighted whole body MRI and skeletal scintigraphy for the detection of bone metastases in patients with prostate or breast carcinoma. *Skeletal Radiol* 2010; **39**(4): 333–43.

43. Nakanishi K, Kobayashi M, Nakaguchi K, *et al.* Whole-body MR imaging for detecting metastatic bone tumor: diagnostic value of diffusion-weighted images. *Magn Reson Med Sci* 2007; **6**(3): 147–55.

44. Ohno Y, Koyama H, Onishi Y, *et al.* Non-small cell lung cancer: whole-body MR examination for M-stage assessment – utility for whole-body diffusion-weighted imaging compared with integrated FDG PET/CT. *Radiology* 2008; **248**(2): 643–54.

45. Takenaka D, Ohno Y, Matsumoto K, *et al.* Detection of bone metastases in non-small cell lung cancer patients: comparison of whole-body diffusion-weighted imaging (DWI), whole-body MR imaging without and with DWI, whole-body FDG-PET/CT, and bone scintigraphy. *J Magn Reson Imaging* 2009; **30**(2): 298–308.

46. Kwee TC, van Ufford HM, Beek FJ, *et al.* Whole-body MRI, including diffusion-weighted imaging, for the initial staging of malignant lymphoma: comparison to computed tomography. *Invest Radiol* 2009; **44**(10): 683–90.

47. Squillaci E, Manenti G, Mancino S, *et al.* Staging of colon cancer: whole-body MRI vs. whole-body PET-CT – initial clinical experience. *Abdom Imaging* 2008; **33**(6): 676–88.

48. Schmidt GP, Baur-Melnyk A, Haug A, *et al.* Whole-body MRI at 1.5T and 3T compared with FDG-PET-CT for the detection of tumor recurrence in patients with colorectal cancer. *Eur Radiol* 2009; **19**(6): 1366–78.

49. Coenegrachts K, Matos C, ter Beek L, *et al.* Focal liver lesion detection and characterization: comparison of non-contrast enhanced and SPIO-enhanced diffusion-weighted single-shot spin echo echo planar and turbo spin echo T2-weighted imaging. *Eur J Radiol* 2009; **72**(3): 432–9.

50. Nakai G, Matsuki M, Inada Y, *et al.* Detection and evaluation of pelvic lymph nodes in patients with gynecologic malignancies using body diffusion-weighted magnetic resonance imaging. *J Comput Assist Tomogr* 2008; **32**(5): 764–8.

51. Sakurada A, Takahara T, Kwee *et al.* Diagnostic performance of diffusion-weighted magnetic resonance imaging in esophageal cancer. *Eur Radiol* 2009; **19**(6): 1461–9.

52. Mürtz P, Krautmacher C, Traber F, *et al.* Diffusion-weighted whole-body MR imaging with background body signal suppression: a feasibility study at 3.0 Tesla. *Eur Radiol* 2007; **17**(12): 3031–7.

53. Kim SH, Lee JM, Lee MW, *et al.* Diagnostic accuracy of 3.0-Tesla rectal magnetic resonance imaging in preoperative local staging of primary rectal cancer. *Invest Radiol* 2008; **43**(8): 587–93.

Chapter 2

Imaging of the kidneys and MR urography at 3T

John R. Leyendecker

Introduction

The use of MR imaging for assessment of the urinary tract is not a new concept. However, MR imaging of the kidneys, ureters, and bladder remains a seldom performed technique at many medical centers, in part due to the dominant role computed tomography (CT) has played for the evaluation of urinary tract neoplasms and stone disease. Growing interest in medical radiation dose reduction coupled with advances in MR imaging technology has stimulated interest in renal MR imaging and MR urography. While contrast resolution has been a major advantage of MR imaging over other imaging modalities for many body applications, the limited temporal and spatial resolution of MR imaging, in addition to its relative insensitivity for detecting calcifications, have impeded the widespread adoption of MR imaging for urinary tract imaging.

Three Tesla MR imaging systems provide a significant improvement in signal-to-noise ratio (SNR) compared with 1.5T systems that translates readily into improvements in spatial resolution, making high-resolution imaging of structures such as the kidneys, renal collecting systems, and bladder possible. Alternatively, imaging times can be reduced while maintaining acceptable SNR. While such improvements in spatial and temporal resolution should portend a bright future for 3T MR imaging of the urinary tract, challenges such as artifact suppression and limited coil technology must be addressed prior to widespread implementation of urinary tract imaging at 3T. Furthermore, data assessing the efficacy of urinary tract imaging at 3T are sparse, and direct comparisons between urinary tract imaging at 1.5T and 3T in humans are currently lacking. This necessitates some degree of speculation based on theory mixed with anecdotal experience when discussing this topic.

Current indications for MR imaging of the urinary tract include the characterization of focal renal lesions, staging of renal cell carcinoma, follow-up after ablative therapy for renal neoplasms, diagnosis and evaluation of urothelial tumors and congenital anomalies (Figures 12.1 and 12.2), and the staging of bladder carcinoma. In this chapter, we will focus our discussion primarily on renal mass characterization and the technique of MR urography at 3T.

MR imaging of the kidney

Kidney protocol

A sample 3T kidney protocol is shown in Table 12.1. Despite the increased SNR available at 3T compared with 1.5T, a phased-array torso coil should be used when possible to optimize SNR and to allow use of parallel imaging. Parallel imaging is important, not only to improve efficiency, but also to lower specific absorption rate (SAR) levels. The use of parallel imaging can also reduce the image blurring intrinsic to very long echo-train spin-echo sequences. If renal imaging is to be performed with bladder imaging (such as in the case of MR urography), a large field-of-view torso coil should be utilized. Unfortunately, coil technology for 3T systems has lagged behind such technology for 1.5T systems, although this gap is narrowing.

Any renal MR imaging protocol should include a minimum of a T1-weighted opposed-phase and in-phase gradient echo sequence(s) (discussed in more detail below), a fat-suppressed T2-weighted sequence, and a multiphase, contrast-enhanced, fat-suppressed

(a)

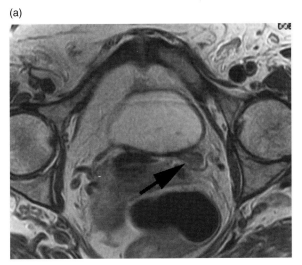

(b)

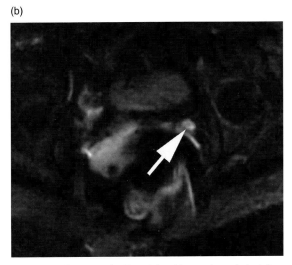

Figure 12.1 Urothelial carcinoma of the left distal ureter imaged at 3T. (a) Transaxial fast spin echo T2-weighted image through the left distal ureter demonstrates a small mass at the ureterovesical junction (arrow). (b) The mass (arrow) demonstrates high signal intensity on diffusion-weighted imaging (b-value = 800 s/mm^2).

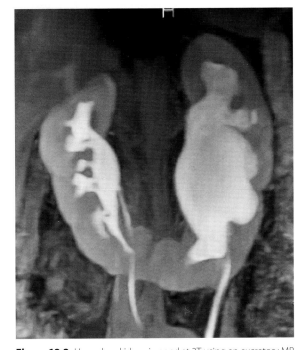

Figure 12.2 Horseshoe kidney imaged at 3T using an excretory MR urography technique (three-dimensional, fat-suppressed, T1-weighted gradient echo sequence; 0.05 mmol/kg intravenous gadobenate dimeglumine; 5 mg intravenous furosemide and 250 mL intravenous normal saline). Left hydronephrosis is present due to a left ureteropelvic junction stricture.

T1-weighted sequence (usually performed as a three-dimensional (3D) gradient echo sequence). Fat suppression is important for T2-weighted imaging,

as it improves conspicuity of cystic lesions as well as inflammation and edema. Many individuals augment the fat-suppressed images with nonsuppressed images performed using a single-shot echo-train spin-echo-type sequence. Fat-suppressed T1-weighted imaging prior to contrast administration is useful for the identification of blood products, which typically appear bright in the subacute phase. For gadolinium-enhanced sequences, the addition of fat suppression improves the conspicuity of enhancing structures by eliminating competing high signal intensity from fat. The role of diffusion-weighted imaging is under investigation, but some form of single-shot spin-echo echo planar diffusion-weighted sequence is available on most MR systems and can be performed if desired.

Renal mass characterization

MR imaging offers significant advantages over ultrasound and CT for the characterization of solid and cystic renal masses. Specifically, a sonographic window is not required, and MR imaging provides superior tissue contrast resolution. Furthermore, MR imaging is exquisitely sensitive to contrast enhancement with gadolinium-based contrast agents (GBCAs), aiding the detection of enhancing septa and nodules. Unfortunately, MR imaging has typically lagged behind these other modalities in spatial resolution. High-resolution imaging of the kidneys requires a sufficient level of signal relative to noise while compensating for

Table 12.1 Sample generic 3T kidney protocol

Sequence	Comments
Single-shot echo-train spin-echo T2W - Coronal	- Maintaining a relatively short TE will improve SNR - Parallel imaging reduces SAR and blurring
Opposed-phase and in-phase T1W - Axial	- If feasible, use a dual-echo sequence with TEs as close to 1.1 ms and 2.2 ms as possible - Opposed-phase and in-phase images can be obtained as separate acquisitions if necessary. - Reducing flip angle, increasing bandwidth, and shortening TR help get TE as low as possible for opposed-phase image.
Fat-suppressed T2W - Axial	- Can perform as respiratory-triggered or breath-hold sequence
- Diffusion-weighted SE-EPI - Axial - b-value = 1000 s/mm^2	- Optional. The role of diffusion-weighted imaging of the kidneys is still being defined, but may be of benefit in patients who cannot receive contrast
- Multiphase, fat-suppressed, contrast-enhanced gradient echo T1W - Axial or coronal	- Pre-contrast, corticomedullary phase, and nephrographic phase - For preoperative imaging, coronal arterial phase images can be helpful to define vascular anatomy
Consider fat-suppressed T1W imaging in additional planes	

T1W = T1-weighted, T2W = T2-weighted, SE-EPI = spin-echo echo planar imaging, TE = echo time, SNR = signal-to-noise ratio, SAR = specific absorption rate, TR = repetition time.

respiratory motion of the kidneys. These requirements limit the spatial resolution achievable on many MR systems. The 3T systems provide additional signal necessary to advance the limits of spatial resolution, making the potential benefits of MR imaging more compelling.

Spatial resolution is particularly important for characterization of cystic renal neoplasms, as one of the primary goals of imaging is to detect septa and enhancing components that might elevate the likelihood that a mass is malignant. At the present time, the most widely used classification system of cystic renal lesions remains some permutation of the system proposed by Bosniak [1]. While initially applied primarily to CT, this system translates reasonably well to MR imaging. The successful implementation of this classification system requires accurate assessment of such features as the cyst wall, internal septa, and nodules for thickness, irregularity, and enhancement. It has been shown that MR imaging can detect additional features compared with CT that may result in an upgrade

in lesion classification [2]. As a result, one might expect that the improvements in spatial resolution afforded by imaging at 3T will aid in even more accurate lesion characterization, potentially reducing the number of indeterminate masses and patients subjected to indefinite imaging follow-up (Figure 12.3). Unfortunately, such potential benefits remain theoretical.

The characterization of renal lesions involves more than simply delineating morphology. Other features of a renal mass, such as signal intensity, the presence of intracellular lipid and macroscopic fat, and enhancement and diffusion characteristics, can also influence the differential diagnosis. When analyzing a renal lesion, one often begins with the signal intensity on T1- and T2-weighted images, which when combined with enhancement characteristics, often provides valuable information regarding the diagnosis. A unilocular lesion that is uniformly hyperintense (similar to cerebrospinal fluid) on T2-weighted images, uniformly hypointense (relative to renal cortex) on T1-weighted

(a)

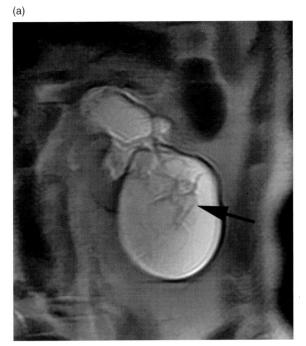

(b)

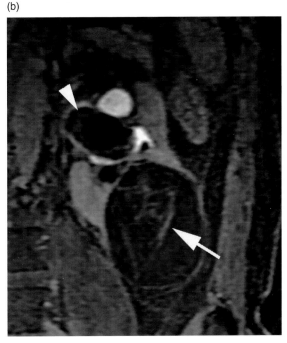

Figure 12.3 Bosniak class 3 lesion imaged at 3T. (a) Coronal T2-weighted single-shot fast spin echo image through the left kidney demonstrates a cystic lesion with fine internal septa (arrow). (b) Coronal excretory phase, fat-suppressed, T1-weighted 3D gradient echo image shows enhancing internal septa (arrow). Note that the lesion bulges into the renal pelvis (arrowhead), allowing a presumptive diagnosis of multilocular cystic nephroma.

images, and nonenhancing is, for all practical purposes, a simple cyst. A unilocular lesion that is uniformly hyperintense (relative to renal cortex) on T1-weighted images, variable on T2-weighted images, and nonenhancing is either a hemorrhagic or proteinaceous cyst. Hemorrhagic cysts often demonstrate a type of "hematocrit" effect, with higher signal intensity material layering dependently on T1-weighted images. Many papillary renal cell carcinomas are hypointense or isointense to renal parenchyma on T2-weighted images, enhance less than renal cortex, and demonstrate restricted diffusion on high b-value diffusion-weighted images (Figure 12.4).

Because tissue relaxation rates differ at 1.5T and 3T, transitioning to higher field strength might be expected to affect the relative signal characteristics of renal lesions. This is of particular concern, because the change in T1 value from 1.5T to 3T is tissue dependent, with renal parenchyma experiencing as much as a 73% increase in T1 value [3]. The T1 of lipids, on the other hand, increases by approximately 20%. As a result, there is a very real difference in image contrast on a T1-weighted image

performed at 3T compared with a similar type of image performed at 1.5T. While these differences affect how the image looks, they do not appear to significantly affect renal lesion characterization. Because the T1 relaxation times of cortex and medulla do not change by the same relative amount between 1.5T and 3T, a slightly lower degree of corticomedullary differentiation might be noticed at 3T compared with 1.5T if imaging parameters are similar (Figure 12.5) [4]. T2 values do not vary sufficiently between 1.5T and 3T to be of clinical concern for renal mass characterization.

The presence of macroscopic fat is an important discriminator when characterizing renal lesions. The presence of macroscopic fat within a renal mass virtually assures a diagnosis of angiomyolipoma, with exceptions being extremely rare. Large foci of macroscopic fat can be readily identified by comparing T1-weighted images performed with and without the application of fat suppression. The improved spectral resolution provided at 3T compared with lower field strengths means that chemically selective fat suppression techniques work very well at 3T.

(a)

(b)

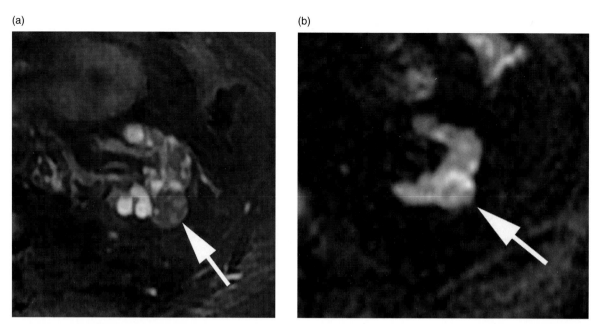

Figure 12.4 Papillary renal cell carcinoma imaged at 3T. (a) Transaxial fat-suppressed T2-weighted image of the left kidney shows a predominately low-signal-intensity mass (arrow). Multiple renal cysts are also present in this dialysis patient. (b) Diffusion-weighted image (b-value = 500 s/mm^2) at the same level shows the mass (arrow) to have intermediate to high signal intensity relative to the normal renal parenchyma. In general, b-values higher than 500 s/mm^2 are recommended for renal imaging to reduce the signal intensity of normal renal parenchyma and simple cysts.

(a)

(b)

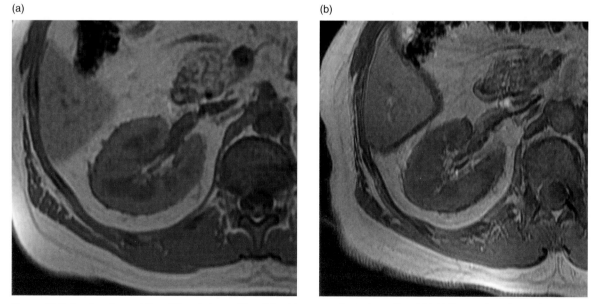

Figure 12.5 Renal corticomedullary differentiation on T1-weighted images performed at 1.5T and 3T. (a) Transaxial gradient echo T1-weighted image of the right kidney performed at 1.5T shows reasonably good corticomedullary differentiation. (b) Image performed at 3T in the same patient using similar imaging parameters (image is no longer in phase due to similar echo time [TE]) shows poor distinction between cortex and medulla.

Of greater implication for 3T imaging is the dependence of opposed-phase and in-phase echo times on field strength. At 1.5T, a dual gradient echo sequence with opposed-phase and in-phase echo times of approximately 2.2 ms and 4.4 ms is a standard part of most renal mass protocols. The purpose of

(a)

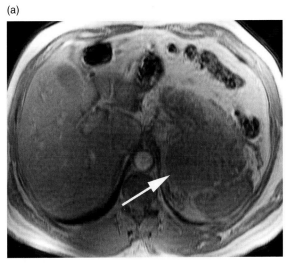

(b)

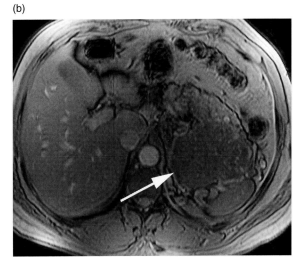

Figure 12.6 Clear cell carcinoma imaged at 3T with in-phase and opposed-phase echo times during separate breath-holds. (a) Transaxial in-phase T1-weighted gradient echo image of the left kidney shows a large renal mass (arrow). The first in-phase echo was collected at a TE of approximately 2.1 ms. (b) Opposed-phase image (TE was approximately 3.2 ms) shows subtle signal loss in the mass (arrow) due to the presence of intracellular lipid. The adjacent spleen serves as a useful reference standard. Note that breath-holding was consistent between acquisitions.

this type of sequence is to provide breath-hold T1-weighted images and to detect intracellular lipid in renal and adrenal masses. The presence of intracellular lipid in a renal mass is implied at 1.5T when areas of signal loss are identified on opposed-phase images relative to in-phase. Subtle areas of ill-defined signal loss are highly correlated with clear cell subtype of renal cell carcinoma, while more profound signal loss (typically greater than 25% on 1.5T systems) is associated with some angiomyolipomas. Dual-echo imaging can be performed as a stand-alone sequence or with fat-only and water-only Dixon reconstructions, the latter of which can serve as fat-suppressed T1-weighted images. At 3T, the first opposed-phase echo time shortens to approximately 1.1 ms, while the first in-phase echo time occurs at approximately 2.2 ms. At first glance, this may be seen as an advantage, as the shorter echo times reduce the effects of T2* decay. Unfortunately, some 3T MR systems in use are not capable of obtaining images at the first opposed-phase and in-phase echo times as part of a dual-echo sequence. Obtaining opposed-phase and in-phase images as separate breath-hold acquisitions can help alleviate this problem, but spatial misregistration between data sets can make direct comparisons between images difficult (Figure 12.6). Some manufacturers have dealt with this issue by designing a dual-echo sequence that collects the first in-phase echo followed by the third opposed-phase echo. This approach has two major limitations. First, the distinction between lipid and hemosiderin becomes difficult, as the opposed-phase image also has a longer echo time (Figure 12.7). Second, it may be difficult to distinguish between signal loss resulting from the intermixture of water and lipid and signal loss related to T2* decay (which occurs even in the absence of hemosiderin). In addition, signal loss thresholds established for opposed-phase and in-phase imaging at 1.5T to distinguish between renal cell carcinoma and lipid-poor angiomyolipoma may not be directly applicable to renal imaging at 3T. To prevent confusion caused by obtaining an opposed-phase image with a relatively long echo time, the first opposed-phase echo time can be approximated on older platforms by decreasing the flip angle, increasing the bandwidth, and reducing the TR [5].

Contrast enhancement remains a critical element in the characterization of renal masses. The presence of enhancement within a renal lesion excludes the diagnosis of simple or hemorrhagic cyst. The presence of enhancing nodules within a cystic lesion greatly increases the likelihood that the lesion is malignant. The pattern of enhancement is also of importance. For example, papillary renal cell carcinomas typically demonstrate significantly less enhancement than other subtypes of renal cell carcinoma [6].

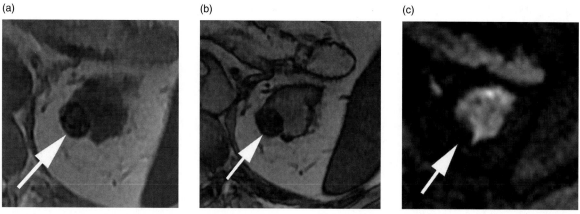

Figure 12.7 Hemosiderin-containing papillary renal cell carcinoma imaged with a dual-echo T1-weighted gradient echo sequence at 3T. This is a second tumor in the same patient as Figure 12.4. (a) Transaxial in-phase image acquired at TE of 2.4 ms shows a mass in the upper pole of the left kidney (arrow) that contains multiple small foci of low signal intensity (hemosiderin). (b) Opposed-phase image acquired as part of the same dual-echo sequence (TE = 5.8 ms) shows signal loss in the mass (arrow) relative to (a). By acquiring the opposed-phase image with a longer TE, the distinction between signal loss from lipid and hemosiderin becomes difficult. (c) Diffusion-weighted image shows profound signal loss within the mass (arrow) caused by iron-related susceptibility artifact.

While the relaxivity of GBCAs decreases as field strength increases, this is not a major source of concern for renal imaging. While absolute GBCA relaxivity is lower at 3T than at 1.5T, the conspicuity of enhancement (contrast-to-noise ratio, CNR) may actually be better at 3T based on data obtained in the central nervous and vascular systems. In the abdomen, relative renal enhancement has been shown to be significantly higher at 3T compared with 1.5T during the hepatic arterial phase using an identical contrast agent and injection protocol [7]. As a result, the difference in contrast agent relaxivity between 1.5T and 3T does not appear to be problematic for renal imaging.

Additional challenges of renal imaging at 3T

Several additional imaging artifacts that can interfere with renal lesion characterization are exacerbated at 3T. Susceptibility artifacts are increased at 3T, and when severe, can obscure focal lesions or large areas of the kidney and interfere with some forms of fat suppression. Potential sources of susceptibility artifact include surgical clips (including clips dropped at the time of cholecystectomy, which often settle in the hepatorenal fossa), bowel gas, spinal orthopedic hardware, and concentrated gadolinium. This latter source can be eliminated by imaging prior to the excretory phase, but the former sources cannot be

easily removed. The deleterious effects of bowel gas can be ameliorated by having the patient fast in advance of the examination, although this is rarely done for purposes of renal imaging. At the time of imaging, susceptibility artifact can be reduced by optimizing shimming and using a higher receiver bandwidth (at the expense of SNR) and a short echo time. Techniques that fill k-space in a radial and partially overlapping manner can also reduce susceptibility artifact and may be useful for diffusion-weighted imaging. Most currently available diffusion-weighted imaging sequences are echo planar-based, making them particularly sensitive to susceptibility differences. This commonly results in signal loss or geometric distortion in the kidney when gas-filled colon or metallic artifacts are nearby. The use of parallel imaging can reduce this effect. Additionally, the presence of hemosiderin within a renal neoplasm can interfere with diffusion-weighted imaging and calculation of apparent diffusion coefficient (ADC) values (Figure 12.7). Diffusion-weighted imaging at 3T also suffers from more pronounced motion and blurring artifacts than similar sequences at 1.5T [8].

The precessional frequency difference between fat and water protons increases from 1.5T to 3T, exacerbating chemical shift artifact of the first kind resulting from spatial misregistration of fat protons relative to water protons. This manifests as bands of high or low signal intensity along fat–water interfaces in the frequency-encoding direction. This artifact could potentially

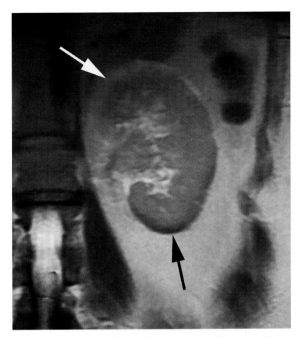

Figure 12.8 Chemical shift artifact (arrows) manifesting in the frequency-encoding direction along the left kidney on a coronal single-shot fast spin echo sequence at 3T. This artifact could simulate perinephric fluid/edema at the upper pole or obscure small abnormalities along the renal capsule.

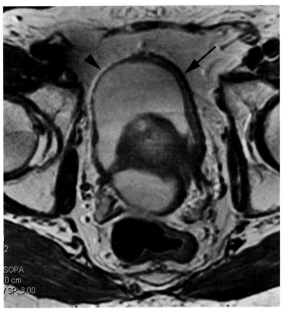

Figure 12.9 Chemical shift artifact causing spurious bladder wall thickening on a transaxial T2-weighted image through the pelvis (arrow). Note that the opposite bladder wall has a high-signal-intensity band running alongside (arrowhead). The receiver bandwidth was intentionally set low to help with localization of fiducial markers in the prostate gland (not shown).

obscure small abnormalities along the renal capsule, simulate perinephric fluid, or create artificial cyst or bladder wall thickening (Figures 12.8 and 12.9). We have also seen this artifact interfere with chemical shift artifact of the second kind ("India ink" artifact) (Figure 12.10). Increasing receiver bandwidth reduces the severity of chemical shift artifact (of the first kind) at the expense of reduced SNR. Fortunately, fat-suppressed sequences are routinely performed for characterization of renal masses, reducing the diagnostic impact of this artifact.

Whole-body MR systems at 3T are notorious for producing "shading" artifacts related to B1 inhomogeneity. Long echo train sequences such as fast/turbo spin echo and single-shot fast/turbo spin echo seem to be particularly susceptible to shading artifacts that manifest as spatial variations in signal intensity across the image. When mild, such artifacts can simply be an annoyance. However, if present at the site of a renal cyst, misclassification of a simple cyst as a complicated cyst might result or thin septa might be obscured (Figure 12.11). When severe, shading artifacts can obscure lesions or regions of interest. Fortunately, MR system manufacturers are well aware of

this limitation of abdominal imaging at 3T, resulting in improved image quality on newer systems.

Future opportunities for renal imaging at 3T

Many advanced MR applications have been shown to benefit from the shift from 1.5T to 3T. The potential for increased SNR at 3T provides for opportunities to image less abundant nuclei such as sodium and map their distribution in the kidney [9]. Improved spectral resolution may enhance interest in MR spectroscopy of the kidney. Blood oxygen level-dependent MR imaging has also been shown to benefit from the shift from 1.5T to 3T, with improvements in discrimination of R2* values between cortex and medulla [10]. Improvements in SNR and CNR during diffusion tensor imaging of the kidney at 3T have been demonstrated without changes in ADC values compared with 1.5T [11]. Maximum signal intensity during gadolinium-enhanced perfusion imaging of the kidney is increased at 3T compared with 1.5T without a change in mean transit time or time to peak [12].

(a) 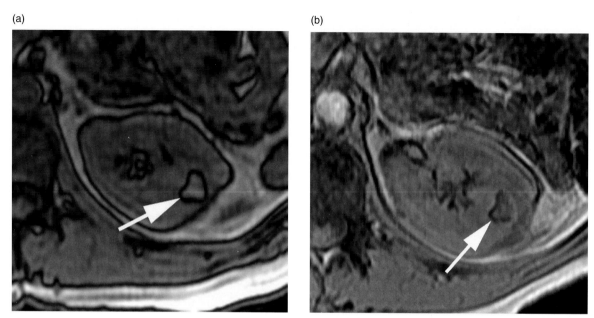 (b)

Figure 12.10 Chemical shift artifact of the first kind interfering with chemical shift artifact of the second kind at 3T. (a) Transaxial opposed-phase T1-weighted gradient echo image through the left kidney acquired at 1.5T shows an angiomyolipoma (arrow) clearly outlined by "India ink" artifact. This artifact is helpful in identifying the composition of the mass as fat-containing. (b) The same kidney imaged at an opposed-phase echo time at 3T fails to demonstrate the "India ink" artifact as clearly surrounding the mass (arrow) due to the presence of enhanced chemical shift artifact of the first kind.

(a) 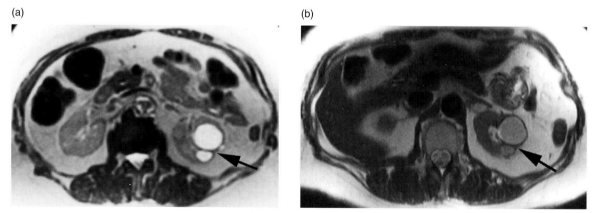 (b)

Figure 12.11 Shading artifact at 3T due to B1 inhomogeneity. (a) Transaxial single-shot fast spin echo image acquired at 1.5T shows two adjacent simple cysts in the left kidney (arrow). Mild shading is present in the central portions of the image, but the cysts are homogeneously very bright. (b) Single-shot fast spin echo image of the same patient acquired at 3T shows considerable shading in the central portions of the image. Note that the renal cysts (arrow) are not as conspicuously high in signal intensity on this image.

MR urography

MR urography protocol

With a few exceptions, MR urography can be performed at 3T in a manner similar to MR urography performed at lower field strengths. The additional signal provided by the higher field strength can be used to obtain high-resolution images of the renal collecting systems and bladder. For most indications, we perform a comprehensive protocol designed to evaluate the

Table 12.2 Sample comprehensive 3T MR urography protocol

Sequence	Comments
Intravenous hydration	- Optional. 250 mL normal saline if no contraindication exists
Single-shot echo-train spin-echo T2W - Coronal - Abdomen and pelvis	- Maintaining a relatively short TE will improve SNR - Parallel imaging reduces SAR and blurring
Opposed-phase and in-phase T1W - Axial - Abdomen and pelvis	- If possible, use a dual-echo sequence with TEs as close to 1.1 ms and 2.2 ms as possible - Opposed-phase and in-phase images can be obtained as separate acquisitions if necessary - Reducing flip angle, increasing bandwidth, and shortening TR help get TE as low as possible for opposed-phase image
Fat-suppressed T2W - Axial - Abdomen and pelvis	- Can perform as respiratory-triggered or breath-hold sequence - For bladder cancer staging, perform without fat suppression
Administer furosemide Thick-slab T2W MR urogram	- 5 to 10 mg intravenously for adults if no contraindication exists - Repeat multiple times to visualize all of ureters
Fat-suppressed, unenhanced gradient echo T1W - Axial (can do coronal for abdomen if desired) - Abdomen and pelvis	- Will likely need to perform abdomen and pelvis as separate acquisitions if imaging in the transaxial plane
Fat-suppressed, contrast-enhanced gradient echo T1W - Axial (can do coronal for abdomen if desired) - Abdomen	- Two breath-hold acquisitions with brief time to breath between. This can provide arterial and corticomedullary phase images
Fat-suppressed, contrast-enhanced gradient echo T1W - Axial - Pelvis	- Perform immediately after preceding sequence before urine within bladder enhances and causes mixing artifact
Fat-suppressed, excretory phase gradient echo T1W - Axial, coronal, and/or sagittal - Abdomen and pelvis	- Additional high-resolution images can be obtained through limited regions if desired

T1W = T1-weighted, T2W = T2-weighted, TE = echo time, SNR = signal-to-noise ratio, SAR = specific absorption rate, TR = repetition time.

kidneys, ureters, and bladder sufficiently to detect and stage renal and urothelial neoplasms, evaluate congenital anomalies, or assess the location and cause of obstructive uropathy (Table 12.2). As with renal imaging, a phased array torso coil should be used. Ideally, the coil should be capable of including the kidneys, ureters, and bladder within a single coronal field-of-view. As we have already discussed the characterization of renal masses, we will focus the following discussion on dedicated MR urographic techniques.

T2-weighted MR urography involves the use of long echo train, heavily T2-weighted sequences

(a)

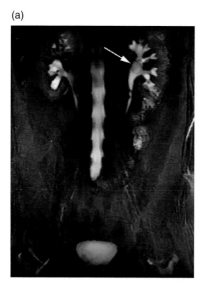

(b)

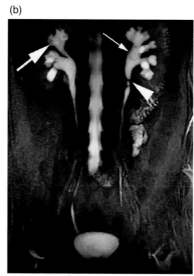

Figure 12.12 T2-weighted MR urography at 3T. (a) Coronal heavily T2-weighted image through the kidneys, ureters, and bladder performed immediately after intravenous administration of furosemide (5 mg) shows relatively poor distension of the renal collecting systems and bladder. The upper pigtail of a ureteral stent is seen (thin arrow). (b) Repeat image performed several minutes after furosemide administration shows improved distension of the renal collecting systems (arrow), improved visualization of the ureters, and persistent narrowing of the left ureteropelvic junction (arrowhead). Note that the stent is still visible (thin arrow).

similar to those used for MR cholangiopancreatography (Figure 12.12). Long effective echo times and fat suppression are used to improve conspicuity of fluid-containing structures relative to background tissues. A T2-weighted MR urography study can be performed as a thin-section 3D respiratory-triggered sequence that can be manipulated to create volume-rendered or maximum-intensity-projection images in multiple projections. Alternatively, images can be obtained as single thick slabs acquired in multiple projections as separate acquisitions. Images are typically obtained in the coronal plane with a field of view that includes the kidneys, ureters, and bladder. As with conventional intravenous urography, oblique imaging or multiplanar reconstructions of the intra-renal collecting systems can be helpful to better define anatomy. Ureteral and collecting system distension can be improved by hydrating the patient before the examination and administering a low dose (5–10 mg IV for adults) of furosemide (Figure 12.12). A full urinary bladder can also improve distension of the upper tracts, provided the patient can tolerate such an approach [13]. For T2-weighted urography, intravenous hydration is preferable to oral hydration to prevent the obscuring effects of fluid within bowel.

Advanced administration of a negative oral contrast agent can aid in reducing unwanted signal from bowel, but the use of iron-based agents is discouraged due to the enhanced susceptibility effects at 3T. To reduce the susceptibility-related effects of bowel gas,

which are also enhanced at 3T, it might be preferable to have patients fast in advance of the examination. Bowel-related susceptibility effects are most problematic in the regions of the distal ureters and bladder dome (Figure 12.13).

A thick-slab T2-weighted MR urogram can be performed in a few seconds or less. Repeat imaging is easily performed and effective at visualizing the ureters in varying degrees of distension to confirm the presence of fixed narrowings, obstructions, and filling defects. When using this technique, time must be provided between acquisitions to permit tissues to recover longitudinal magnetization between excitations and to prevent saturation of signal. Because T2-weighted MR urography is quick and easy to perform and does not require administration of intravenous contrast material or ionizing radiation, it is ideally suited for imaging pregnant women. However, there is not proven benefit to imaging pregnant women at field strengths higher than 1.5T, and the safety of imaging at 3T in such a setting has not been carefully studied. Furthermore, satisfactory images might be more difficult to obtain in the setting of pregnancy due to standing wave and conductivity effects [14]. Therefore, we do not currently recommend performing MR urography on pregnant women at 3T.

As with MR urography performed at 1.5T, when T2-weighted techniques are combined with gadolinium-enhanced imaging, the T2-weighted images must be

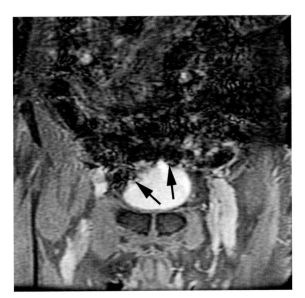

Figure 12.13 Susceptibility artifact related to bowel. This coronal, fat-suppressed T1-weighted gradient echo excretory phase image shows severe susceptibility artifact along the bladder dome (arrows) due to adjacent bowel. The patient had been given an oral iron-based MR contrast agent to eliminate signal in the bowel. Because of artifacts such as this, we no longer use such agents for MR urography at 3T.

obtained before concentrated excreted contrast material accumulates within the collecting systems, significantly diminishing signal from urine. Excretory MR urography is not recommended in patients with severe renal insufficiency due to the risk of nephrogenic systemic fibrosis (NSF) and the inability of severely impaired kidneys to adequately excrete administered contrast material.

Excretory MR urography using an intravenous GBCA is usually better at demonstrating nonobstructed ureters or a communication between the renal collecting system and a fluid collection than T2-weighted techniques. However, the administration of a standard 0.1-mmol/kg dose of an extracellular GBCA eventually lowers the signal intensity of urine due to the T2* effects of concentrated excreted contrast. Hydrating the patient and/or administering a low dose of diuretic such as furosemide prevents excessive concentration of the contrast material within the urinary tract while improving contrast distribution and ureteral distension in patients without urinary tract obstruction [15, 16]. T1-weighted 3D gradient echo sequences, with or without fat suppression, provide high-resolution MR urographic images following gadolinium-based contrast administration. The

coronal plane provides the greatest anatomical coverage in the shortest time, although additional planes can occasionally be useful. Coronal imaging is facilitated by use of a multichannel torso coil that can simultaneously image the abdomen and pelvis while employing parallel imaging to shorten acquisition times. At a field strength of 3T using parallel imaging, the entire collecting system can be imaged with 1-mm to 2-mm through-plane resolution in the coronal plane during a single breath-hold (Figure 12.14). The ability to improve spatial resolution remains the biggest advantage of higher field strength imaging for MR urography. Unfortunately, ureteral peristalsis, which contributes to blurring of the ureter, remains a problem for imaging with a 3D sequence, and there is currently no evidence to suggest that imaging at 3T can provide sufficient temporal resolution to eliminate peristalsis-related artifacts while preserving spatial resolution. Ultimately, it can be expected that this issue will be addressed by T1-weighted sequences with higher temporal resolution or use of two-dimensional (2D) sequences. Nonetheless, a comparison of T1-weighted excretory MR urography performed at 1.5T with that performed at 3T in an animal model using a 3D gradient echo sequence showed that image quality and SNR were improved at the higher field strength [17].

Clinical applications

MR urography is highly accurate for determining the level of urinary tract obstruction. GBCA-enhanced 3D gradient echo (excretory) MR urography combined with T2-weighted techniques can detect up to 90% of ureteral stones [18]. Signs of acute calculus urinary tract obstruction include persistent ureteral dilation above a filling defect and high-signal-intensity perinephric edema on T2-weighted images. Persistence of the corticomedullary phase of enhancement and delayed excretion of contrast media can be present when obstruction is severe. At the time of this writing, it is unknown whether imaging at 3T can improve detection of ureteral calculi, although the improved spatial resolution and enhanced susceptibility artifact associated with higher field strength should be expected to provide some benefit.

Obstructing urothelial carcinoma is well demonstrated with T2-weighted and excretory MR urography techniques. The site of obstruction is often readily visible on T2-weighted images, although specificity is enhanced with the addition of contrast

(A)

(B)

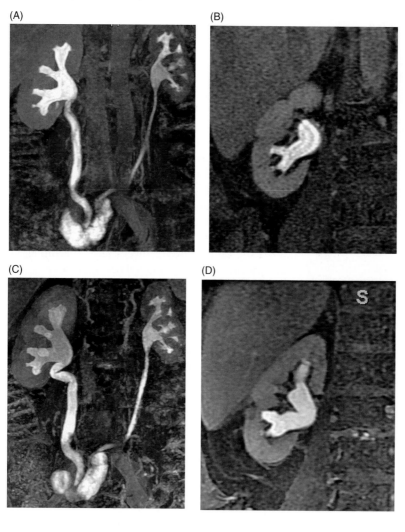

(C)

(D)

Figure 12.14 Excretory MR urography at 1.5T and 3T in the same patient with prior cystectomy and ileal conduit formation for bladder carcinoma. In each case, images were acquired using a coronal 3D fat-suppressed T1-weighted sequence after intravenous hydration and administration of 0.05 mmol/kg gadobenate dimeglumine. Partition thickness was 2 mm for each. (A) Maximum-intensity-projection reconstruction of images obtained at 1.5T. (B) Coronal source image obtained at 1.5T. (C) Maximum intensity projection of images obtained at 3T. (D) Coronal source image obtained at 3T. S = superior.

material. Intravenous GBCA can also aid in demonstrating the extent of the tumor. When urothelial carcinoma is discovered, additional foci of tumor should be sought. Fat-suppressed contrast-enhanced sequences are also helpful for assessing extrinsic processes that involve the ureter, such as prostate or uterine carcinoma or retroperitoneal fibrosis. The feasibility of using MR urography to detect small urothelial carcinomas has been demonstrated, although data comparing sensitivity between 1.5T and 3T are currently lacking [19]. As with detection of calculi, the higher spatial resolution and/or SNR of 3T should be beneficial for urothelial tumor detection.

CT urography will likely continue to be the test of choice for evaluation of patients with hematuria, although MR urography may play a role in young

patients or patients with mild to moderate renal insufficiency. MR imaging is sensitive and specific for blood clots, which typically appear bright on T1-weighted images and fail to enhance after administration of intravenous contrast agents. This appearance is not significantly altered at a field strength of 3T. MR urography has been shown to have a high negative predictive value for urothelial neoplasms and compares favorably with retrograde pyelography [20]. However, there have been no published data assessing the sensitivity and specificity of 3T MR urography in the evaluation of patients with hematuria.

MR urography can accurately assess congenital urinary tract anomalies. In such cases, high spatial resolution can be critical to demonstrating small crossing vessels in the setting of ureteropelvic junction obstruction or determining the precise site of insertion of an ectopic ureter. In these cases, higher field strength can potentially be of benefit.

Conclusion

Imaging of the urinary tract benefits from the increased SNR afforded by 3T MR systems, primarily by leveraging the gain in SNR for higher spatial resolution. However, with this added SNR comes an array of challenges that require minor pulse sequence modifications and familiarity with new or exacerbated artifacts. While many urinary tract abnormalities will continue to be adequately assessed at 1.5T, as 3T technology matures, it is likely that 3T imaging will become the standard for detection and characterization of small renal and urothelial lesions. Furthermore, advanced MR applications, such as spectroscopy, multinuclear imaging, and perfusion imaging and diffusion tensor imaging appear to benefit from increases in field strength, providing additional potential for urinary tract imaging at 3T.

References

1. Bosniak MA. The current radiological approach to renal cysts. *Radiology* 1986; **158**: 1–10.

2. Israel GM, Hindman N, Bosniak MA. Evaluation of cystic renal masses: comparison of CT and MR imaging by using the Bosniak classification system. *Radiology* 2004; **231**: 365–71.

3. Stanisz GJ, Odrobina EE, Pun J, *et al.* T1, T2 relaxation and magnetization transfer in tissue at 3T. *Magn Reson Med* 2005; **54**: 507–12.

4. de Bazelaire CM, Duhamel GD, Rofsky NM, Alsop DC. MR imaging relaxation times of abdominal and pelvic tissues measured in vivo at 3.0 T: preliminary results. *Radiology* 2004; **230**: 652–9.

5. Cornfeld D, Weinreb J. Simple changes to 1.5-T MRI abdomen and pelvis protocols to optimize results at 3 T. *AJR Am J Roentgenol* 2008; **190**: W140–50.

6. Sun MR, Ngo L, Genega EM, *et al.* Renal cell carcinoma: dynamic contrast-enhanced MR imaging for differentiation of tumor subtypes – correlation with pathologic findings. *Radiology* 2009; **250**: 793–802.

7. Goncalves Neto JA, Altun E, Elazzazi M, *et al.* Enhancement of abdominal organs on hepatic arterial phase: quantitative comparison between 1.5- and 3.0-T magnetic resonance imaging. *Magn Reson Imaging* 2010; **28**: 47–55.

8. Mürtz P, Krautmacher C, Träber F, *et al.* Diffusion-weighted whole-body MR imaging with background

body signal suppression: a feasibility study at 3.0 Tesla. *Eur Radiol* 2007; **17**: 3031–7.

9. Maril N, Rosen Y, Reynolds GH, *et al.* Sodium MRI of the human kidney at 3 Tesla. *Magn Reson Med* 2006; **56**: 1229–34.

10. Gloviczki ML, Glockner J, Gomez SI, *et al.* Comparison of 1.5 and 3 T BOLD MR to study oxygenation of kidney cortex and medulla in human renovascular disease. *Invest Radiol* 2009; **44**: 566–71.

11. Notohamiprodjo M, Dietrich O, Horger W, *et al.* Diffusion tensor imaging (DTI) of the kidney at 3 tesla-feasibility, protocol evaluation and comparison to 1.5 Tesla. *Invest Radiol* 2010; **45**: 245–54.

12. Michaely HJ, Kramer H, Oesingmann N, *et al.* Intraindividual comparison of MR-renal perfusion imaging at 1.5 T and 3.0 T. *Invest Radiol* 2007; **42**: 406–11.

13. Coville JA, Killeen RP, Buckley O, *et al.* Does a full bladder aid upper tract visualization in magnetic resonance urography? *Australas Radiol* 2007; **51**: 362–4.

14. Merkle EM, Dale BM, Paulson EK. Abdominal MR imaging at 3T. *Magn Reson Imaging Clin N Am* 2006; **14**: 17–26.

15. Nolte-Ernsting CC, Bucker A, Adam GB, *et al.* Gadolinium-enhanced excretory MR urography after low-dose diuretic injection: comparison with conventional excretory urography. *Radiology* 1998; **209**: 147–57.

16. Ergen FB, Hussain HK, Carlos RC, *et al.* 3D excretory MR urography: improved image quality with intravenous saline and diuretic administration. *J Magn Reson Imaging* 2007; **25**: 783–9.

17. Reiger M, Nolte-Ernsting C, Adam G, Kemper J. Intraindividual comparison of image quality in MR urography at 1.5 and 3 Tesla in an animal model. *Rofo* 2008; **180**: 915–21.

18. Sudah M, Vanninen R, Partanen K, *et al.* MR urography in evaluation of acute flank pain: T2-weighted sequences and gadolinium-enhanced three-dimensional FLASH compared with urography. *AJR Am J Roentgenol* 2001; **176**: 105–12.

19. Takahashi N, Kawashima A, Glockner JF, *et al.* Small (2-cm) upper-tract urothelial carcinoma: evaluation with gadolinium-enhanced three dimensional spoiled gradient-recalled echo MR urography. *Radiology* 2008; **247**: 451–7.

20. Lee KS, Zeikus E, DeWolf WC, Rofsky NM, Pedrosa I. MR urography versus retrograde pyelography/ureteroscopy for the exclusion of upper urinary tract malignancy. *Clin Radiol* 2010; **65**: 185–92.

MR imaging and MR-guided biopsy of the prostate at 3T

Katarzyna J. Macura and Jurgen J. Fütterer

Introduction

Prostate cancer is a major public health and socio-economic problem throughout the world. Prostate cancer is the most frequently diagnosed cancer in men. The 2009 report from the American Cancer Society projected 192 280 new cases of prostate cancer in the USA in 2009. With an estimated 27 360 deaths in the USA in 2009, prostate cancer is the second-leading cause of cancer death in men [1]. The high incidence of prostate cancer, combined with earlier detection and stage migration towards the smaller cancer volumes at the time of diagnosis, and the slow natural progression and heterogeneous biologic behavior of the disease make the management of prostate cancer a very complex and controversial issue. There is a wide discrepancy between the number of men diagnosed and those dying from prostate cancer. Incidence rates for prostate cancer have increased substantially over the past 20 years, in large part reflecting changes in prostate cancer screening with the prostate-specific antigen (PSA) blood test. In addition to PSA, screening for prostate cancer involves digital rectal examination (DRE) and transrectal ultrasonography (TRUS) with biopsy. Although elevated PSA levels can be suggestive of malignancy, benign conditions such as benign prostatic hyperplasia or prostatitis can also lead to PSA elevation [2]. It was demonstrated that only 25–40% of men with PSA above the 4 ng/ml threshold will be diagnosed with cancer, leading to about 60–75% of men in the PSA range 4–10 ng/ml undergoing an unnecessary biopsy [3]. In about 14% of men with prostate cancer, diagnosis can be established on the basis of DRE alone [4]. About 15% of men over the age of 60 have prostate cancer that is clinically silent, i.e., not detectable on DRE or with a PSA level of less than 4 ng/ml [5]. Thus, TRUS-guided core prostate biopsies are being used routinely to systematically sample the entire gland in patients with abnormal DRE and/or elevated PSA in the search for prostate cancer. Since prostate cancer is an age-related disease, the increasing life expectancy will result in further increase of both the incidence of and the deaths related to prostate cancer [6].

To date, the histopathologic examination of biopsy tissue remains the gold standard for diagnosing prostate cancer. The widely used TRUS provides real-time visualization of the prostate gland, but most prostate cancers are isoechoic and therefore invisible, resulting in TRUS having a positive predictive value (PPV) of only 15.2% [7]. Although the systematic sextant biopsy approach has improved the detection of prostate cancer, the sensitivity and specificity of TRUS in diagnosing impalpable prostate cancer still remains low: the number of false negatives in a single sextant biopsy session reported ranges between 30% and 45% [8, 9]. Current clinical standards for TRUS-guided prostate biopsy include systematic minimum 12-core sampling to yield higher accuracy in prostate cancer detection. Prostate cancer has multiple foci in more than 85% of cases [10]. Additionally, the intra-glandular anatomical localization of prostate cancer is often incorrect on sextant biopsy, when compared to final prostatectomy results, likely due to a combination of sampling error and technical problems in localizing the specimen site during biopsy [11, 12]. About 65% of the biopsy-positive cores predict the correct Gleason score found at radical prostatectomy. This poses a serious challenge in patients' management, because accurate tumor detection, localization, and staging may critically influence the choice of treatment. Currently available treatment options include radical

Body MR Imaging at 3 Tesla, ed. Ihab R. Kamel and Elmar M. Merkle. Published by Cambridge University Press.
© Cambridge University Press 2011.

(prostatectomy, hormone ablation, radiotherapy) and local/focal, minimally invasive therapies (cryosurgery, radiofrequency ablation, focused ultrasound). As long as prostate cancer is confined to the prostate (there is no extracapsular tumor extension, no seminal vesicle invasion, or no metastatic spread to lymph nodes or bones) treatment of the disease has a curative intent. Some patients with low-volume, low-risk prostate cancer may also be candidates for active surveillance. There is growing demand for patient-specific therapies that can minimize treatment morbidity while maximizing treatment benefit. Therefore, emerging imaging techniques that can aid safer and more individualized management of patients with prostate cancer have become the focus of intense research and have been rapidly transitioning into the clinical care.

Magnetic resonance (MR) imaging of the prostate is such a technique, as due to its superior soft tissue contrast resolution, high spatial resolution, multiplanar capability it allows detailed assessment of the prostate morphology together with the functional assessment of prostate tissue biochemical profile, perfusion, and intracellular and intercellular environments. MR imaging at a standard magnetic field strength of 1.5T has been shown to add incremental value to the management of prostate cancer to improve cancer staging, to assess biologic tumor potential, to aid treatment planning, to evaluate therapy response, to diagnose local recurrence, and to guide targeted biopsies [13].

With the growing availability of 3T whole-body MR scanners, imaging of the prostate at 3T benefits from the increased signal-to-noise ratio (SNR) and the potential for significant improvements in spatial, spectral, and temporal resolution. The typical imaging sequences used for morphologic evaluation of the prostate include T2-weighted (T2W) imaging and T1-weighted (T1W) imaging. For functional molecular evaluation of the prostatic tissue, newer MR imaging sequences are used for the assessment of: (1) Brownian motion of water molecules by diffusion-weighted imaging (DWI), (2) biochemical tissue composition by MR spectroscopic imaging (MRSI), and (3) prostate tissue perfusion by dynamic contrast-enhanced MR imaging (DCE-MRI). The ability to localize prostate cancer with MR imaging provides an opportunity to utilize MR guidance for prostate biopsy [14–17]. Accurate characterization of prostate cancer based on MR imaging findings and MR-guided tissue sampling may become essential not only for initial diagnosis and assessment of prognosis, but

also at different times in the course of the disease as MR imaging can guide biopsy procedures to confirm cancer presence and to assess tumor biology, can guide localized treatment procedures to reduce morbidity, and can guide an active surveillance (watchful waiting) approach, when patients opt to monitor the disease without treatment.

In this chapter we focus on the high-magnetic-field MR imaging techniques for morphologic and functional assessment of the prostate gland when used for the diagnosis, localization, and staging of prostate cancer. We also highlight the advancements in MR-guided prostate biopsy.

Application of endorectal coil: is it needed at 3T?

The need for using an endorectal coil at 3T has been controversial. Initially, the imaging of the prostate at 3T was performed with the use of only a pelvic phased-array coil [18]. Sosna *et al.* found no significant difference in image quality between torso phased-array 3T imaging and endorectal 1.5T imaging of the prostate [19]. Bloch *et al.* documented the feasibility of MR imaging of the prostate with a combination of endorectal and pelvic phased-array coils [20]. This resulted in excellent anatomical detail with good T2 contrast and high-quality multiplanar reconstructions with clear visualization of small anatomical structures. Similar to the diagnostic gains on imaging at 1.5T, prostate cancer localization and staging was documented to be significantly improved at 3T with the use of an endorectal coil as compared with an external surface array coil [21]. In this study, the authors found a significant improvement of image quality and staging accuracy when using an endorectal coil versus a body-array coil in the same group of patients evaluated at 3T. With endorectal coil imaging, the area under the receiver operating curve (AUC) for localization of prostate cancer was significantly increased from 0.62 to 0.68. Also, endorectal imaging significantly increased the AUC for staging; sensitivity for detection of locally advanced disease by experienced readers was increased from 7% to a range of 73–80% whereas a high specificity of 97–100% was maintained. Extracapsular tumor extension as small as 0.5 mm at histopathologic examination could be accurately detected only with endorectal imaging. However, significantly more motion artifacts were present on endorectal imaging. All other image quality characteristics improved significantly with endorectal imaging. Similar results for endorectal staging were confirmed in a different study, in which 3T endorectal MR imaging was investigated and the authors reported a high staging accuracy of 94% and specificity of 96% [22]. In this study, two of three histopathology-proven cases of minimal capsular invasion were only visible on endorectal MR imaging. Therefore, it has been concluded that when the imaging of the prostate is ordered for local staging, it should be performed with an endorectal coil at 3T.

The application of endorectal coil allows imaging with an increased spatial resolution for morphologic assessment with T2W and T1W imaging, with increased temporal resolution for DCE-MRI, and also with increased spectral resolution for MRSI [23]. For MR imaging at 3T with an endorectal coil, the spatial resolution can be increased to 0.18 mm, compared with 0.55 mm at 1.5T, and the pixel size can be reduced to 0.13 mm^2, compared with 1.21 mm^2 at 1.5T [23].

The application of an endorectal coil comes with many challenges at 3T. The increased susceptibility and sensitivity to the signal intensity inhomogeneity due to the nonuniform endorectal coil sensitivity profile mandates its proper positioning to optimize the anatomical coverage of the receiving signal from the prostate gland. Therefore, the accuracy of coil placement relative to the prostate is an important aspect in prostate MR imaging to achieve clear visualization of all parts of the prostate, from the gland base proximally to the apex distally. The evaluation of the initial scout images is crucial in confirming the proper positioning of the coil in the rectum, with the coverage of the prostate base and seminal vesicles at the proximal aspect of the coil and inferior coverage of the prostate apex at the distal end of the coil. Additionally, proper positioning in the right-to-left orientation should be confirmed, as rotation of the coil to one side will adversely affect the signal received from the noncovered part of the prostate. To reduce the degradation of images by rectal motion artifacts, the frequency direction should be set at anterior-to-posterior instead of right-to-left direction. For imaging at 1.5T, the endorectal coil could be filled with air. However, due to the more pronounced susceptibility artifacts at 3T, the endo-rectal coil balloon should be filled with liquid per-fluorocarbon (PFC) [24] or barium [25] instead of air to improve the homogeneity of the magnetic

field. A rigid probe can be used as well without the need for instillation with any filling agent and was shown at 1.5T to provide approximately 2.5-fold higher SNR than inflatable coils near the peripheral zone midline and produced less tissue distortion [26]. Development of a rigid coil compatible with 3T may prove to provide similar benefits to those seen at 1.5T.

Morphologic imaging of the prostate: T2-weighted and T1-weighted imaging

Prior to MR scan, an intramuscular injection of spas-molytic agent, e.g., 1 mg glucagon, is advised to reduce the bowel peristalsis and motion artifacts. An endorectal coil is placed following the digital rectal examination and is insufflated with approximately 60–80 mL of a liquid agent, as mentioned above. Sagittal and axial T2W half-Fourier acquisition single-shot turbo spin-echo localizer images are obtained to evaluate the endorectal coil positioning. It is important to perform the prostate MR imaging at least 4 and optimally 6 weeks after prostate biopsy, because the presence of hemorrhage may obscure or mimic prostate cancer on T2W images and blood products may interfere with functional imaging [27]. For T2W MR imaging, the following parameters are suggested: repetition time (TR)/echo time (TE) 3500–5000 ms/124 ms, 2.5- to 3-mm section thickness, 18–20 slices, 200-mm field of view (FOV), and matrix at least 512×512. To reduce the radio-frequency (RF) power deposition, hyperechoes are used [28]. The spin echoes are obtained with a train of low-power pulses with modulated flip angles to produce a full spin echo at the effective TE. At 3T, the T1 relaxation time increases and T2 relaxation time decreases compared with those at 1.5T, as docu-mented by de Bazelaire et al. [29], who found an increase of 21% for T1 relaxation time and a decrease of 16% for T2 relaxation time in the prostate. It was shown that at longer TEs (TE time beyond the T2 relaxation time of the prostate – ie, 74 ± 9 ms), the difference between cancer and healthy prostate tissue was more accentuated, provided the tissue with the shortest T2 still had adequate SNR [21]. In addition to T2W images, an axial T1W to intermediate-weighted sequence is required to detect post-biopsy hemorrhage. The following parameters for T1W imaging can be used: TR/TE 20 ms/4.4 ms, flip angle of 8°, and 250- to 350-mm FOV.

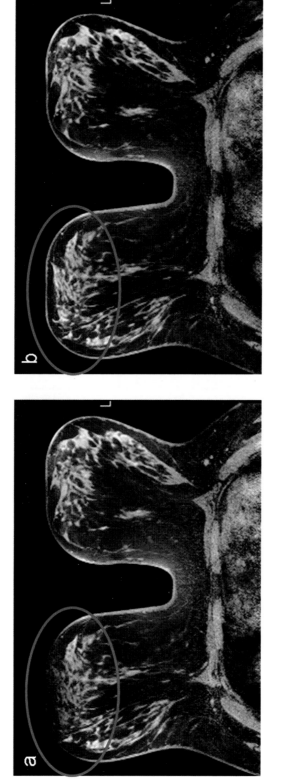

Figure 3.3 Comparison of breast MR images acquired at 3T using a standard rectangular volume shim technique (a) and a "patient-adaptive" image-based shim technique (SmartExam Breast, Philips Healthcare, Best, The Netherlands) (b). Images were acquired using a 3D T1-weighted gradient echo sequence with parallel imaging and active fat suppression, 16-channel coil, and scan time of 2:50 minutes. In this example, improved image quality was obtained at air–tissue interfaces (circled region) using the image-based shim due to improved B0 homogeneity (b).

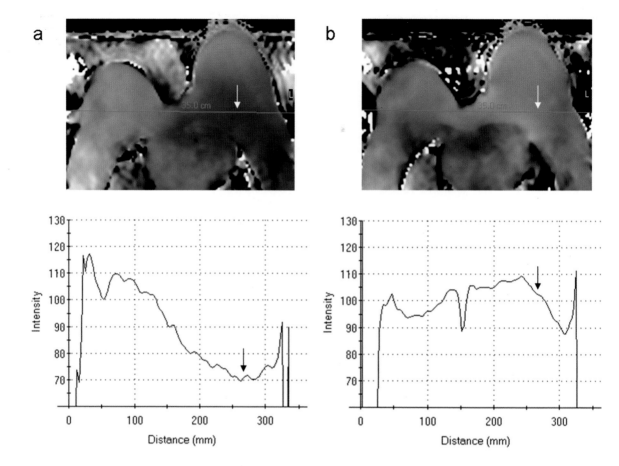

Figure 3.4 Improvement in B1 homogeneity using an adaptive parallel RF transmission technique. B1 maps acquired with conventional single source RF transmission (a) and with parallel transmission (Multi-Transmit, Philips Healthcare, Best, The Netherlands) (b) are compared. Shown below the B1 maps are corresponding flip angle profiles measured across the field of view as indicated by the red line. Signal intensity relates to the delivered excitation, expressed as percent of intended flip angle or B1. B1 maps were calculated using an interleaved dual-TR T1-weighted gradient echo sequence. Improved bilateral B1 homogeneity can be appreciated on both the parallel RF transmission B1 map and corresponding plot (b), particularly in the left breast (arrows). Flip angle variation across the image ranged from 70% to 115% of the intended flip angle with conventional imaging, compared with only 90% to 110% using parallel transmission.

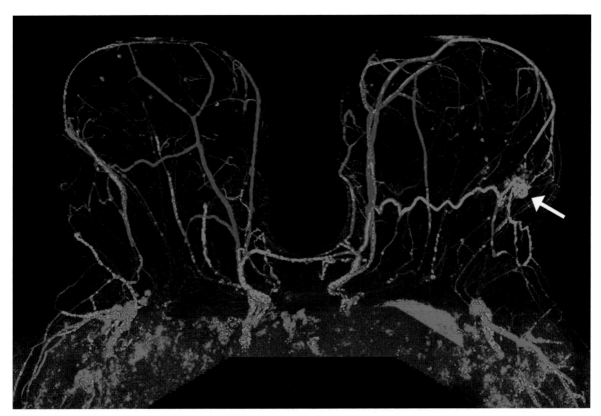

Figure 3.5 Maximum intensity projection (MIP) of dynamic contrast-enhanced breast MR images acquired at 3T. The MIP was created from subtraction images (post-contrast minus pre-contrast) to demonstrate enhancing structures. Delayed phase contrast kinetics are represented in color, with red, green, and blue representing washout, plateau, and persistent enhancement, respectively. In this example case, a lesion with suspicious enhancement characteristics is visible in the left breast (arrow).

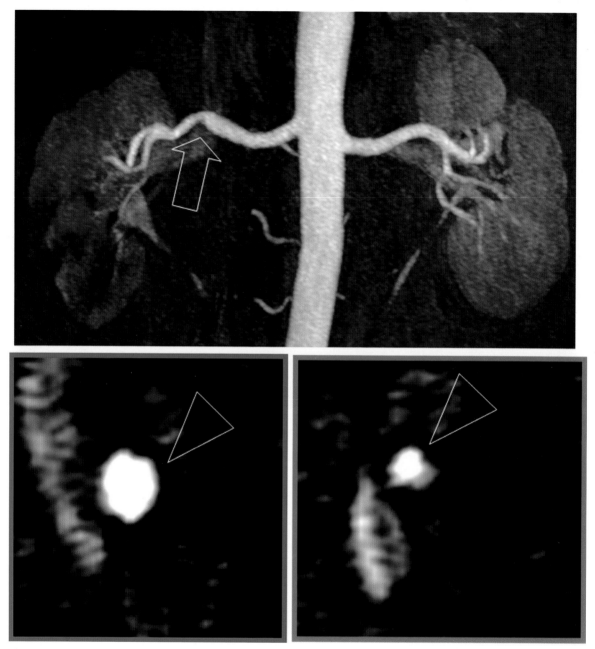

Figure 5.1 Coronal thin maximum-intensity-projection (MIP) view of a patient with 50% right-sided renal artery stenosis (arrow). In this view the stenosis is seen in the diameter view. In the two reformatted views perpendicular to the renal artery at the site of the stenosis (red frame) and in a normal segment (green frame) the normal vessel area as well as the stenotic vessel area (arrowheads) can be accurately measured to calculate the area of stenosis.

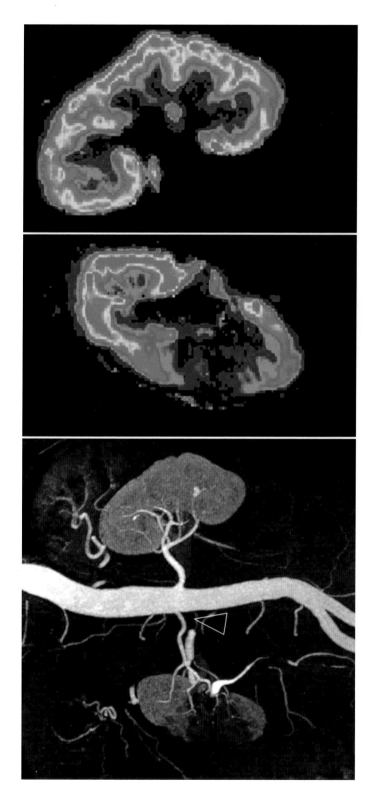

Figure 5.10 In the coronal thin-volume MIP of the renal arteries (left image) two renal arteries on the patient's right side can be seen. The upper vessel appears slender and normal while the lower renal artery cannot be visualized proximally (arrowhead) with post-stenotic dilation. The color-perfusion maps demonstrate normal perfusion on the left side while the right kidney demonstrates a reduced (lower pole) and almost absent (mid portion) plasma flow in the lower half of the organ.

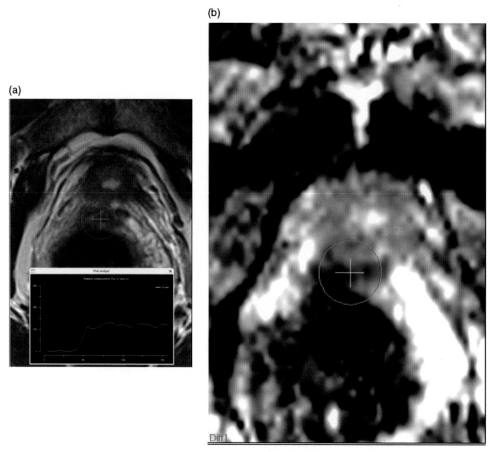

(a)

(b)

Figure 13.3 A 65-year-old man with a PSA level of 28 ng/ml and three previous negative 10-core transrectal ultrasound-guided biopsy sessions. (a) Transverse T2W turbo spin echo MR imaging. Circle annotates a low-signal-intensity lesion at the base of the prostate, which is suspected for prostate cancer. (b) Axial ADC map of a diffusion-weighted MR imaging at the corresponding level of (A). This image was obtained using a single-shot echo planar imaging sequence with diffusion module and fat suppression. The ADC map of the base of the prostate shows restriction (circle), which is a suspect for prostate cancer. (c) Axial parametric map for a DCE-MRI showing the parameter K^{trans}. Early contrast enhancement is shown at the base of the prostate (circle). (d) Sagittal slice of a parametric map for a DCE-MRI showing the parameter washout. Washout of the contrast material is shown at the base of the prostate (circle). Multimodality MR imaging examinations were interpreted as a T2N0M0 cancer. MR-guided biopsy was performed of the cancer-suspected region. A Gleason $4 + 3 = 7$ adenocarcinoma was found.

(c)

(d)

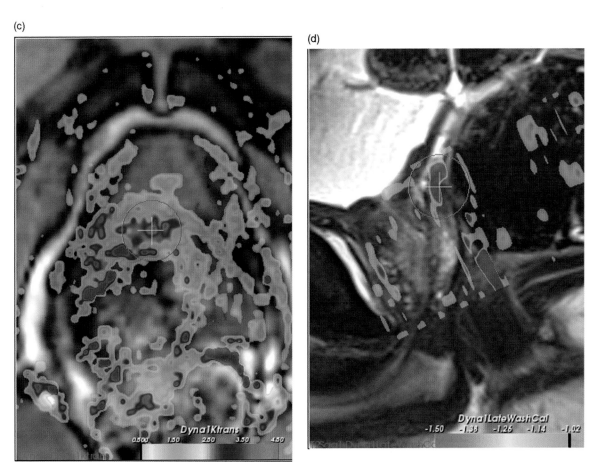

Figure 13.3 *(cont.)*

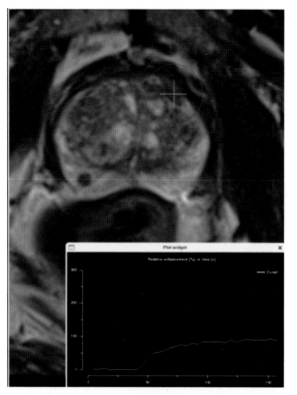

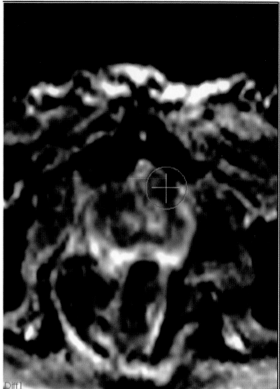

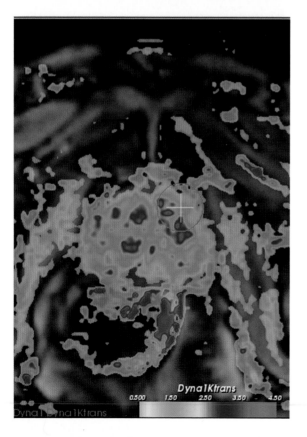

Figure 13.4 A 69-year-old man with a PSA level of 20 ng/ml and five previous negative 12-core transrectal ultrasound-guided biopsy sessions. (a) Axial T2-weighted turbo spin echo MR imaging. Circle annotates a low signal intensity lesion in the left transition zone of the prostate, which is suspected for prostate cancer. (b) Axial ADC map of a diffusion-weighted MR imaging at the corresponding level of (A). This image was obtained using a single-shot echo planar imaging sequence with diffusion module and fat suppression. The ADC map of the base of the prostate shows restriction (circle), which is suspect for prostate cancer in the left base anteriorly. (c) Axial slice of a parametric map for a DCE-MRI showing the parameter K^{trans}. Early contrast enhancement (circle) is shown at the left anterior transition zone of the prostate. Multimodality MR imaging examination was interpreted as a T2N0M0 cancer. MR-guided biopsy was performed of the cancer-suspected region. A Gleason $3 + 3 = 6$ adenocarcinoma was found.

Prostate cancer detection, localization, and staging with T2-weighted imaging

MR imaging findings in prostate cancer were first described in the early 1980s [30]. Later studies established that prostate cancer is characterized by low T2 signal intensity replacing the normally high T2 signal intensity tissue in the peripheral zone [31] (Figures 13.1 and 13.2). However, the presence of reduced T2 signal intensity in the peripheral zone is of limited sensitivity, because some tumors are iso-intense. The finding is also of limited specificity, because there are other possible causes of low T2 signal intensity in the peripheral zone including hemorrhage; prostatitis; scarring; atrophy; and effect of radiotherapy, cryosurgery, and hormonal therapy. Prostate cancer arising in the transition zone of the prostate gland poses additional imaging difficulties [32], because of the heterogeneity of signal in the central gland. Studies at 1.5T, even when using high-resolution endorectal MR imaging, documented low sensitivity and specificity, and high interobserver variability in the detection of prostate cancer [32–35]. At 3T, Turkbey et al. [36] demonstrated that conventional T2W sequences had the highest sensitivity for detection of peripheral zone tumors and transition zone tumors for all Gleason scores; however, T2W images were inferior in specificity to functional imaging with MRSI and DCE-MR imaging. The authors performed multiparametric imaging of the prostate at 3T with endorectal coil for detection of prostate cancer by using T2W imaging, MRSI, and DCE-MRI, using the whole-mount pathologic findings as reference standard. In this prospective, single-institution study of 70 patients with biopsy-proven prostate cancer, sensitivity and specificity values obtained for T2W imaging of the peripheral zone and transition zone, with stringent approach, were 0.42 (95% confidence interval [CI]: 0.36, 0.47) and 0.83 (95% CI: 0.81, 0.86), and for the alternative neighboring approach, sensitivity and specificity values were 0.73 (95% CI: 0.67, 0.78) and 0.89 (95% CI: 0.85,0.93), respectively.

Staging prostate cancer

The role of T2W imaging in tumor staging has been evaluated. MR imaging is being used to detect the presence and location of extracapsular tumor extension (ECE) and seminal vesicle invasions (SVI). On endorectal MR imaging, criteria for ECE include asymmetry of the neurovascular bundle, tumor encasement of the neurovascular bundle, bulging prostate gland contour (Figures 13.1 and 13.2), an irregular or spiculated margin, obliteration of the rectoprostatic angle, capsular retraction, a tumor-capsule interface greater than 1 cm, and a breach of the capsule with evidence of direct tumor extension [32]. Multivariate feature analysis has shown that the MR imaging findings most predictive of ECE are: focal irregular capsular bulge, asymmetry or invasion of the neurovascular bundles, and obliteration of the rectoprostatic angle [37]. The features of SVI on endorectal MR imaging include focal low signal intensity within the seminal vesicle, enlarged low-signal-intensity seminal vesicle, enlarged low-signal-intensity ejaculatory ducts, obliteration of the angle between the prostate and the seminal vesicle, and demonstration of direct tumor extension from the base of the prostate into and around the seminal vesicle [32]. In spite of well-defined MR imaging criteria for organ-confined versus extraglandular tumor extension, MR imaging has been reported to have a wide range of sensitivities (13–95%) and specificities (49–97%) for ECE detection with a similarly wide range of sensitivities (23–80%) and specificities (81–99%) for SVI detection [32]. Therefore, the overall accuracy of MR imaging in staging prostate cancer has ranged from 54% to 93% [32, 38–41], concerning for limitations of conventional morphologic MR imaging of the prostate. Despite the initial technologic advancements, the accuracy results for staging prostate cancer for conventional anatomical 1.5T MR imaging were not optimal as documented in two meta-analysis studies, where a maximum pooled sensitivity and specificity were 71–74% [42, 43]. With introduction of imaging at 3T, initial results showed improved staging accuracy, especially with the application of endorectal coil [22], as discussed above. As reported by Turkbey et al. [36], for local staging at 3T, the sensitivity, specificity, false-positive and false-negative rates, and the accuracy of MR imaging for extracapsular tumor extension and seminal vesicle invasion were 78.2% and 80%, 80.9% and 97%, 19.1% and 3.7%, 21.7% and 20%, and 80% and 95.7%, respectively.

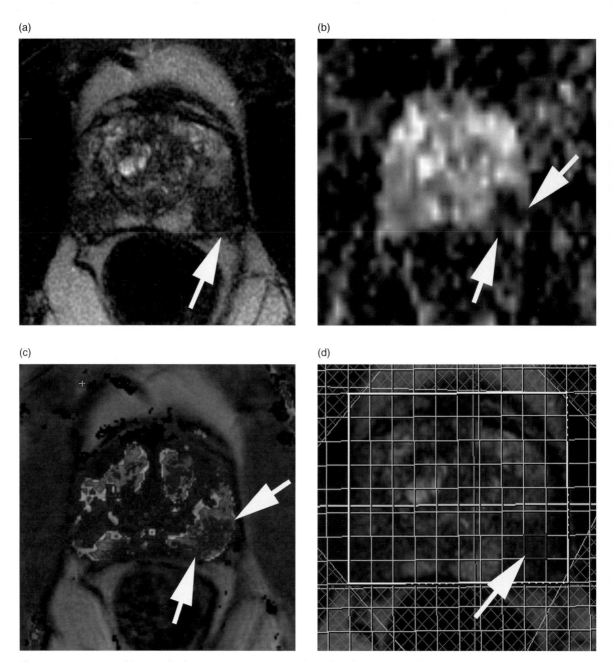

Figure 13.1 A 55-year-old man with Gleason 9 prostate cancer involving the left posterolateral base and mid gland. MR imaging of the prostate was performed with body matrix coil at 3.T. (a) Axial T2-weighted image (TR/TE 5660 ms/149 ms) shows hypointense tumor in the left mid posterolateral peripheral zone (arrow). Note irregularity of the capsule and established extracapsular tumor extension (ECE) on the left. There is also contralateral tumor present in the peripheral zone. (b) Apparent diffusion coefficient (ADC) map shows significantly restricted diffusion in the left peripheral zone tumor (arrows), ADC value 0.7×10^{-3} mm^2/s. (c) DCE-MR imaging computer-aided dectection (CAD) axial image shows mapping of the highest permeability (K^{trans}) corresponding to the left tumor (arrows). (d) MRSI grid overlying the T2-weighted image shows voxel of interest (arrow) in the region of abnormal decreased T2 signal on the left. (e) Spectrum corresponding to the voxel of interest in (d) shows elevated choline (Cho) at 3.2 ppm. (f) MRSI grid overlying the T2-weighted image shows voxel adjacent to the tumor with normal high T2 signal (arrow). (g) Spectrum corresponding to the voxel of interest in (f) shows normal level of choline (Cho) at 3.2 ppm. Note well-defined creatine (Cr) peak at 3.05 ppm and citrate (Ci) at 2.6 ppm that has a tall central peak doublet split into two smaller peaks on either side, which are not usually resolved in vivo at 1.5T. At 1.5T citrate resonance appears as a singlet, whereas at 3T the spectral resolution increases twofold, more clearly revealing the complex shape of the citrate signals that can appear with either positive or negative inner lines and nonzero satellite peaks. Copyrights Elsevier, Seminars in Roentgenology 2008. Reproduced with permission from Macura KJ. Multiparametric magnetic resonance imaging of the prostate: current status in prostate cancer detection, localization, and staging. *Semin Roentgenol* 2008; **43**(4): 303–13.

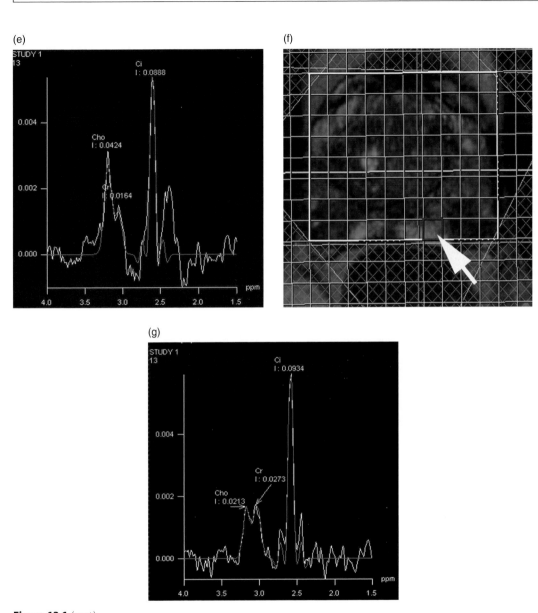

Figure 13.1 (*cont.*)

Functional imaging of the prostate: diffusion-weighted imaging

DWI provides image contrast through measurement of the diffusion properties of random thermal (Brownian) motion of water molecules. The microscopic motion includes both molecular diffusion of water and microcirculation of blood in the capillary network. The diffusion properties of tissue are associated with the amount of interstitial free water and permeability. Generally, cancer tends to have more restricted diffusion than normal tissue because it has higher cell densities and excesses of intra- and intercellular membranes [44–46] (Figures 13.1–13.4). Reduced diffusion of water in prostate cancer has been attributed to increased cellularity of malignant lesions [47] that restricts water motion in a reduced extracellular space [48].

The amount of diffusion is determined by the diffusion coefficient. However, because the measurement of the diffusion coefficient in vivo may be affected by many factors, such as temperature, blood

(a)

(b)

(c)

(d)

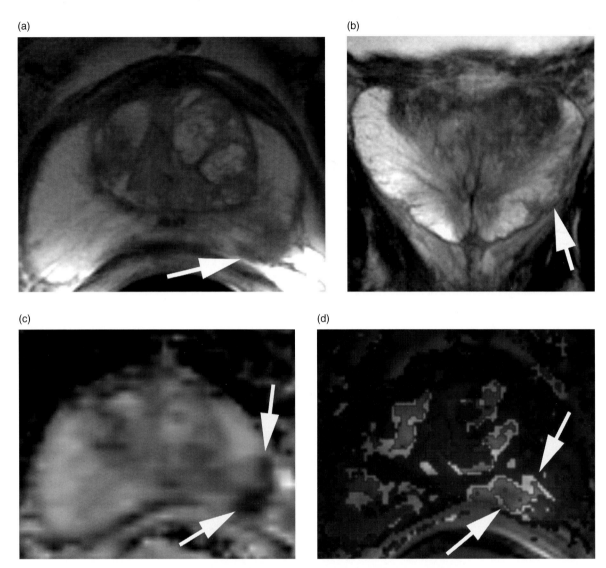

Figure 13.2 A 65-year-old man with PSA 4.5 ng/ml. MR imaging of the prostate was performed with endorectal coil and body matrix coil at 3.T. (a) Axial T2-weighted image (TR/TE 3400 ms/109 ms) of the prostate at mid gland level shows a hypointense lesion in the left lateral posterior peripheral zone with associated capsular retraction and irregularity suggestive of extracapsular tumor extension (arrow). (b) Coronal T2-weighted image (TR/TE 3400 ms/109 ms) shows left mid peripheral zone tumor with capsular irregularity (arrow). (c) ADC map shows a focus of significantly restricted diffusion in the left peripheral zone lesion (arrows), ADC value 0.5×10^{-3} mm^2/s, suggestive of a high-grade (at least Gleason 7) prostate cancer. (d) DCE-MRI CAD axial image shows increased permeability (K^{trans}) in the left peripheral zone tumor (arrows). (e) MRSI grid overlying the T2-weighted image shows voxel of interest (arrow) in the region of abnormal decreased T2 signal on the left. (f) Spectrum corresponding to the voxel of interest in (E) shows significantly elevated choline (Cho) at 3.2 ppm and decreased citrate (Ci) at 2.6 ppm, a signature of prostate cancer. (g) MRSI grid overlying the T2-weighted image shows voxel of interest (arrow) on the right in the region of normal T2 signal. (h) Spectrum corresponding to the voxel of interest in (g) shows normal low choline (Cho) peak at 3.2 ppm, creatine (Cr) peak at 3.09 ppm and a tall doublet citrate (Ci) peak at 2.6 ppm. Copyrights Elsevier, Seminars in Roentgenology 2008. Reproduced with permission from Macura KJ. Multiparametric magnetic resonance imaging of the prostate: current status in prostate cancer detection, localization, and staging. *Semin Roentgenol* 2008; **43**(4): 303–13.

(e)

(f)

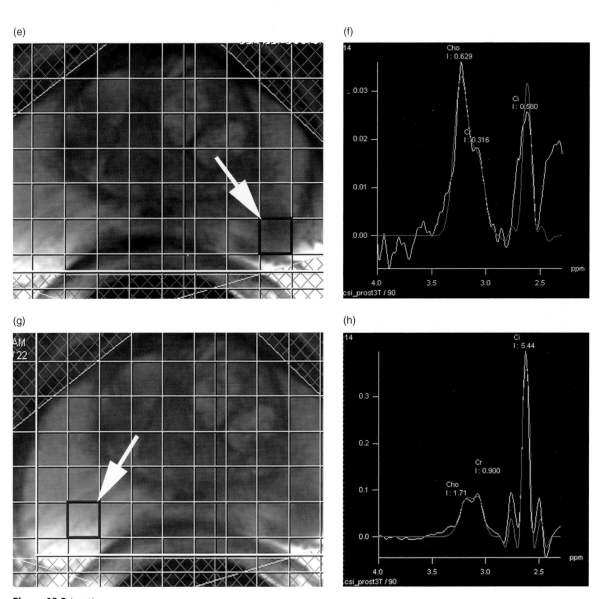

(g)

(h)

Figure 13.2 (cont.)

perfusion, magnetic susceptibility in the tissue, or other kinds of motion, apparent diffusion coefficient (ADC) rather than diffusion coefficient is used clinically. The ADC quantifies the combined effects of both diffusion and capillary perfusion. An important parameter for DWI scanning is the b-value, which specifies the sensitivity of diffusion. As the b-value increases, the amount of diffusion weighting increases, and sensitivity to diffusion increases. At high b-value, DWI represents the molecular diffusion of water almost exclusively. However, as the b-value increases, it prolongs the gradient RF pulse, thus increasing the

TE value, and the quality of the diffusion-weighted images is seriously degraded and the SNR decreases accordingly [49, 50]. The smaller the b-value, the higher the quality and SNR of the diffusion-weighted images, but T2 shine-through effect and perfusion of the tissue increase their influence on DWI. Traditionally, for prostate MR imaging a b-value of 0 and 1000 s/mm^2 or above has been used.

DWI is a challenging technique because as it measures molecular motion it is also sensitive to bulk motion and therefore requires ultrafast imaging techniques. With the implementation of fast gradient

(a)

(b)

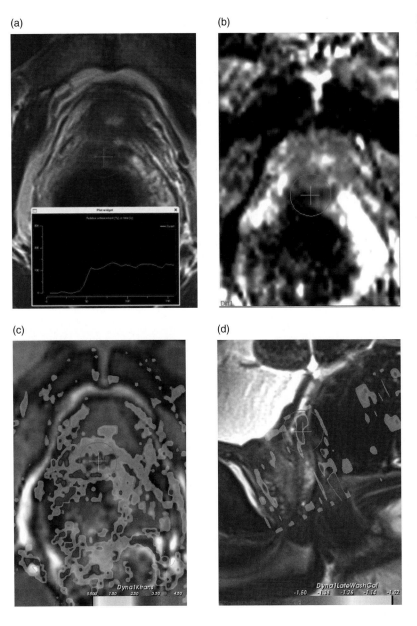

(c)

(d)

Figure 13.3 A 65-year-old man with a PSA level of 28 ng/ml and three previous negative 10-core transrectal ultrasound-guided biopsy sessions. (a) Transverse T2W turbo spin echo MR imaging. Circle annotates a low-signal-intensity lesion at the base of the prostate, which is suspected for prostate cancer. (b) Axial ADC map of a diffusion-weighted MR imaging at the corresponding level of (A). This image was obtained using a single-shot echo planar imaging sequence with diffusion module and fat suppression. The ADC map of the base of the prostate shows restriction (circle), which is a suspect for prostate cancer. (c) Axial parametric map for a DCE-MRI showing the parameter K^{trans}. Early contrast enhancement is shown at the base of the prostate (circle). (d) Sagittal slice of a parametric map for a DCE-MRI showing the parameter washout. Washout of the contrast material is shown at the base of the prostate (circle). Multimodality MR imaging examinations were interpreted as a T2N0M0 cancer. MR-guided biopsy was performed of the cancer-suspected region. A Gleason $4 + 3 = 7$ adenocarcinoma was found. See plate section for color version.

coils, single-shot echo planar imaging (EPI) emerged as a technique of choice for diffusion measurements in intra-abdominal organs as well as the prostate gland. Gibbs *et al.* successfully investigated T2 relaxation rates and diffusion-weighted images of the human prostate using a pelvic phased-array coil at 1.5T [51]. Another study used a pelvic phased-array coil to image the prostate gland of patients with biopsy-proven cancer and demonstrated significant differences in the ADCs between malignant peripheral zone tissue and nonmalignant tissue [52]. The study concluded that prostate cancer causes restricted diffusion of water relative to that of normal tissue, resulting in decreased signal of malignant lesions on ADC maps. Hosseinzadeh *et al.* showed that DWI of the prostate was possible with the use of an endorectal coil [53]. As shown, ADC values of malignant prostate tissue are lower than in the healthy peripheral zone [54]. The ADC value of the healthy peripheral zone is also higher compared with that of the central gland.

(a)

(b)

(c)

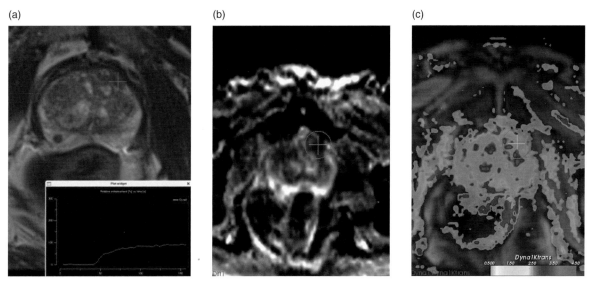

Figure 13.4 A 69-year-old man with a PSA level of 20 ng/ml and five previous negative 12-core transrectal ultrasound-guided biopsy sessions. (a) Axial T2-weighted turbo spin echo MR imaging. Circle annotates a low signal intensity lesion in the left transition zone of the prostate, which is suspected for prostate cancer. (b) Axial ADC map of a diffusion-weighted MR imaging at the corresponding level of (A). This image was obtained using a single-shot echo planar imaging sequence with diffusion module and fat suppression. The ADC map of the base of the prostate shows restriction (circle), which is suspect for prostate cancer in the left base anteriorly. (c) Axial slice of a parametric map for a DCE-MR imaging showing the parameter K^{trans}. Early contrast enhancement (circle) is shown at the left anterior transition zone of the prostate. Multimodality MR imaging examination was interpreted as a T2N0M0 cancer. MR-guided biopsy was performed of the cancer-suspected region. A Gleason $3 + 3 = 6$ adenocarcinoma was found. See plate section for color version.

Sato *et al.* compared the ADC values of normal and cancerous tissue in both peripheral and transition zones at 1.5T [55]. The ADC values of prostate cancer in both zones were significantly lower than those of benign tissue in the corresponding zone. Average values of the ADC (10^{-3} mm²/s) calculated from the DWI data acquired with a single-shot DWI EPI sequence at 1.5T within normal peripheral zone, central gland, and prostate cancer were as follows: peripheral zone 1.992 ± 0.208, central gland 1.518 ± 0.126, prostate cancer 1.214 ± 0.254 [56].

To date, only a few studies have been published on DWI of the prostate at 3T [57–62]. Pickles *et al.* were the first to report the application of DWI of the prostate at 3T while using a phased-array coil and parallel imaging, a single-shot DWI EPI technique with b = 0 and 500 s/mm² to determine the utility of ADC values in differentiating tumor from normal peripheral zone tissue [61]. ADC values were significantly lower for tumor ($1.38 \pm 0.32 \times 10^{-3}$ mm²/s) than for benign peripheral zone ($1.95 \pm 0.50 \times 10^{-3}$ mm²/s). However, a considerable overlap of ADC values and variability was noted between tissue types and among subjects. Kim *et al.* assessed both the peripheral and transition zones and used whole-mount

section histopathology as the standard of reference [57]. They imaged patients at 3T using a phased-array coil, with a single-shot DWI EPI technique with b = 0 and b = 1000 s/mm². They found that the ADC values of malignant tissues were significantly lower than those of benign tissues in the peripheral zone and transition zone. The ADC values of malignant tissues in the peripheral zone were $1.32 \pm 0.24 \times 10^{-3}$ mm²/s versus benign tissue $1.97 \pm 0.25 \times 10^{-3}$ mm²/s, and in the transition zone were $1.37 \pm 0.29 \times 10^{-3}$ mm²/s versus $1.79 \pm 0.19 \times 10^{-3}$ mm²/s. For tumor diagnosis, cutoff values of 1.67×10^{-3} mm²/s for peripheral zone and 1.61×10^{-3} mm²/s for transition zone resulted in sensitivities and specificities of 94% and 91% and 90% and 84%, respectively [57]. The cutoff values for ADC to differentiate cancer from benign tissue may vary between different vendors' hardware and imaging parameters. However, cancer typically yields ADC values $< 1.0 \times 10^{-3}$ mm²/s. Almost all studies of DWI focused on ADC measurements as a biomarker for healthy and cancerous prostate tissue. However, Manenti *et al.* performed a feasibility study for 3T diffusion tensor imaging (DTI) and fiber tracking in prostate cancer patients and reported good delineation of the prostate anatomical structures such as the capsule outline, peripheral and central gland borders, prostate cancer extension, and capsule infiltration [62].

The advantages of DWI are short acquisition time and high contrast resolution between tumors and normal tissue. Studies that investigated combining T2-weighted and DWI MR imaging for localizing prostate cancer revealed that sensitivity in the detection of significant cancer (Gleason score ≥ 6 and diameter > 4 mm) suggests that DWI MR imaging has the potential to increase the specificity of prostate cancer detection [48], as well as to support prediction of tumor aggressiveness [63].

Functional imaging of the prostate: magnetic resonance spectroscopic imaging

MRSI is based on the chemical shift imaging principle, where the very slight differences in the Larmor frequencies of protons in different molecules allow detection of specific metabolites resonating at a predictable range of frequencies. Proton spectroscopy (^{1}H MRSI) is the most widely used technique because it can be implemented with standard MR systems and clinically used coils. As a three-dimensional (3D) technique, MRSI can provide spectra from a grid of contiguous volumes, allowing metabolic information to be obtained from a voxel corresponding to a specific anatomical area of the prostate. Therefore, MRSI and conventional MR imaging can be used together to perform a combined metabolic and morphologic evaluation of the prostate in a single study [64].

In order to be used for evaluating prostate cancer, MRSI requires good spatial resolution (below 1 cm^3) [65], high SNR, efficient water and fat suppression techniques, and an optimal TE for detection of metabolites. MRSI studies of the human prostate at 1.5T have demonstrated that the levels of the prostate metabolites (polyamines, choline, creatine, and citrate) are important specific markers for differentiating prostate malignancies from healthy peripheral zone [64–70]. Choline resonates at 3.25 ppm (parts per minute), creatine at 3.05 ppm and citrate at 2.62 ppm, so the relative concentration of chemical compounds can be inferred from the metabolite peaks [65]. On MRSI, the prostate cancer signature is characterized by elevated levels of choline, related to high turnover of phospholipid in cell membranes

during cellular proliferation [65], decrease in polyamines [70], and decrease in citrate, a metabolite which is normally synthesized and released in large amounts in the healthy prostate tissue [65]. Since choline and creatine resonances overlap at 1.5T, it was proposed that a ratio of choline plus creatine over citrate would be used to diagnose prostate cancer [65]. Peripheral zone voxels where the ratio of choline plus creatine over citrate is at least two standard deviations above the average ratio in the normal peripheral zone of the prostate are considered likely representative of cancer at 1.5T. When the same ratio is more than three standard deviations above the average (above 0.86), voxels are considered highly suggestive of cancer [65, 71]. MRSI was shown to be useful in detecting transitional zone cancer as well; however, the metabolite ratios vary due to the overlap between cancer and benign tissue in the transitional zone [72].

Several studies showed improved performance of MR imaging when MRSI was combined with the anatomical information provided by endorectal MR imaging at 1.5T for the assessment of cancer location within the prostate and cancer volume [64, 73–79], extracapsular tumor extension [80, 81], and cancer aggressiveness [82–83].

At 1.5T, MRSI of the prostate without an endorectal coil is feasible using the spine-array surface coil at 1.5T [84]. However, spectral quality and SNR are inferior to those obtained in examinations performed with endorectal coils.

For MRSI, increased magnetic field strength provides two advantages, smaller voxel size and improved separation of metabolite peaks. With the increased SNR, the spectral voxel size at 3T is 0.15 cm^3 while the MRSI voxel size at 1.5T is approximately 0.30 cm^3 [85]. Smaller voxel size reduces volume averaging effects with periprostatic fat, seminal vesicles, postbiopsy hemorrhage, and periurethral tissues. At 1.5T, the choline, polyamine, and creatine peaks blend into a single peak. At 3T, the creatine and the choline peaks are distinct (Figures 13.1 and 13.2) and the ratio of choline to citrate is easier to measure. The ability to identify a separate choline peak at 3T may increase the specificity of MRSI, especially when combined with increased spatial resolution, allowing differentiation of smaller tumor foci from normal tissue. The susceptibility artifacts are more pronounced at 3T, for endorectal coil imaging the endorectal coil balloon should be filled with liquid PFC [24] or barium [25] instead of air. It has been demonstrated that at 3T, diagnostic MRSI with good spectral resolution can be performed with external body coils [86].

An adequate suppression of lipid signals and a locally homogeneous magnetic field strength are essential. Scheenen *et al.* [87] suggested using short TEs (75 ms); however, problems with lipid contamination can occur. A short repetition time of 750 ms partially saturates choline signals but increases the SNR per unit time for citrate. At 3T, the spectral shape of citrate is different from that at 1.5T, which may impair its detection [88]. At 1.5T, the choline, polyamine, and creatine peaks blend into a single peak. Therefore, criteria for identifying suspicious spectra involve qualitative assessment of the peaks' height and measuring the ratio of choline plus creatine to citrate, because separating the choline peak from creatine peak can be difficult, and creatine levels are relatively unchanged between normal and malignant tissue [65]. At 3T, the creatine and the choline peaks are distinct and the ratio of choline to citrate is easier to measure and has been used for differentiating malignant from benign prostate tissue, as reported by Turkbey *et al.* [36]. Authors defined the mean healthy choline–citrate ratio value at 0.13, SD 0.081; voxels were considered abnormal when the choline–citrate ratio was 3 or more SD above the mean healthy tissue value.

Challenges with MRSI include acquiring high-quality spectral data with voxels in which there is good SNR and no partial volume effects, and post-processing of the prostatic spectra. While MRSI shows promise as a problem-solving modality with high specificity, it suffers from low sensitivity. False-positive results with MRSI can be seen with seminal vesicle contamination, when the signal from seminal vesicles contributes to the voxels acquired over the prostate, in prostatitis, as well as in focal prostate atrophy [89]. Significant number of spectral voxels acquired may contain non-diagnostic levels of metabolites due to poor SNR related to suboptimal shimming and artifacts from motion. Postbiopsy hemorrhage can also degrade spectral analysis, as demonstrated at 1.5T by Qayyum *et al.* [90]. However, it was also shown at 1.5T that MRSI may improve diagnostic accuracy of cancer in the presence of postbiopsy hemorrhage, when findings on T2W images are non diagnostic [91].

Functional imaging of the prostate: dynamic contrast-enhanced MR imaging

Fast T1W DCE-MRI for imaging of the prostate has gained attention in recent years as it allows monitoring the uptake of an intravascular contrast with good spatial resolution and is a powerful technique to study prostate cancer microvascularity and angiogenesis [92–101]. Three major factors determine the behavior of contrast media in the prostate: blood perfusion, transport of contrast agent across vessel walls, and diffusion of contrast medium in the interstitial space [101]. Physiologic processes such as tissue perfusion and microvessel permeability, and the extracellular leakage space can be characterized qualitatively by the evaluation of kinetic enhancement curves or quantitatively by applying complex compartmental modeling techniques [102]. Qualitative assessment is usually based on the gestalt review of shape of the signal intensity–time curve (i.e., progressive fill-in, plateau, wash out), semiquantitative curve-fitting algorithms (calculation of the maximum enhancement and time-to-peak) or more complicated pharmacokinetic modeling approaches that quantify the tumor blood flow and capillary permeability [103] (Figures 13.1–13.4). Examples of modeling parameters in quantitative analysis include the contrast leakage space (v_e), efflux rate constant (k_{ep}), and the influx transfer constant (K^{trans}). These parameters are connected by the equation: $v_e = K^{trans}/k_{ep}$ [104]. Preliminary results showed improved accuracy in prostate cancer detection and localization with DCE-MRI [100, 101]. There has been limited experience with the use of DCE-MRI in staging prostate cancer [105, 106] and detection of capsular penetration and SVI. Using DCE-MRI in staging prostate cancer yielded significant improvement in staging performance for the less-experienced readers but had no benefit for the experienced reader according to the study by Fütterer *et al.* [106]. Typically, high-spatial-resolution T2W imaging remains the standard sequence for staging; however, DCE-MRI may draw the radiologist's attention to suspicious regions with abnormal perfusion to facilitate the assessment of T2 images. Challenges for the DCE-MRI technique include inadequate differentiation of prostatitis from prostate cancer in the peripheral zone and in distinguishing between benign prostatic hyperplasia and transition zone tumors, due to lack of validated thresholds for differentiation of cancer from benign tissue.

At 1.5T, DCE-MRI has limitations in temporal and spatial resolution; therefore, a tradeoff between the two has to be considered for optimization of prostate cancer detection usually by applying a high spatial resolution and intermediate temporal resolution. The use of 3T MR imaging enables the increase in temporal resolution up to 1–2 seconds. The T1 relaxation time of the tissues is prolonged at 3T compared with 1.5T. The relaxivity properties of gadolinium chelate are not significantly different at 1.5 from those at 3T. Longer T1 relaxation time of tissues and increased SNR improve contrast between tumor and normal tissue [107]. Kim *et al.* described the first localization results of prostate cancer by DCE-MRI at 3T [108]. They reported superior prostate cancer localization results for DCE-MRI compared with T2W imaging; however, this result did not achieve statistical significance. The depiction of tumor borders was statistically superior compared with anatomical MR images. In a study by Ocak *et al.* [109], the authors reported that for prostate MR imaging performed at 3T using an endorectal coil, pathologically confirmed cancers in the peripheral zone of the prostate were characterized by their low signal intensity on T2-weighted scans and by their early enhancement, early washout, or both on dynamic contrast-enhanced MR images. The overall sensitivity, specificity, PPV, and negative predictive value (NPV) of T2W imaging were 94%, 37%, 50%, and 89%, respectively. The sensitivity, specificity, PPV, and NPV of DCE-MRI were 73%, 88%, 75%, and 75%, respectively. K^{trans}, k_{ep}, and AUGC (the area under the gadolinium concentration curve) in the first 90 seconds after injection were significantly higher ($p < 0.001$) in cancer than in normal peripheral zone. The v_e parameter was not significantly associated with prostate cancer. The authors concluded that at 3T prostate MR imaging using an endorectal coil produces high-quality T2W images; however, specificity for prostate cancer is improved by also performing DCE-MRI and using pharmacokinetic parameters, particularly K^{trans} and k_{ep}, for analysis. In a follow-up work, as reported by Turkbey *et al.* [36], sensitivity for DCE-MRI (0.18) or MRSI (0.13) was lower than that of T2W imaging. However, specificity for DCE-MRI (0.96) and MRSI (0.97) was higher than that for T2W imaging. The addition of DCE-MRI and MRSI to the prostate imaging protocol increased the accuracy and predictive value of conventional T2W imaging for accurately localizing peripheral zone prostate cancers. The authors concluded that larger tumors with higher Gleason scores are more reliably detected at 3T imaging. On DCE-MRI, color-coded parametric maps reflecting

wash-in K^{trans}, k_{ep} (washout) were obtained with a two-compartmental pharmacokinetic model. Color-coded maps were assessed qualitatively, as quantitative values were not used due to significant inter-patient variations.

MR-guided biopsy of the prostate

The advantage of MR imaging lies in the fact that all the features of prostate cancer described above can be used in combination in order to localize prostate cancer. Therefore, contemporary prostate MR imaging protocols are multiparametric. Multiparametric approaches to MR imaging of the prostate have shown increased diagnostic accuracy in the detection of prostate cancer. At 1.5T, combined DWI and DCE-MRI provided better sensitivity in detecting prostate cancer, as reported by Kozlowski *et al.* [110], and combined DWI and MR spectroscopy increased the specificity for prostate cancer detection while retaining the sensitivity compared with MR spectroscopy alone or DWI alone [111]. Various protocols for a combined MRSI and DCE-MRI have been evaluated in multiple patient cohorts [79, 112, 113]. At 3T, Turbey *et al.* showed the benefit of adding functional techniques MRSI and DCE-MRI to the standard T2W imaging in order to increase MR imaging specificity for the detection and localization of prostate cancer [36]. With these multi-modality approaches, an opportunity emerges for precise targeting of specific regions within the prostate that are deemed suspicious for harboring cancer.

MR-guided prostate biopsy potentially can increase prostate cancer detection, as tissue samples can be obtained from previously determined cancer-suspicious regions. As has been shown, MR-guided biopsy is technically feasible and can be performed on a routine basis. This technique is typically used in patients with at least one or more previous negative TRUS-guided prostate biopsy sessions. Transrectal MR-guided prostate biopsy has shown promising cancer detection rates of between 38% and 59% [14–17]. Beyersdorff *et al.* performed an MR-guided biopsy in 12 patients with elevated PSA levels and histologic analysis showed prostate cancer in five patients and prostatitis in six [14]. Anastasiadis *et al.* found prostate cancer in 15 out of 27 (55.5%) patients who underwent MR-guided biopsy following at least one prior negative TRUS-guided prostate biopsy [15]. Engelhard *et al.* studied 37 patients with previous negative prostate biopsies and concluded that suspicious lesions with a diameter of 10 mm could be successfully targeted with MR guidance [16]. Prostate cancer was detected in 14 out of 37 (38%) patients. As reported by Hambrock *et al.* [17], the tumor detection rate of multimodal MR imaging-guided biopsy at 3T was 59% (40 of 68 cases) using a median of four cores. The tumor detection rate was significantly higher than that of TRUS-guided prostate biopsy in all patient subgroups except in those with PSA greater than 20 ng/ml, prostate volume greater than 65 cc and PSA density greater than 0.5 ng/ml/cc, in which similar rates were achieved. These are promising data and demonstrate the potential clinical value of MR-guided biopsies. A limitation of MR-guided biopsy is that multiparametric MR imaging for localization and the MR-guided biopsy are performed in two different sessions, as image analysis and tumor localization demands post-processing that is time-consuming. Another disadvantage is the movement of the prostate during the biopsy procedure. An alternative approach has been proposed where MR imaging findings have been used to direct biopsies under TRUS guidance with the overall success rate of MR imaging-directed TRUS-guided biopsy of 25%, which was higher compared with a 9% success rate achieved without MR guidance [114]. Experimental fusion of high-resolution endorectal MR images and TRUS data has been used to perform MR-guided TRUS biopsy [115] and to perform target-directed transperineal ultrasound-guided prostate biopsy [116]. Also, new robotic devices are being implemented for MR-guided instrumentation to allow precise targeting of specific areas in the prostate for diagnostic and therapeutic interventions [117].

Example protocol for MR-guided biopsy at 3T

After the diagnostic multiparametric MR examination (preferably within 2 weeks), patients undergo an MR-guided biopsy using a pelvic phased-array coil and dedicated US Food and Drug Administration (FDA)-approved MR biopsy device (Invivo, Schwerin, Germany) [118]. All patients receive oral antibiotics prophylaxis, 500 mg (CIPROXIN, Bayer, Leverkusen, Germany) the evening before, on the morning of the biopsy, as well as 6 hours post biopsy. The prostate biopsies are performed with the patient in the prone position. Pelvic phased-array coils are placed on the patient's back as well as beneath the hips and pelvis. Chlorhexidine/lidocaïne gel (Instillagel, FARCO-PHARMA GmbH, Köln, Germany) is used to facilitate insertion of the needle guider (filled with gadolinium) and local anesthesia rectally. The needle guider is then attached to the arm of the MR biopsy device. The needle guide can be adjusted in height, rotated, and moved forward and backward for optimal positioning depending on the patient's anatomy (Figure 13.5).

Two sequences T2W (TR 3500 ms/TE 116 ms, flip angle 180°, slice thickness 3 mm, in-plane resolution 0.7×0.7 mm^2, number of slices 15) and DWI EPI (TR/TE 2400 ms/81 ms; 3-mm slice thickness; 204×204-mm^2 field of view and 136×136 matrix, b-values of 0, 50, 500, and 800 s/mm^2) are used to relocate the cancer-suspicious regions that were identified on pre-biopsy MR scan (Figures 13.3 and 13.4). The axial T2W and DWI slices have a similar angulation relative to the dorsal surface of the prostate as during the localization MR session. After relocation of the desired target – cancer-suspicious region – adjustments are made to the biopsy device to aim the needle guide exactly towards this region. In-between adjustments, fast T2W true FISP (true fast imaging with steady-state free precession) images (TR/TE 4.48ms/2.24 ms; flip angle 70°; 228×228 mm^2 field of view, 228×228 matrix, slice thickness 3 mm) can be obtained. After reaching the correct position, tissue samples with an 18-gauge MR-compatible biopsy gun with tissue core sampling length of 20 mm, are taken. After obtaining a biopsy, fast T2W axial and sagittal images are obtained with the needle left *in situ* to verify correct needle position relative to the targeted cancer-suspicious region.

Conclusion

For prostate cancer detection and localization the combined conventional MR imaging, providing anatomical detail, and functional MR imaging approach, providing additional metabolic/perfusion information, have shown promising results. With the increasing experience and standardization of imaging protocols at 3T, true gains in SNR will be fully translated into superior diagnostic performance. Imaging at 3T offers the potential for significant improvements in both spatial and spectral resolution, as well as in imaging speed. The most significant advantages of 3T for prostate imaging are likely to become apparent for functional MR imaging techniques, such as DWI, MRSI, and DCE-MRI. The combination of diagnostic multiparametric MR imaging and MR-guided biopsy of the prostate may positively impact

A
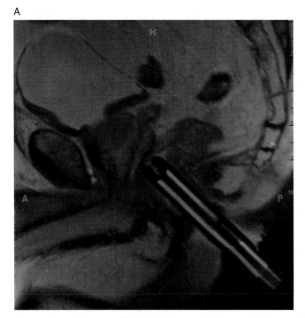

B
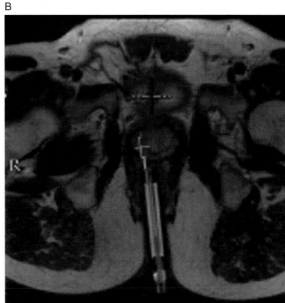

Figure 13.5 MR-compatible biopsy device placement and planning for MR-guided transrectal biopsy. (a) Sagittal T2-weighted turbo spin echo MR image shows endorectal placement of the needle guide. (b) Axial oblique T2-weighted MR image displayed in a planning window shows the biopsy trajectory to reach the right apex abnormality.

patients' management through increase in tumor detection rate and precision of cancer localization, through improvement in cancer staging, and through guidance in selection of optimal treatment strategies.

References

1. American Cancer Society. *Cancer Facts & Figures 2009*. Atlanta, American Cancer Society, 2009.

2. Bosch JL, Bohnen AM, Groeneveld FP. Validity of digital rectal examination and serum prostate specific antigen in the estimation of prostate volume in community-based men aged 50 to 78 years: the Krimpen Study. *Eur Urol* 2004; **46**: 753–9.

3. Catalona WJ, Smith DS, Ratliff TL, *et al.* Measurement of prostate-specific antigen in serum as a screening test for prostate cancer. *N Engl J Med* 1991; **324**: 1156–61.

4. Okotie OT, Roehl KA, Han M, *et al.* Characteristics of prostate cancer detected by digital rectal examination only. *Urology* 2007; **70**(6): 1117–20.

5. Thompson IM, Pauler DK, Goodman PJ, *et al.* Prevalence of prostate cancer among men with a prostate-specific antigen level < or =4.0 ng per milliliter. *N Engl J Med* 2004; **350**(22): 2239–46.

6. Jemal A, Siegel R, Ward E, *et al.* Cancer statistics, 2009. *CA Cancer J Clin* 2009; **59**(4): 225–49.

7. Mettlin C. Preliminary findings from the American Cancer Society National Prostate Cancer Detection Project. *Proceedings of the 5th International Symposium on Transrectal Ultrasound in the Diagnosis and Management of Prostate Cancer*, Chicago IL, 1990. pp. 84–5.

8. Levine MA, Ittman M, Melamed J, *et al.* Two consecutive sets of transrectal ultrasound guided sextant biopsies of the prostate for the detection of prostate cancer. *J Urol* 1998; **159**: 471–6.

9. Steven D, McCabe K, Peretsman S, *et al.* Prostate rebiopsy is a poor surrogate of treatment efficacy in localized prostate cancer. *J Urol* 1998; **159**: 1606–08.

10. Byar DP, Mostofi FK. Carcinoma of the prostate: prognostic evaluation of certain pathologic features in 208 radical prostatectomies. Examined by the step-section technique. *Cancer* 1972; **30**(1): 5–13.

11. Obek C, Louis P, Civantos F, *et al.* Comparison of digital rectal examination and biopsy results with the radical prostatectomy specimen. *J Urol* 1999; **161**: 494–8.

12. Salomon L, Colombel M, Patard JJ, *et al.* Value of ultrasound-guided systematic sextant biopsies in prostate tumor mapping. *Eur Urol* 1999; **35**: 289–93.

13. Wang L. Incremental value of magnetic resonance imaging in the advanced management of prostate cancer. *World J Radiol* 2009; **1**(1): 3–14.

14. Beyersdorff D, Winkel A, Hamm B, *et al.* MR imaging-guided prostate biopsy with a closed MR unit at 1.5 T: initial results. *Radiology* 2005; **234**: 576–81.

15. Anastasiadis AG, Lichy MP, Nagele U, *et al.* MRI-guided biopsy of the prostate increases diagnostic performance in men with elevated or increasing PSA

levels after previous negative TRUS biopsies. *Eur Urol* 2006; **50**: 738–48.

16. Engelhard K, Hollenbach HP, Kiefer B, *et al.* Prostate biopsy in the supine position in a standard 1.5-T scanner under real time MR-imaging control using a MR-compatible endorectal biopsy device. *Eur Radiol* 2006; **16**: 1237–43.

17. Hambrock T, Somford DM, Hoeks C, *et al.* Magnetic resonance imaging guided prostate biopsy in men with repeat negative biopsies and increased prostate specific antigen. *J Urol* 2010; **183**(2): 520–8.

18. Kim HW, Buckley DL, Peterson DM, *et al.* In vivo prostate magnetic resonance imaging and magnetic resonance spectroscopy at 3 Tesla using a transceive pelvic phased array coil: preliminary results. *Invest Radiol* 2003; **38**: 443–51.

19. Sosna J, Pedrosa I, Dewolf WC, *et al.* MR imaging of the prostate at 3 Tesla: comparison of an external phased-array coil to imaging with an endorectal coil at 1.5 Tesla. *Acad Radiol* 2004; **11**: 857–62.

20. Bloch BN, Rofsky NM, Baroni RH, *et al.* 3 Tesla magnetic resonance imaging of the prostate with combined pelvic phased-array and endorectal coils; initial experience. *Acad Radiol* 2004; **11**(8): 863–7.

21. Heijmink SW, Fütterer JJ, Hambrock T, *et al.* Prostate cancer: body-array versus endorectal coil MR imaging at 3 T – comparison of image quality, localization, and staging performance. *Radiology* 2007; **244**: 184–95.

22. Futterer JJ, Heijmink SW, Scheenen TW, *et al.* Prostate cancer: local staging at 3-T endorectal MRI – early experience. *Radiology* 2006; **238**: 184–91.

23. Futterer JJ, Scheenen TW, Huisman HJ, *et al.* Initial experience of 3 Tesla endorectal coil magnetic resonance imaging and 1H-spectroscopic imaging of the prostate. *Invest Radiol* 2004; **39**: 671–80.

24. Hailton G, Middelton M, Choi S, *et al.* Improved MR spectral analysis for a PFC-filled endo-rectal prostate surface coil compared to an air-filled coil. *Proceedings 15th Scientific Meeting, International Society for Magnetic Resonance in Medicine*, Berlin, 2007. p. 1400.

25. Rosen Y, Bloch BN, Lenkinski RE, *et al.* 3T MR of the prostate: reducing susceptibility gradients by inflating the endorectal coil with a barium sulfate suspension. *Magn Reson Med* 2007; **57**: 898–904.

26. Noworolski SM, Crane JC, Vigneron DB, Kurhanewicz J. A clinical comparison of rigid and inflatable endorectal-coil probes for MRI and 3D MR spectroscopic imaging (MRSI) of the prostate. *J Magn Reson Imaging* 2008; **27**: 1077–82.

27. Ikonen S, Kivisaari L, Vehmas T, *et al.* Optimal timing of post-biopsy MRI of the prostate. *Acta Radiol* 2001; **42**: 70–3.

28. Hennig J, Scheffler K. Hyperechoes. *Magn Reson Med* 2001; **46**: 6–12.

29. de Bazelaire CM, Duhamel GD, Rofsky NM, Alsop DC. MRI relaxation times of abdominal and pelvic tissues measured in vivo at 3.0 T: preliminary results. *Radiology* 2004; **230**: 652–9.

30. Hricak H, Williams RD, Spring DB, *et al.* Anatomy and pathology of the male pelvis by magnetic resonance imaging. *AJR Am J Roentgenol* 1983; **141**: 1101–10.

31. Bezzi M, Kressel HY, Allen KS, *et al.* Prostatic carcinoma: staging with MRI at 1.5T. *Radiology* 1988; **168**: 339–46.

32. Hricak H, Choyke PL, Eberhardt SC, *et al.* Imaging prostate cancer: a multidisciplinary perspective. *Radiology* 2007; **243**: 28–53.

33. Rifkin MD, Zerhouni EA, Gatsonis CA, *et al.* Comparison of magnetic resonance imaging and ultrasonography in staging early prostate cancer. Results of a multi-institutional cooperative trial. *N Engl J Med* 1990; **323**: 621–6.

34. Schnall MD, Pollack HM. Magnetic resonance imaging of the prostate gland. *Urol Radiol* 1990; **12**: 109–14.

35. Schiebler ML, Yankaskas BC, Tempany C, *et al.* MR imaging in adenocarcinoma of the prostate: interobserver variation and efficacy for determining stage C disease. *AJR Am J Roentgenol* 1992; **158**: 559–62.

36. Turkbey B, Pinto PA, Mani H, *et al.* Prostate cancer: value of multiparametric MRI at 3 T for detection – histopathologic correlation. *Radiology* 2010; **255**(1): 89–99.

37. Yu KK, Hricak H, Alagappan R, *et al.* Detection of extracapsular extension of prostate carcinoma with endorectal and phased-array coil MRI: multivariate feature analysis. *Radiology* 1997; **202**: 697–702.

38. Outwater EK, Petersen RO, Siegelman ES, *et al.* Prostate carcinoma: assessment of diagnostic criteria for capsular penetration on endorectal coil MR images. *Radiology* 1994; **193**: 333–9.

39. Bernstein MR, Cangiano T, D'Amico A, *et al.* Endorectal coil magnetic resonance imaging and clinicopathologic findings in T1c adenocarcinoma of the prostate. *Urol Oncol* 2000; **5**: 104–7.

40. May F, Treumann T, Dettmar P, *et al.* Limited value of endorectal magnetic resonance imaging and transrectal ultrasonography in the staging of clinically localized prostate cancer. *BJU Int* 2001; **87**: 66–9.

41. Cornud F, Flam T, Chauveinc L, *et al.* Extraprostatic spread of clinically localized prostate cancer: factors predictive of pT3 tumor and of positive endorectal MRI examination results. *Radiology* 2002; **224**: 203–10.

42. Sonnad SS, Langlotz CP, Schwartz JS. Accuracy of MR imaging for staging prostate cancer: a metaanalysis to examine the effect of technologic change. *Acad Radiol* 2001; **8**: 149–57.

43. Engelbrecht MR, Jager GJ, Laheij RJ, *et al.* Local staging of prostate cancer using magnetic resonance imaging: a meta-analysis. *Eur Radiol* 2002; **12**: 2294–302.

44. Tien RD, Felsberg GJ, Friedman H, *et al.* MR imaging of high-grade cerebral gliomas: value of diffusion-weighted echoplanar pulse sequences. *AJR Am J Roentgenol* 1994; **162**: 671–7.

45. Sugahara T, Korogi Y, Kochi M, *et al.* Usefulness of diffusion-weighted MRI with echo-planar technique in the evaluation of cellularity in gliomas. *J Magn Reson Imaging* 1999; **9**: 53–60.

46. Castillo M, Smith JK, Kwock L, *et al.* Apparent diffusion coefficients in the evaluation of high-grade cerebral gliomas. *AJNR Am J Neuroradial* 2001; **22**: 60–4.

47. Anderson AW, Xie J, Pizzonia J, *et al.* Effects of cell volume fraction changes on apparent diffusion in human cells. *Magn Reson Imaging* 2000; **18**: 689–95.

48. Desouza NM, Reinsberg SA, Scurr ED, *et al.* Magnetic resonance imaging in prostate cancer: the value of apparent diffusion coefficients for identifying malignant nodules. *Br J Radiol* 2007; **80**: 90–5.

49. Ichikawa T, Haradome H, Hachiya J, *et al.* Diffusion-weighted MRI with a single-shot echoplanar sequence: detection and characterization of focal hepatic lesions. *AJR Am J Roentgenol* 1998; **170**: 397–402.

50. Ichikawa T, Haradome H, Hachiya J, *et al.* Diffusion-weighted MR imaging with single-shot echo-planar imaging in the upper abdomen: preliminary clinical experience in 61 patients. *Abdom Imaging* 1999; **24**: 456–61.

51. Gibbs P, Tozer DJ, Liney GP, *et al.* Comparison of quantitative T2 mapping and diffusion-weighted imaging in the normal and pathologic prostate. *Magn Reson Med* 2001; **46**: 1054–58.

52. Bashar I. In vivo measurement of the apparent diffusion coefficient in normal and malignant prostatic tissues using echo-planar imaging. *J Magn Reson Imaging* 2002; **16**: 196–200.

53. Hosseinzadeh K, Schwarz SD. Endorectal diffusion-weighted imaging in prostate cancer to differentiate malignant and benign peripheral zone tissue. *J Magn Reson Imaging* 2004; **20**: 654–61.

54. Issa B. In vivo measurement of the apparent diffusion coefficient in normal and malignant prostatic tissues using echo-planar imaging. *J Magn Reson Imaging* 2002; **16**: 196–200.

55. Sato C, Naganawa S, Nakamura T, *et al.* Differentiation of noncancerous tissue and cancer lesions by apparent diffusion coefficient values in transition and peripheral zones of the prostate. *J Magn Reson Imaging* 2005; **21**: 258–62.

56. Kozlowski P, Chang SD, Goldenberg SL. Diffusion-weighted MR imaging in prostate cancer – comparison between single-shot fast spin echo and echo planar imaging sequences. *Magn Reson Imaging* 2008; **26**: 72–6.

57. Kim CK, Park BK, Han JJ, *et al.* Diffusion-weighted imaging of the prostate at 3 T for differentiation of malignant and benign tissue in transition and peripheral zones: preliminary results. *J Comput Assist Tomogr* 2007; **31**: 449–54.

58. Gibbs P, Pickles MD, Turnbull LW. Repeatability of echo-planar-based diffusion measurements of the human prostate at 3T. *Magn Reson Imaging* 2007; **25**: 1423–9.

59. Miao H, Fukatsu H, Ishigaki T. Prostate cancer detection with 3-T MRI: comparison of diffusion-weighted and T2-weighted imaging. *Eur J Radiol* 2007; **61**: 297–302.

60. Gibbs P, Pickles MD, Turnbull LW. Diffusion imaging of the prostate at 3.0 Tesla. *Invest Radiol* 2006; **41**: 185–8.

61. Pickles MD, Gibbs P, Sreenivas M, Turnbull LW. Diffusion-weighted imaging of normal and malignant prostate tissue at 3.0T. *J Magn Reson Imaging* 2006; **23**: 130–4.

62. Manenti G, Carlani M, Mancino S, *et al.* Diffusion tensor magnetic resonance imaging of prostate cancer. *Invest Radiol* 2007; **42**: 412–19.

63. Desouza NM, Riches SF, Vanas NJ, *et al.* Diffusion-weighted magnetic resonance imaging: a potential non-invasive marker of tumour aggressiveness in localized prostate cancer. *Clin Radiol* 2008; **63**(7): 774–82.

64. Scheidler J, Hricak H, Vigneron DB, *et al.* Prostate cancer: localization with three-dimensional proton MR spectroscopic imaging – clinicopathologic study. *Radiology* 1999; **213**: 473–80.

65. Kurhanewicz J, Vigneron DB, Hricak H, *et al.* Three-dimensional H-1 MR spectroscopic imaging of the in situ human prostate with high (0.24–0.7-cm³) spatial resolution. *Radiology* 1996; **198**: 795–805.

66. Denis LJ, Murphy GP, Schroeder FH. Report of the consensus workshop on screening and global strategy for prostate cancer. *Cancer* 1995; **75**: 1187–207.

67. Coakley FV, Qayyum A, Kurhanewicz J. Magnetic resonance imaging and spectroscopic imaging of prostate cancer. *J Urol* 2003; **170**: S69–75.

68. Liney GP, Turnbull LW, Knowles AJ. In vivo magnetic resonance spectroscopy and dynamic contrast

enhanced imaging of the prostate gland. *NMR Biomed* 1999; **12**: 39–44.

69. Kurhanewicz J, Swanson MG, Nelson SJ, *et al.* Combined magnetic resonance imaging and spectroscopic imaging approach to molecular imaging of prostate cancer. *J Magn Reson Imaging* 2002; **16**: 451–63.

70. Shukla-Dave A, Hricak H, Moskowitz C, *et al.* Detection of prostate cancer with MR spectroscopic imaging: an expanded paradigm incorporating polyamines. *Radiology* 2007; **245**: 499–506.

71. Males RG, Vigneron DB, Star-Lack J, *et al.* Clinical application of BASING and spectral/spatial water and lipid suppression pulses for prostate cancer staging and localization by in vivo 3D 1H magnetic resonance spectroscopic imaging. *Magn Reson Med* 2000; **43**: 17–22.

72. Zakian KL, Eberhardt S, Hricak H, *et al.* Transition zone prostate cancer: metabolic characteristics at 1H MR spectroscopic imaging – initial results. *Radiology* 2003; **229**: 241–7.

73. Wefer AE, Hricak H, Vigneron DB, *et al.* Sextant localization of prostate cancer: comparison of sextant biopsy, magnetic resonance imaging and magnetic resonance spectroscopic imaging with step section histology. *J Urol* 2000; **164**: 400–4.

74. Hasumi M, Suzuki K, Taketomi A, *et al.* The combination of multivoxel MR spectroscopy with MR imaging improve the diagnostic accuracy for localization of prostate cancer. *Anticancer Res* 2003; **23**: 4223–7.

75. Portalez D, Malavaud B, Herigault G, *et al.* Predicting prostate cancer with dynamic endorectal coil MR and proton spectroscopic MRI. *J Radiol* 2004; **85**: 1999–2004.

76. Squillaci E, Manenti G, Mancino S, *et al.* MR spectroscopy of prostate cancer. Initial clinical experience. *J Exp Clin Cancer Res* 2005; **24**: 523–30.

77. Vilanova JC, Barcelo J. Prostate cancer detection: MR spectroscopic imaging. *Abdom Imaging* 2007; **32**: 253–61.

78. Jung JA, Coakley FV, Vigneron DV, *et al.* Prostate depiction at endorectal MR spectroscopic imaging: investigation of a standardized evaluation system. *Radiology* 2004; **233**: 701–8.

79. Futterer JJ, Heijmink SW, Scheenen TWJ, *et al.* Prostate cancer localization with dynamic contrast-enhanced MR imaging and proton MR spectroscopic imaging. *Radiology* 2006; **241**: 449–58.

80. Yu KK, Scheidler J, Hricak H, *et al.* Prostate cancer: prediction of extracapsular extension with endorectal MR imaging and three-dimensional proton MR spectroscopic imaging. *Radiology* 1999; **213**: 481–8.

81. Wang L, Hricak H, Kattan MW, *et al.* Prediction of organ-confined prostate cancer: incremental value of MR imaging and MR spectroscopic imaging to staging nomograms. *Radiology* 2006; **238**: 597–603.

82. Kurhanewicz J, Vigneron DB, Males RG, *et al.* The prostate: MR imaging and spectroscopy. Present and future. *Radiol Clin North Am* 2000; **38**: 115–38.

83. Zakian KL, Sircar K, Hricak H, *et al.* Correlation of proton MR spectroscopic imaging with Gleason score based on step-section pathologic analysis after radical prostatectomy. *Radiology* 2005; **234**: 804–14.

84. Lichy MP, Pintaske J, Kottke R, *et al.* 3D proton MR spectroscopic imaging of prostate cancer using a standard spine coil at 1.5 T in clinical routine: a feasibility study. *Eur Radiol* 2005; **15**: 653–60.

85. Chen A, Xu D, Sotto C, *et al.* High resolution MRSI and DTI of prostate cancer at 3T. *Proceedings 15th Scientific Meeting International Society for Magnetic Resonance in Medicine*, Berlin, 2007. p. 2887.

86. Scheenen TW, Heijmink SW, Roell SA, *et al.* Three-dimensional proton MR spectroscopy of human prostate at 3 T without endorectal coil: feasibility. *Radiology* 2007; **245**: 507–16.

87. Scheenen TW, Gambarota G, Weiland E, *et al.* Optimal timing for in vivo 1H-MR spectroscopic imaging of the human prostate at 3.0T. *Magn Reson Med* 2005; **53**: 1268–74.

88. Rouviere O, Hartman RP, Lyonnet D. Prostate MR imaging at high-field strength: evolution or revolution? *Eur Radiol* 2006; **16**: 276–84.

89. Prando A, Billis A. Focal prostatic atrophy: mimicry of prostatic cancer on TRUS and 3D-MRSI studies. *Abdom Imaging* 2009; **34**: 271–5.

90. Qayyum A, Coakley FV, Lu Y, *et al.* Organ-confined prostate cancer: effect of prior transrectal biopsy on endorectal MRI and MR spectroscopic imaging. *AJR Am J Roentgenol* 2004; **183**: 1079–83.

91. Kaji Y, Kurhanewicz J, Hricak H, *et al.* Localizing prostate cancer in the presence of post-biopsy change on MR images: role of proton MR spectroscopic imaging. *Radiology* 1998; **206**: 785–90.

92. Liney GP, Turnbull LW, Knowles AJ. In vivo magnetic resonance spectroscopy and dynamic contrast enhanced imaging of the prostate gland. *NMR Biomed* 1999; **12**: 39–44.

93. Jager GJ, Ruijter ET, van de Kaa CA, *et al* Dynamic TurboFLASH subtraction technique for contrast-enhanced MR imaging of the prostate: correlation with histopathologic results. *Radiology* 1997; **203**: 645–52.

94. Jager GJ, Ruijter ET, van de Kaa CA, *et al.* Local staging of prostate cancer with endorectal MRI: correlation with histopathology. *AJR Am J Roentgenol* 1996; **166**: 845–52.

95. Barentsz JO, Engelbrecht M, Jager GJ, *et al.* Fast dynamic gadolinium-enhanced MR imaging of urinary bladder and prostate cancer. *J Magn Reson Imaging* 1999; **10**: 295–304.

96. Namimoto T, Morishita S, Saitoh R, *et al.* The value of dynamic MR imaging for hypointensity lesions of the peripheral zone of the prostate. *Comput Med Imaging Graph* 1998; **22**: 239–45.

97. Padhani AR, Gapinski CJ, Macvicar DA, *et al.* Dynamic contrast enhanced MRI of prostate cancer: correlation with morphology and tumour stage, histological grade and PSA. *Clin Radiol* 2000; **55**: 99–109.

98. Padhani AR, Hayes C, Landau S, *et al.* Reproducibility of quantitative dynamic MRI of normal human tissues. *NMR Biomed* 2002; **15**: 143–53.

99. Engelbrecht MR, Huisman HJ, Laheij RJ, *et al.* Discrimination of prostate cancer from normal peripheral zone and central gland tissue by using dynamic contrast-enhanced MRI. *Radiology* 2003; **229**: 248–54.

100. Buckley DL, Roberts C, Parker GJ, *et al.* Prostate cancer: evaluation of vascular characteristics with dynamic contrast-enhanced T1-weighted MR imaging – initial experience. *Radiology* 2004; **233**: 709–15.

101. Alonzi R, Padhani AR, Allen C. Dynamic contrast enhanced MRI in prostate cancer. *Eur J Radiol* 2007; **63**: 335–50.

102. d'Arcy JA, Collins DJ, Padhani AR, *et al.* Informatics in Radiology (infoRAD): Magnetic Resonance Imaging Workbench: analysis and visualization of dynamic contrast-enhanced MR imaging data. *Radiographics* 2006; **26**: 621–32.

103. Tofts PS, Brix G, Buckley DL, *et al.* Estimating kinetic parameters from dynamic contrast-enhanced T(1)-weighted MRI of a diffusable tracer: standardized quantities and symbols. *J Magn Reson Imaging* 1999; **10**: 223–32.

104. Tofts PS. Modeling tracer kinetics in dynamic Gd-DTPA MRI. *J Magn Reson Imaging* 1997; **7**: 91–101.

105. Hara N, Okuizumi M, Koike H, *et al.* Dynamic contrast-enhanced magnetic resonance imaging (DCE-MRI) is a useful modality for the precise detection and staging of early prostate cancer. *Prostate* 2005; **62**: 140–7.

106. Fütterer JJ, Engelbrecht MR, Huisman HJ, *et al.* Staging prostate cancer with dynamic contrast-enhanced endorectal MR imaging prior to radical prostatectomy: experienced versus less experienced readers. *Radiology* 2005; **237**: 541–9.

107. Nobauer-Huhmann IM, Ba-Ssalamah A, Mlynarik V, *et al.* Magnetic resonance imaging contrast enhancement of brain tumors at 3 tesla versus 1.5 tesla. *Invest Radiol* 2002; **37**: 114–19.

108. Kim CK, Park BK, Kim B. Localization of prostate cancer using 3T MRI: comparison of T2-weighted and dynamic contrast-enhanced imaging. *J Comput Assist Tomogr* 2006; **30**: 7–11.

109. Ocak I, Bernardo M, Metzger G, *et al.* Dynamic contrast-enhanced MRI of prostate cancer at 3 T: a study of pharmacokinetic parameters. *AJR Am J Roentgenol* 2007; **189**(4): 849.

110. Kozlowski P, Chang SD, Jones EC, *et al.* Combined diffusion-weighted and dynamic contrast-enhanced MRI for prostate cancer diagnosis – correlation with biopsy and histopathology. *J Magn Reson Imaging* 2006; **24**: 108–13.

111. Reinsberg SA, Payne GS, Riches SF, *et al.* Combined use of diffusion-weighted MRI and 1H MR spectroscopy to increase accuracy in prostate cancer detection. *AJR Am J Roentgenol* 2007; **188**: 91–8.

112. Van Dorsten FA, Van der Graaf M, Engelbrecht MR, *et al.* Combined quantitative dynamic contrast-enhanced MR imaging and (1)H MR spectroscopic imaging of human prostate cancer. *J Magn Reson Imaging* 2004; **20**: 279–87.

113. Noworolski SM, Henry RG, Vigneron DB, *et al.* Dynamic contrast-enhanced MRI in normal and abnormal prostate tissue as defined by biopsy, MRI, and MRSI. *Magn Reson Med* 2005; **53**: 249–55.

114. Kumar V, Jagannathan NR, Kumar R, *et al.* Transrectal ultrasound-guided biopsy of prostate voxels identified as suspicious of malignancy on three-dimensional (1)H MR spectroscopic imaging in patients with abnormal digital rectal examination or raised prostate specific antigen level of 4–10 ng/ml. *NMR Biomed* 2007; **20**(1): 11–20.

115. Singh AK, Kruecker J, Xu S, *et al.* Initial clinical experience with real-time transrectal ultrasonography-magnetic resonance imaging fusion-guided prostate biopsy. *BJU Int* 2008; **101**(7): 841–5.

116. Kaplan I, Oldenburg NE, Meskell P, *et al.* Real time MRI-ultrasound image guided stereotactic prostate biopsy. *Magn Reson Imaging* 2002; **20**(3): 295–9.

117. Stoianovici D, Song D, Petrisor D, *et al.* "MRI Stealth" robot for prostate interventions. *Minim Invasive Ther Allied Technol* 2007; **16**(4): 241–8.

118. Yakar D, Hambrock T, Hoeks C, Barentsz JO, Fütterer JJ. Magnetic resonance-guided biopsy of the prostate: feasibility, technique, and clinical applications. *Top Magn Reson Imaging* 2008; **19**(6): 291–5.

Female pelvic imaging at 3T

Darcy J. Wolfman and Susan M. Ascher

Introduction

Magnetic resonance (MR) imaging is a well-established modality for the evaluation of the female pelvis. Accepted clinical applications at 1.5T include staging of gynecologic malignancies, evaluation of congenital uterine anomalies, evaluation pre and post uterine artery embolization, evaluation of adnexal masses, and problem-solving difficult cases. As 3T MR imaging systems become increasingly available for routine clinical use, female pelvic imaging applications are emerging. This chapter will discuss 3T female pelvic imaging to include the advantages and disadvantages, commonly used sequences, and current clinical applications.

Advantages and disadvantages of female pelvic imaging at 3T

There are several advantages of imaging the female pelvis at 3T, including higher spatial resolution and increased chemical shift.

The signal-to-noise ratio (SNR) at 3T MR imaging should theoretically be improved by a factor of 2 over the SNR at 1.5T. However, tissue characteristics, such as T1 and T2 relaxation time, and sequence parameters, such as receiver bandwidth, affect the intrinsic SNR. Even given these factors, there is a significant gain in SNR at 3T compared with 1.5T [1]. This improvement in SNR contributes to a higher spatial resolution or, with the use of parallel imaging, increased temporal resolution and a decrease in imaging time [2] (Figure 14.1). These improvements in imaging should theoretically improve the diagnostic accuracy of female pelvic MR imaging.

Chemical shift is more pronounced at 3T than at 1.5T secondary to the increase in proton precessional frequency. The most clinically relevant benefit of this is better frequency-selective fat suppression. Fat suppression is important in female pelvic imaging for the evaluation of ovarian masses; for example, distinguishing an ovarian dermoid cyst from an ovarian endometrioma or hemorrhagic cyst.

Another potential benefit of the increase in chemical shift at 3T is more effective spectroscopy [3]. Better spectral separation may enable better visualization of previously described metabolites and may allow for detection of different metabolites. Spectroscopy at 3T has been used to evaluate ovarian masses with promising results, however, more research with larger sample size is needed [4].

Although MR imaging at 3T does provide distinct advantages over MR imaging at 1.5T, these advantages come at a price. Increased radiofrequency (RF) power deposition at 3T must be addressed. Several artifacts are also of particular concern when imaging the female pelvis at 3T, including motion artifact and susceptibility artifact.

RF pulses with four times higher energy (B1) are needed to excite protons at 3T compared with 1.5T. Increase in B1 results in increased RF heating and higher specific absorption ratio (SAR). This excessive heating can lead to tissue damage. Additionally, an increase in SAR deposition reduces the number of slices per repetition time (TR) that can be performed and lengthens examination times at 3T. Currently, the US Food and Drug Administration (FDA) set SAR limits of no more than 4 W/kg averaged over the entire body for a period of 15 minutes or more and no more than 8 W/kg for any gram of tissue within the head or torso for 5 minutes or longer [5]. There are multiple solutions to this issue, and a full discussion is beyond the scope of this chapter. In our institution, parallel imaging is used to reduce SAR for female pelvic imaging at 3T.

Body MR Imaging at 3 Tesla, ed. Ihab R. Kamel and Elmar M. Merkle. Published by Cambridge University Press.
© Cambridge University Press 2011.

(a)

(b)

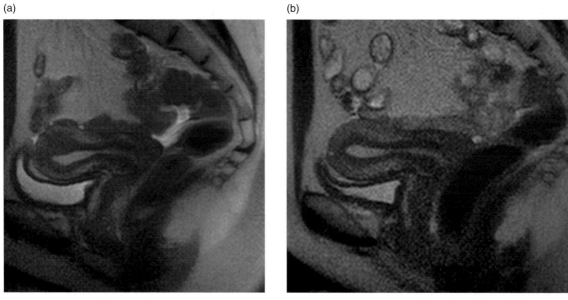

Figure 14.1 Normal female pelvis at 3T MR imaging. Sagittal T2-weighted images of a normal uterus in the same patient demonstrate improved spatial resolution at 3T (a) compared with 1.5T (b).

Susceptibility artifacts are caused by local field distortions and are increased with increasing magnet field strength. Thus, these artifacts are more pronounced at 3T compared with 1.5T. Susceptibility artifacts can cause signal loss with gradient echo (GRE) sequences and are particularly prominent at gas–soft tissue interfaces and with metallic devices and surgical clips. Susceptibility artifacts can be decreased by local shimming, decreasing voxel size, using a shorter TE and minimizing echo train lengths. Again, a full discussion is beyond the scope of this chapter.

Motion artifact is increased at 3T (Figure 14.2). When imaging the female pelvis, respiratory motion is negligible, however, bowel motion is significant. Several solutions can be used to decrease bowel motion artifact. When using fast spin echo (FSE) sequences, the echo acquisition time can be shortened by decreasing the echo train length, increasing the bandwidth, and using parallel imaging [6]. Alternatively, the SNR can be increased by increasing the echo train length, decreasing the bandwidth, and turning off parallel imaging [7]. Further, placing the frequency direction in the anterior–posterior direction reduces motion from the anterior pelvic wall. To decrease bowel motion, antiperistaltic agents can be administered; however, we do not routinely administer these agents for female pelvic imaging at our institution.

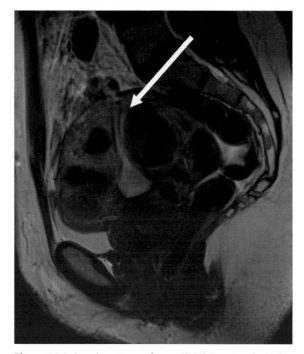

Figure 14.2 Bowel motion artifact at 3T MR imaging. Sagittal T2-weighted high-resolution image of the uterus with bowel motion artifact obscuring the endometrium at the uterine fundus (arrow).

(a)

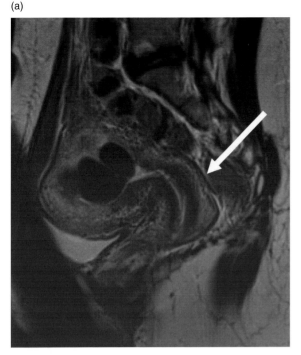

(b)

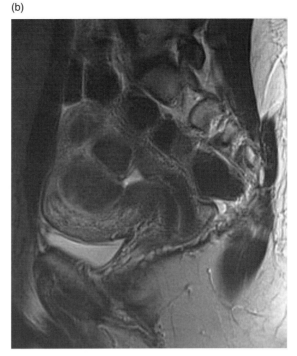

Figure 14.3 Improved zonal anatomy at 3T MR imaging. Sagittal T2-weighted high-resolution images of the female pelvis in the same patient at 3T (a) and 1.5T (b). Note the improved visualization of the cervical zonal anatomy at 3T (white arrow in a).

Sequences for female pelvic imaging at 3T

Female pelvic MR imaging at 3T should utilize similar sequences as those used at 1.5T including: (1) single-shot FSE (SSFSE) T2-weighted sequences, (2) high-resolution T2-weighted FSE sequence, (3) T1-weighted two-dimensional (2D) GRE in- and out-of-phase sequences, and (4) 3D T1-weighted GRE sequence with fat suppression pre- and post-gadolinium contrast administration.

At our institution, patient preparation for 3T female pelvic MR imaging is identical to 1.5T female pelvic MR imaging. Patients are asked to fast for 4 hours prior to the examination and empty their bladder immediately prior to imaging. Some centers routinely use antiperistaltic agents to decrease bowel motion during female pelvic MR imaging. Endoluminal contrast agents, both endovaginal and endorectal, are useful for specific imaging protocols, such as dynamic pelvic floor imaging.

T2-weighted sequences provide the foundation of female pelvic imaging. The SSFSE T2-weighted sequences should be performed in three orthogonal planes with a small field of view. The high-resolution T2-weighted FSE sequence provides detailed anatomy of the uterus and ovaries and should be performed in the sagittal plane routinely. For staging gynecologic malignancies, we add an orthogonal high-resolution T2-weighted FSE. Morakkabti-Spitz, *et al.* showed that MR images of the female pelvis obtained at 3T are comparable in diagnostic quality to those at 1.5T with a similar spatial resolution [8]. High-resolution T2-weighted images of the female pelvis at 3T have been shown to provide significantly better delineation of small anatomical detail and a superior image for the evaluation of the cervix, ovary, and vagina [9, 10] (Figure 14.3).

A 3D T2-weighted turbo spin echo (TSE) sequence with high sampling frequency (SPACE) has been described at 1.5T as an alternative to the high-resolution T2-weighted FSE sequence [11]. A volumetric data set is generated allowing for reconstruction of high-resolution T2-weighted images in any plane. Time of acquisition at 1.5T is over 10 minutes, which can be prohibitive in a clinical setting. However, acquisition times of 6 minutes have been reported at 3T, which would make using this sequence more clinically feasible [12].

T1-weighted GRE in- and out-of-phase images are most useful in female pelvic imaging for adnexal lesion characterization. Because of the increase in chemical shift at 3T, echo times (TEs) for in- and out-of-phase imaging are more closely spaced, making acquisition of both during a single acquisition difficult. Images are optimized by obtaining the out-of-phase images at a shorter TE than in-phase images. T1-weighted GRE sequences also require a longer TR at 3T than at 1.5T in order to maintain T1 contrast.

Although the increase in chemical shift at 3T compared with 1.5T causes problems with T1-weighted GRE in- and out-of-phase imaging, this same increase in chemical shift allows for improved fat suppression when using a fat-suppressed T1-weighted GRE sequence, given sufficient B0 homogeneity.

Diffusion-weighted imaging (DWI) at 3T would allow for higher b-values and thinner slices than at 1.5T, potentially improving image quality and diagnostic value. One study by Namimoto *et al.* evaluated the use of DWI at 3T for distinguishing uterine sarcoma from uterine fibroids with promising results [13].

Clinical applications of female pelvic imaging at 3T

Gynecologic malignancy

MR imaging at 1.5T is considered the study of choice for the staging of cervical, endometrial, and ovarian cancer. Limited research at 3T has revealed it to be at least equivalent to imaging at 1.5T MR imaging and research using new techniques may improve staging accuracy at 3T compared with 1.5T.

Cervical cancer appears as an iso T2-weighted signal mass with contrast enhancement greater than normal cervical stroma. MR imaging at 1.5T has been shown to be superior to both CT and clinical examination for the staging of cervical cancer with an overall staging accuracy of 77–93% [14]. An intact area of low T2-weighted signal intensity, representing normal peripheral fibrous cervical stroma, is a reliable indication that the tumor is confined to the cervix (stage IB) [15]. Criteria for parametrial tumor invasion (stage IIB) include an irregular cervical margin, prominent parametrial strands, eccentric parametrial enlargement, and/or tumor extension through the fibrocervical stroma into the parametria or cardinal-

uterosacral ligaments on T2-weighted images; and/or loss of the parametrial fat planes on T1-weighted images [16]. Pelvic sidewall extension (stage IIIB) is diagnosed on T2-weighted images by tumor extending beyond the lateral margins of the cardinal ligaments and loss of the normal low signal of the pyriformis, levator ani, and/or obturator internus muscles [17]. Hydronephrosis also indicates stage IIIB disease. Segmental loss of the normal bladder or rectal wall indicates stage IVA disease and is best seen on T2-weighted or T1-weighted fat-suppressed post-contrast images.

The increase in SNR at 3T MR imaging should theoretically improve the staging accuracy of cervical carcinoma compared with 1.5T MR imaging (Figure 14.4). Hori *et al.* demonstrated that 3T MR imaging had a high accuracy for the diagnosis of parametrial invasion and vaginal invasion in cervical carcinomas. However, this accuracy was not significantly better then 1.5T MR imaging [18]. Further research in this area is needed and correlation with the revised International Federation of Gynecology and Obstetrics (FIGO) staging criteria for cervical carcinoma is also needed.

Endometrial cancer is most accurately staged with MR imaging, and MR imaging staging criteria at 1.5T using the FIGO staging criteria have been well described. Overall accuracy of staging endometrial cancer with 1.5T MR imaging ranges from 70% to 94% and is best accomplished with both high-resolution T2-weighted images and dynamic T1-weighted fat-suppressed post-contrast images [19]. The tumors themselves have variable appearance, but most often appear as a homogeneous high T2-weighted signal intensity mass with increased contrast enhancement in the arterial phase compared to the normal endometrium, making identification of even small lesions possible. Endometrial cancer that is confined to the endometrium (stage IA) respects the junctional zone, if present, and demonstrates a sharp, smooth tumor–myometrial interface. Disruption of the junctional zone and/or an irregular tumor–myometrial interface indicates myometrial invasion. If there is less than half myometrial invasion, the tumor is still staged as IA; with equal to or more than half myometrial invasion the tumor is stage IB. Widening and expansion of the cervical canal with associated heterogeneity of the cervical stroma indicates cervical invasion by the endometrial tumor (stage II). Tumor involvement of the uterine serosa and/or

(a)

(b)

(c)

(d)

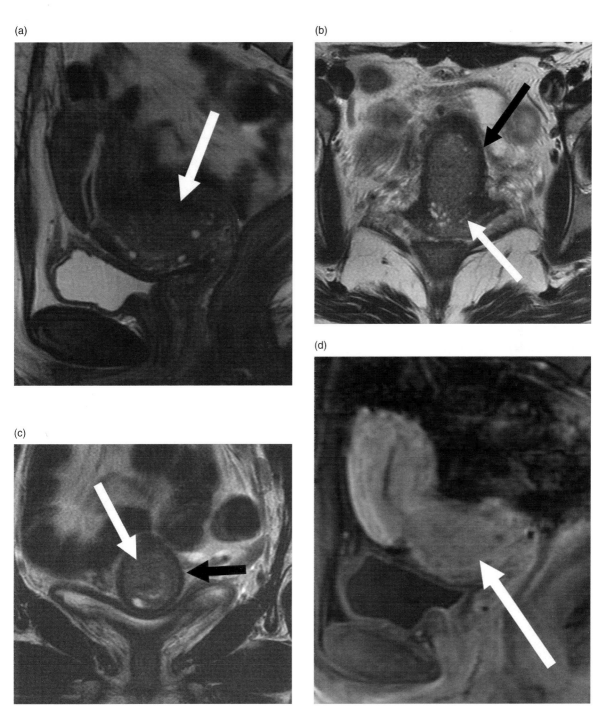

Figure 14.4 Cervical cancer at 3T MR imaging. Sagittal (a), axial (b), and coronal (c) T2-weighted images and sagittal post-contrast image (d) of the female pelvis demonstrating an iso T2-weighted enhancing cervical mass (white arrows in a, b, c, and d). Note the intact low T2-weighted signal fibrous cervical stroma surrounding the mass (black arrows in b and c). Images courtesy of Oguz Akin, MD, Department of Radiology, Memorial Sloan-Kettering Cancer Center, New York, USA.

(a)

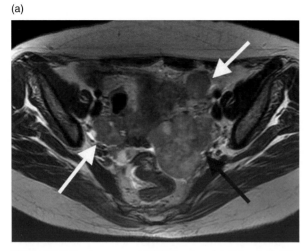

(b)

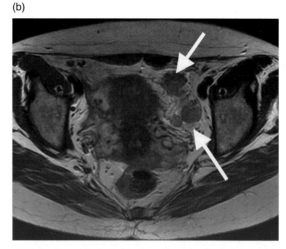

Figure 14.5 Ovarian cancer at 3T MR imaging. Axial T2-weighted images of the female pelvis demonstrate a primary ovarian mass (black arrow in a) and multiple peritoneal implants (white arrows in a and b). Images courtesy of Evis Sala, MD, University Department of Radiology, Addenbrooke's Hospital, Cambridge, UK.

adnexa indicates stage IIIA disease. Vaginal invasion with focal disruption of the normal low T2 signal wall or parametrial involvement is classified as stage IIIB. Pathologically enlarged pelvic lymph nodes (stage IIIC1) and para-aortic lymph nodes (stage IIIC2) are diagnosed in the usual fashion on MR imaging. Focal disruption of the normally low T2 signal wall of the bladder or rectum signifies stage IVA disease.

MR imaging at 3T, in theory, may further improve the accuracy of staging endometrial carcinoma. Recent work has demonstrated that staging at 3T MR imaging is highly accurate in the staging of endometrial carcinoma, but not significantly improved compared with 1.5T MR imaging [20]. Another study by Lin *et al.* evaluated the use of T2-weighted images combined with DWI at 3T with promising results [21]. More research in this area is needed.

MR imaging is useful for the staging of ovarian cancer and, at 1.5T, has an overall accuracy of 75–78%, which is comparable to computed tomography (CT), the gold standard [22]. Stage II disease is defined as direct extension into or implants on the uterus and/or fallopian tubes (stage IIA) or other pelvic organs, such as the rectum, bladder, or peritoneum (stage IIB). This finding is depicted on MR imaging as a tumor–normal structure interface of greater than 90% or direct soft tissue extension into the structure with associated irregular margins. Tumor spread outside of the pelvis, including capsular implants on the liver, is stage III disease and is best identified on MR using dynamic T1-weighted fat-

suppressed post-contrast images. Using this technique, lesions as small as 1 cm can be identified [23].

With the improved SNR of 3T MR imaging compared with 1.5T, the staging accuracy of ovarian cancer may improve. Recently, it was shown that accurate staging of ovarian cancer at 3T MR imaging is possible compared with surgical staging [24] (Figure 14.5) Sala *et al.* documented the feasibility of using DWI at 3T MR imaging to aid in the staging of ovarian cancer [25]. The increase in chemical shift at 3T may allow for better spectroscopy than at 1.5T and this is of particular interest in ovarian cancer evaluation. A study by Stanwell *et al.*, showed that spectroscopy of ovarian masses at 3T can be performed with acceptable spectral quality and good SNR [26]. More research in this area is needed, but initial results are promising.

Pelvic floor dysfunction

Functional disorders of the pelvic floor are a common problem in women and often affect quality of life. There are three compartments of the pelvic floor in women, anterior, middle, and posterior. The anterior compartment is composed of the bladder and urethra; the middle compartment the vagina and uterus; and the posterior compartment the anus and rectum. Dysfunction of the pelvic floor is often a complex problem involving multiple compartments and patient symptoms are dependent on the compartments involved. Dynamic imaging involves evaluation of

(a)

(b)

(c)

(d)

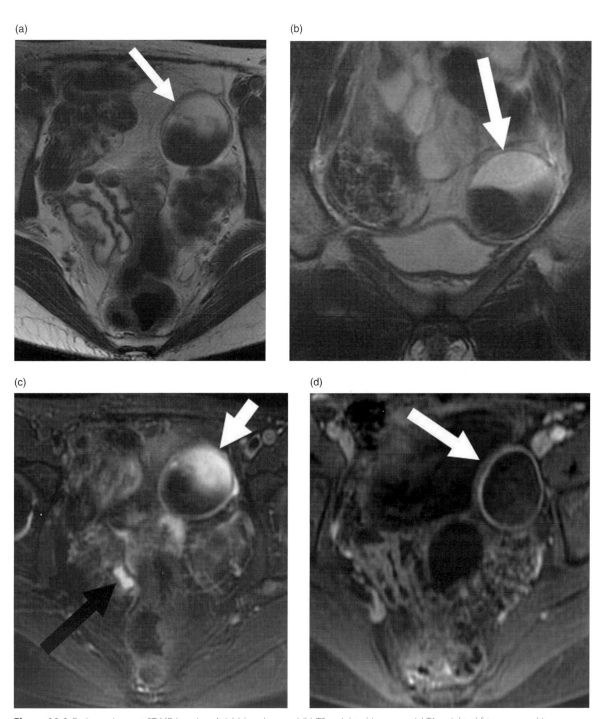

Figure 14.6 Endometrioma at 3T MR imaging. Axial (a) and coronal (b) T2-weighted images, axial T1-weighted fat-suppressed image (c), and axial post-contrast image (d) demonstrating an endometrioma (white arrows). Note the small endometrial implant seen on the T1-weighted fat-suppressed image (black arrow in C). Images courtesy of Oguz Akin, MD, Department of Radiology, Memorial Sloan-Kettering Cancer Center, New York, USA.

the pelvic structures at rest, with squeezing, with straining, and with defecation. MR imaging at 1.5T is becoming more frequently used for the evaluation of pelvic floor disorders because of the multiplanar imaging capability, lack of ionizing radiation, and ability to visualize the pelvic floor musculature. Morakkabati-Spitz et al. recently documented the feasibility of dynamic female pelvic floor imaging at 3T and showed that the overall image quality and diagnostic accuracy was comparable to 1.5T [27]. More research is needed to determine if there is any added benefit to performing dynamic female pelvic floor imaging at 3T compared with 1.5T.

Adnexal mass

Endometriosis is a benign disease caused by ectopic endometrial tissue outside of the uterus. Female pelvic MR imaging is useful for the diagnosis and staging of endometriosis. The diagnosis of deep endometriosis is especially important for pre-surgical planning and allows surgeons to plan the most appropriate surgery. Hottat et al. showed that female pelvic MR imaging at 3T improved the specificity, sensitivity, negative predictive value (NPV), positive predictive value (PPV), and accuracy for the diagnosis of deep endometriosis compared with female pelvic MR imaging at 1.5T [28]. Most importantly, they showed an improvement in NPV from 89% with 1.5T to 93.3% with 3T for the diagnosis of deep endometriosis (Figure 14.6).

The combination of improvement in fat suppression and spatial resolution at 3T should theoretically improve the ability to diagnose dermoid cysts, especially small lesions. Our experience has shown this to be the case; however, this has yet to be shown in the literature.

Conclusion

Female pelvic MR imaging at 3T is now routinely being used in clinical practice and provides for fast imaging and very high spatial resolution compared with 1.5T MR imaging. Currently, 3T female pelvic MR imaging has been shown to be advantageous for the evaluation of deep endometriosis and comparable to 1.5T for staging of gynecologic malignancies and dynamic pelvic floor imaging. Further research holds promise for future applications in female pelvic imaging including DWI and spectroscopy.

References

1. Schindera ST, Merkle EM, Dale BM, et al. Abdominal magnetic resonance imaging at 3T: what is the ultimate gain in signal-to-noise ratio? Acad Radiol 2006; 13: 1236–43.

2. Martin DR, Friel HT, Danrad R, et al. Approach to abdominal imaging at 1.5Tesla and optimization at 3.0 Tesla. Magn Reson Imaging Clin N Am 2005; 13: 241–54, v–vi.

3. Katz-Brull R, Rofsky NM, Lenkinski RE. Breathhold abdominal and thoracic proton MR spectroscopy at 3T. Magn Reson Med 2003; 50: 461–7.

4. Stanwell P, Russell P, Carter J, et al. Evaluation of ovarian tumors by proton magnetic spectroscopy at three Tesla. Invest Radiol 2008; 43(10): 745–51.

5. FDA Guidance of Industry and FDA Staff. Criteria for significant risk investigations of magnetic resonance diagnostic devices. http://www.fda.gov/downloads/MedicalDevices/DeviceRegulationandGuidance/GuidanceDocuments/ucm072688.pdf. Accessed April 22, 2010.

6. Hussain S, van den Bos I, Oliveto J, et al. MR imaging of the female pelvis at 3T. Magn Reson Imaging Clin N Am 2007; 14: 537–44.

7. Cornfeld D, Weinred J. Simple changes to 1.5-T MRI abdomen and pelvis protocols to optimize results at 3 T. AJR Am J Roentgenol 2008; 190: W140–50.

8. Morakkabati-Spitz N, Gieseke J, Kuhl C, et al. 3.0-T high-field magnetic resonance imaging of the female pelvis: preliminary experiences. Eur Radiol 2005; 15: 639–44.

9. Morakkabati-Spitz N, Gieseke J, Kuhl C, et al. MRI of the pelvis at 3 T: very high spatial resolution with sensitivity encoding and flip-angle sweep technique in clinically acceptable scan time. Eur Radiol 2006; 16: 634–41.

10. Kataoka M, Kido A, Koyama T, et al. MRI of the female pelvis at 3T compared to 1.5T: evaluation of high-resolution T2-weighted and HASTE images. J Magn Reson Imaging 2007; 25: 527–34.

11. Lichy MP, Wietek BM, Mugler JP 3rd, et al. Magnetic resonance imaging of the body trunk using a single-slab, 3-dimensional, T2-weighted turbo-spin-echo sequence with high sampling frequency (SPACE) for high spatial resolution imaging: initial clinical experiences. Invest Radiol 2005; 40: 754–60.

12. Lim RP, Lee VS, Bennett GL, et al. Imaging the female pelvis at 3.0 T. Top Magn Reson Imaging 2006; 17: 427–43.

13. Namimoto T, Yamashita Y, Awai K, et al. Combined use of T2-weighted and diffusion-weighted 3-T MR imaging for differentiating uterine sarcomas from benign leiomyomas. Eur Radiol 2009; 19(11): 2756–64.

14. Ozsarlako O, Tjalma W, Schepens E, *et al.* The correlation of preoperative CT, MR imaging, and clinical (FIGO) staging with histopathology findings in primary cervical carcinoma. *Eur Radiol* 2003; **13**(10): 2338–45.

15. Mitchell DG, Snyder B, Coakley F, *et al.* Early invasive cervical cancer: tumor delineation by magnetic resonance imaging, computed tomography, and clinical examination, verified by pathologic results, in the ACRIN 6651/GOG 183 Intergroup Study. *J Clin Oncol* 2006; **24**(36): 5687–94.

16. Togashi K, Nishimura D, Sagoh T, *et al.* Carcinoma of the cervix: staging with MR imaging. *Radiology* 1989; **171**: 245–51.

17. Hricak H, Lacey CG, Sandles LG, *et al.* Invasive cervical carcinoma: comparison of MR imaging and surgical findings. *Radiology* 1988; **166**: 623–31.

18. Hori M, Kim T, Murakami T, *et al.* Uterine cervical carcinoma: preoperative staging with 3.0T-MRI imaging – comparison with 1.5T MR imaging. *Radiology* 2009; **251**(1): 96–104.

19. Hricak H, Rubinstein LV, Gherman GM, Karstaedt N. MR imaging evaluation of endometrial carcinoma: results of an NCI cooperative study. *Radiology* 1991; **179**: 829–32.

20. Hori M, Kim T, Murakami T, *et al.* MR imaging of endometrial carcinoma for preoperative staging at 3.0T: comparison with imaging at 1.5T. *J Magn Reson Imaging* 2009; **30**(3): 621–30.

21. Lin G, Ng KK, Chang CJ, *et al.* Myometrial invasion in endometrial cancer: diagnostic accuracy of diffusion-weighted 3.0-T MR imaging–initial experience. *Radiology* 2009; **250**(3): 784–92.

22. Stevens SK, Hricak H, Stern JL. Ovarian lesions: detection and characterization with gadolinium-enhanced MR imaging at 1.5T. *Radiology* 1991; **181**: 481–8.

23. Semelka RC, Lawrence PH, Shoenut JP, *et al.* Primary ovarian cancer: prospective comparison of contrast-enhanced CT and pre- and post-contrast, fat-suppressed MR imaging with histologic correlation. *J Magn Reson Imaging* 1993; **3**: 99–106.

24. Booth SJ, Turnbull LW, Poole DR, *et al.* The accurate staging of ovarian cancer using 3T magnetic resonance imaging–a realistic option. *BJOG* 2008; **115**(7): 894–901.

25. Sala E, Priest AN, Kataoka M, *et al.* Apparent diffusion coefficient and vascular signal fraction measurements with magnetic resonance imaging: feasibility in metastatic ovarian cancer at 3 Tesla: technical development. *Eur Radiol* 2010; **20**(2): 491–6.

26. Stanwell P, Russell P, Carter J, *et al.* Evaluation of ovarian tumors by proton magnetic resonance spectroscopy at three Tesla. *Invest Radiol* 2008; **43**(10): 745–51.

27. Morakkabati-Spitz N, Gieseke J, Willinek WA, *et al.* Dynamic pelvic floor MR imaging at 3 T in patients with clinical signs of urinary incontinence-preliminary results. *Eur Radiol* 2008; **18**: 2620–27.

28. Hottat N, Larrousse C, Anaf V, *et al.* Endometriosis: contribution of 3.0-T pelvic MR imaging in preoperative assessment–initial results. *Radiology* 2009; **253**: 126–34.

Index